MEASUREMENT IN NURSING RESEARCH

MEASUREMENT IN NURSING RESEARCH

CAROLYN FEHER WALTZ, R.N., PH.D., F.A.A.N.
Professor and
Coordinator for Evaluation
University of Maryland
School of Nursing
Baltimore, Maryland

ORA L. STRICKLAND, R.N., PH.D., F.A.A.N.
Associate Professor and
Doctoral Program Evaluator
University of Maryland
School of Nursing
Baltimore, Maryland

ELIZABETH R. LENZ, R.N., PH.D.
Associate Professor and
Director of the Doctoral Program
University of Maryland
School of Nursing
Baltimore, Maryland

F. A. DAVIS COMPANY • Philadelphia

Library of Congress Cataloging in Publication Data

Waltz, Carolyn Feher.
　Measurement in nursing research.

　Includes bibliographies and index.
　1. Nursing—Research.　I. Strickland, Ora.　II. Lenz, Elizabeth R.,
1943-　　.　III. Title. [DNLM: 1. Nursing.　2. Research.　3. Statistics.
WY 20.5 W241m]
RT81.5.W36　1984　　　610.73′072　　　83-14360
ISBN 0-8036-9046-0

PREFACE

This book is intended to serve as a comprehensive text for nurses who are consumers or developers of nursing measures. It is designed to introduce nurses to the theories and principles of sound measurement practices and to present a pragmatic account of the process involved in designing, testing, and selecting instruments and other devices for the measurement of nursing variables in a variety of clinical, educational, and research settings.

Our own experiences in teaching measurement to nurses and other health professionals as well as our involvement in constructing and employing measurement practices in a variety of nursing situations guided the selection of topics and examples. This process of selection resulted in the inclusion of measurement content, strategies, and techniques with direct applicability for nurses in a variety of roles including those of student, educator, clinician, researcher, administrator, and consultant. For example, students in basic and advanced nursing programs as well as graduate nurses who seek to develop or expand their skill in measurement in order to contribute to the further documentation and explication of the outcomes of nursing practice should have a direct use for this book.

The development of sound measurement practices is germane to the further development and advancement of nursing as a profession. Yet measurement, to date, has not been given the attention it warrants. Measurement per se has not been viewed as vital content in most nursing education programs, and too much of the measurement encountered in nursing practice and in the literature lacks rigor and precision. For this reason, this book seeks to meet the needs of a large and diversified nursing audience. Hence, we do not assume that most readers have an extensive background in measurement or statistics. Rather, the discussions begin by assuming little background in these areas and subsequently develop, explain in detail, and illustrate by example the concepts and principles that are operationally important to the content presented. In this manner, it is possible for the less sophisticated reader to develop the level of knowledge necessary to understand the content, such as triangulation and the multi-trait multi-method approach, that is included for the benefit of the more advanced reader.

The focus is on increasing the reader's ability to employ measures that are operationalized within the context of a conceptual framework for nursing, derived from a sound measurement perspective, and adequately tested for reliability and validity using appropriate techniques. Major nursing theories and concepts available for operationalizing nursing variables are examined. Both classical and nonclassical approaches to measurement are included, and step-by-step procedures for developing and testing norm-referenced and criterion-referenced tools and procedures with particular utility for the measurement of nursing variables are presented. Content in this area focuses on the essential considerations to be made in selecting such measures as well as the specific steps to be undertaken in designing and testing them. Attention is given to places where readers may locate tools. Extant tools and procedures employed in nursing are examined, and approaches to evaluating existing tools are suggested. In addition, issues to be addressed in the measurement of nursing variables, such as the use of standardized approaches and borrowed tools, measurement of state-trait characteristics, process/outcome measurement, and ethics, are explored.

Throughout the book references to additional sources are provided for readers who desire to pursue further the topics presented. References have been selected so that the material is readily available in most libraries, and whenever possible, comprehensive summaries of literature in an area or significant sources are cited rather than a myriad of individual books and articles.

CFW
OLS
ERL

CONTENTS

1

INTRODUCTION

This chapter introduces the reader to some terms and ideas basic to the content in subsequent chapters and provides an overview of the types of measures.

OPERATIONALIZING NURSING CONCEPTS

Concepts have been defined in numerous ways by different authors. Simply defined, a concept is a thought, notion, or idea. It is an abstraction. Nursing concepts then are thoughts, notions, or ideas about nursing or nursing practice. *Phenomena* are observable facts or events. To render nursing concepts measurable it is necessary to translate them into phenomena. When one operationalizes a nursing concept, one translates an abstract concept into concrete observable events or phenomena. For example, the concept attitude is frequently operationalized as a tendency to respond in a consistent manner to a certain category of stimuli (Campbell, 1963). If the stimulus is a ten-item questionnaire regarding the antagonistic patient, and the subject responds positively to the majority of the ten items, one would infer from the responses that the subject's attitude toward the antagonistic patient is positive.

Variables are quantities that may assume successive values; they are changeable. The process whereby one decides how to measure a variable is referred to as instrumentation; that is, *instrumentation* is the process of selecting or developing devices and methods appropriate for measuring an attribute or characteristic of interest. In the example, the ten-item questionnaire was a form of instrumentation selected to measure attitudes toward the antagonistic patient. Instrumentation is a component of the measurement process. *Measurement* is defined as the process of assigning numbers to objects to represent the kind and/or amount of an attribute or characteristic possessed by those objects. This definition of measurement includes what has traditionally been referred to as *qualitative* measurement (i.e., assigning objects to categories that represent the *kind* of characteristic possessed and that are mutually exclusive and exhaustive) as well as *quantitative* measurement (i.e., assigning objects to categories that represent the *amount* of a characteristic possessed).

Nursing concepts are usually difficult to operationalize, that is, render measurable. This is explained in part by the fact that nurses deal with a multiplicity of complex variables in diversified settings, employing a myriad of roles as they collaborate with a variety of others to attain their own and others' goals. Hence, the dilemma that the nurse is apt to encounter in measuring nursing concepts is twofold: First, the significant nursing variables to be measured must somehow be isolated; and second, very ambiguous and abstract notions must be reduced to a set of concrete behavioral indicators. What is available to the nurse who must begin to grapple with this dilemma?

Because nurses are currently being challenged to provide services of broadening scope and diversity in order to keep pace with the rapidly changing health care scene, a great deal of controversy has ensued regarding what functions should be included within the realm of nursing practice. A proliferation of definitions and models for nursing practice is evident in the literature. Although for the most part the definitions of nursing advanced in the literature remain ambiguous and global, in each view the major focus for nursing practice can be placed on a continuum ranging from direct to indirect involvement in patient care. Direct nursing practice involves the continuous, ongoing provision of direct services to patients and clients (e.g., the primary care nurse practitioner provides direct nursing services). Indirect nursing practice is usually characterized by activities on behalf of the patient, that is, working with or through others who are directly responsible for the provision of direct services to patients and clients. Nursing education and nursing administration activities exemplify indirect nursing practice. This scheme for categorizing nursing practice has utility for the nurse who is attempting to operationalize nursing concepts.

More specifically, the first task is to identify a definition of nursing that is consistent with the nurse's own views and beliefs about nursing practice. Similarly, although the extent to which available conceptual frameworks and models for nursing practice have been refined and tested varies, their very existence affords nurses a rich opportunity to select a conceptual framework to guide them in systematically identifying and further explicating concepts and variables germane to nursing and nursing practice concerns within their primary focus. The problems, settings, roles, and purposeful activities undertaken by nurses will differ, depending upon whether their primary focus is direct or indirect nursing practice. Furthermore, the goals for and outcomes likely to result from the application of direct and indirect nursing processes will vary. Although there will be differences within each of these categories of practice, there will also be commonalities in processes and outcomes within each focus. Therefore, if nurses consider their measurement concern within the context of their primary focus, delimit the processes and outcomes that characterize that practice, and then search for behavioral indicators within their primary focus that extend beyond their immediate setting (i.e., that are common across settings similar to their own), they are apt to reduce the abstract concepts emanating from their conceptual framework to behavioral indicators with more universal acceptance than those likely to result from a more esoteric approach. In this manner, nurses will also ultimately make a contribution to the profession by accruing information to add to the body of knowledge about nursing, the specific definition and conceptual framework employed, and its utility as a guide for operationalizing nursing and nursing practice concerns. It should be noted that when nurses whose measurement concern emanates from their ongoing practice fail to step back and rethink the problem from a conceptual point of view, they also have a high probability of investigating and measuring their variables from a limited perspective that overlooks important dimensions of the variables that should be measured.

In a profession like nursing in which the primary concern is with the measurement of process variables, which are dynamic, as well as outcome variables, which are usually static, and in which results of the measurement are likely to be applied to the solution of significant problems across practice settings, two characteristics of measurement—reliability and validity—become of utmost importance. First, devices and methods selected or developed for measuring a variable of interest must demonstrate reliability and validity. *Reliability* in this case refers to the consistency with which a device or method assigns scores to subjects. *Validity* refers to the determination of whether or not a device or method is useful for the purpose for which it is intended, that is, measures what it purports to measure. Second, in addition to the concern with instrument reliability and validity, nurses need to attend to the reliability and validity of the measurement process per se. To increase the probability that the measurement process will yield reliable and valid information, it is necessary whenever possible to employ multiple devices or methods to measure any given variable (all of which have demonstrated instrument reliability and validity) and to obtain information about any given variable from a number of different perspectives or sources. Measurement reliability and validity is thus largely a function of a well-designed and well-executed measurement process. For this reason, the intent of this book is to provide the reader with sound background in the theories, principles, and practices of measurement and instrumentation that are germane to the measurement of nursing concepts.

MEASUREMENT FRAMEWORKS

Just as it is important to identify and employ a nursing conceptual framework for delineating the nursing aspects of a measurement process, it is important to identify and employ a measurement framework to guide the design and interpretation of the measurement per se. The two major frameworks for measurement are the norm-referenced and criterion-referenced approaches.

A *norm-referenced approach* is employed when the interest is in evaluating the performance of a subject relative to the performance of other subjects in some well-defined comparison or norm group. The National League for Nursing Achievement Test Battery is an example of a norm-referenced measure in that a given subject's score takes on meaning when it is considered in light of the scores of other nursing students nationwide who took the same test. Similarly, the results of the application of physiologic measures such as blood pressure readings are often interpreted on the basis of readings (usually ranges of values) considered normal for some well-defined comparison group (e.g., black males over 40 years of age with no significant health problems). It should be noted that the terms norm-referenced and standardized are not synonymous. Standardized tests are one type of norm-referenced measure; there are other types as well. A standardized test, unlike most other norm-referenced measures, is designed by experts for wide use and has prescribed content, well-defined procedures for administration and scoring, and established norms.

A key feature of a norm-referenced measure is variance. The task when using a norm-referenced measure is to construct a device that measures a specific characteristic in such a way that it maximally discriminates among subjects possessing differing amounts of that characteristic, that is, spreads people out along the possible ranges of scores. For example, if the characteristic to be measured is knowledge of human sexuality content, then test items are designed to differentiate between individuals with varying levels of knowledge of the content. The goal is to obtain scores in such a manner that the result is a few high scores, most scores in the middle range, and a few low scores. If this goal is achieved the resulting distribution of scores on the measure should look much like a normal curve. Figure 1-1 illustrates the distribution of scores that one would expect to result from the employment of the hypothetical ten-item norm-referenced measure of human sexuality content.

The sole purpose of a *criterion-referenced measure* is to determine whether or not a subject has acquired a predetermined set of target behaviors. The task in this case is to specify the important target behaviors precisely and to construct a test or measure that discriminates between those subjects who have and those who have not acquired the target behaviors. How well a subject's performance compares with the performance of others is irrelevant when a criterion-referenced framework is employed. Criterion-referenced measures are particularly useful in the clinical area when the concern is with the measurement of process and outcome variables. For example, a criterion-referenced measure of process would require that nurses identify standards for nursing intervention and then compare their subjects' clinical performance with the standards for performance (i.e., predetermined target behaviors) rather than compare subjects' performance with that of other subjects, all of whom may not meet the standards. Similarly, when a criterion-referenced measure is employed to measure patient outcomes, a given patient's status is determined by comparing his or her performance with a set of predetermined criteria (e.g., ECG normal, diastolic pressure below 80, other vital signs stable by four hours postop) or

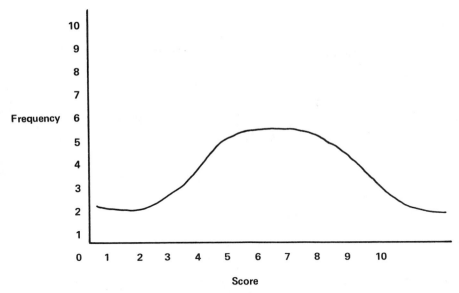

FIGURE 1-1. Distribution of scores on a ten-item norm-referenced test.

target behaviors (e.g., requests for pain medication have ceased by two days postop, verbalizes desire to return to normal activities by third day postop) rather than by comparing his or her performance with that of other patients.

One would expect the distribution of scores resulting from a criterion-referenced measure to look like the one illustrated in Figure 1-2. It should be noted that not only does the distribution of scores resulting from a criterion-referenced measure have less variance or spread than that resulting from a norm-referenced measure, but it also is skewed in shape. In a skewed distribution, scores tend to cluster at one end of the scale; in the example, the high end. A more detailed discussion of score spread (variance) and distribution shape (normal and skewed) is presented in Chapter 3.

Because the design, scoring, interpretation, reliability, and validity testing for norm-referenced and criterion-referenced measures differ, it is important that nurses decide which of the two measurement frameworks they will employ prior to the conduct of any other steps in the measurement process.

TYPES OF MEASURES*

Once nurses have determined their measurement framework, attention turns to the selection of the specific type of measure to be employed. Se-

---

*Portions of the material in this section are adapted with permission from Waltz and Bausell, 1981.

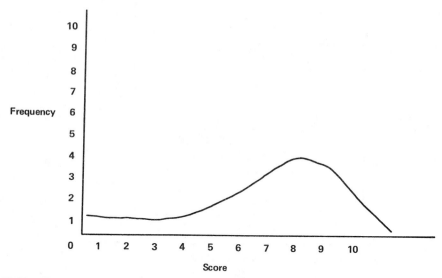

FIGURE 1-2. Distribution of scores on a ten-item criterion-referenced test.

mantics is often a problem for newcomers to the field of measurement. Many different terms are employed to label like measures. For this reason, it is important to consider at this point some of the classification schemes and terms that are used to label the different types of measures available to nurses.

In addition to being categorized as either norm-referenced or criterion-referenced, measuring devices may be classified by (1) what they seek to measure, (2) the manner in which responses are obtained and scored, (3) the type of subject performance they seek to measure, or (4) who constructs them.

WHAT IS MEASURED. In nursing, the concern is usually with measuring cognition, affect, psychomotor skills, and/or physical functioning. *Cognitive* measures assess subjects' knowledge or achievement in a specific content area. Indicators of cognitive behavior usually are obtained via:

1. Achievement tests (objective and essay) that measure the extent to which cognitive objectives have been attained.

2. Self-evaluation measures designed to determine subjects' perceptions of the extent to which cognitive objectives have been met.

3. Rating scales and checklists for judging the qualities of products produced in conjunction with or as a result of an experience.

4. Sentence completion exercises designed to categorize the types of responses and to enumerate their frequencies relative to specific criteria.

5. Interviews to determine the frequencies and levels of satisfactory responses to formal and informal questions raised in a face-to-face setting.

6. Peer utilization surveys to ascertain the frequency of selection or assignment to leadership or resource roles.

7. Questionnaires employed to determine the frequency of responses to items in an objective format or number of responses to categorized dimen-

sions developed from the content analysis of responses to open-ended questions.

8. Anecdotal records and critical incidents to ascertain the frequency of behaviors judged to be highly desirable or undesirable.

9. Review of records, reports, and other written materials (e.g., articles, autobiographical data, awards, citations, honors) to determine the numbers and types of accomplishments of subjects.

The number of cognitive measures employed far exceed the number of other types of measures. Specifically, written multiple choice tests are the most often used, perhaps because they are the most objective of the various cognitive measures and the most reliable, and because they have the greatest utility in measuring all types of knowledge. It should be noted that cognitive measures are not limited to paper and pencil tests and that a variety of other approaches exist that warrant further attention in nursing.

Affective measures seek to determine interests, values, and attitudes. *Interests* are conceptualized as preferences for particular activities. Examples of statements relating to interests are:

I prefer direct nursing practice to indirect nursing practice.
I like to work with student nurses as they give care to patients.
I prefer teaching responsibilities to research responsibilities.
I would enjoy having one day a week to devote to reading about developments in my field.

Values concern preferences for life goals and ways of life, in contrast to interests, which concern preferences for particular activities. Examples of statements relating to values are:

I consider it important to have people respect nursing as a profession.
A nurse's duty to her patient comes before duty to the community.
Service to others is more important to me than personal ambition.
I would rather be a teacher than an administrator.

Attitudes concern feelings about particular social objects, that is, physical objects, types of people, particular persons, or social institutions. Examples of statements relating to attitudes are:

Nursing as a profession is a constructive force in determining health policy today.
Continuing education for nurses should be mandatory for relicensure.
Humanistic care is a right of all patients.
All nurses should be patient advocates.

The feature that distinguishes attitudes from interests and values is that attitudes always concern a particular target or object. In contrast, interests and values concern numerous activities: specific activities in measures of interest and very broad categories of activities in measures of value.

It is extremely difficult to preserve the conceptual differences between interests, values, and attitudes when actually constructing measures of affect. Thus, for the purposes of rendering them measurable, they are all subsumed under the rubric of *acquired behavioral dispositions* (Campbell, 1963) and are defined as tendencies to respond in a consistent manner to a certain category of stimuli. For example, when patients are asked to respond to a questionnaire to indicate their satisfaction with the quality of care received, one is interested in measuring their tendency to consistently respond that they are satisfied or dissatisfied, given a set of questions that ask them about the care they received (the stimuli).

Self-report measures are the most direct approach to the determination of affect. In this type of measure subjects are asked directly what their attitudes, interests, or values are. For example, subjects might be given a list of favorable and unfavorable statements regarding the antagonistic patient and asked to agree or disagree with each. Such a self-report inventory is referred to as an attitude scale. Other indicators of affective behaviors include but are not limited to:

1. Sentence completion exercises designed to obtain ratings of the psychological appropriateness of an individual's responses relative to specific criteria.

2. Interviews.

3. Questionnaires.

4. Semantic differential, Q sort, and other self-concept perception devices.

5. Physiologic measures.

6. Projective techniques, for example, role playing, picture interpretation.

7. Observational techniques and behavioral tests, including measures of congruence between what is reported and how an individual actually behaves in a specific situation.

8. Anecdotal records and critical incidents.

From the empirical evidence that exists concerning the validity of different approaches, it appears that self-report offers the most valid approach currently available. For this reason, at present, most measures of affect are based on self-report and usually employ one of two types of scales: a summated rating scale or a semantic differential scale.

A *scale* is a measuring device composed of:

1. A stem, which is a statement relating to attitudes or an attitudinal object to be rated by the respondent.

2. A series of scale steps.

3. Anchors that define the scale steps.

Table 1-1 presents examples of the components of a scale.

There are different types of anchors that can be employed: numbers, percentages, degrees of agreement-disagreement, adjectives (e.g.,

TABLE 1-1 The components of a scale

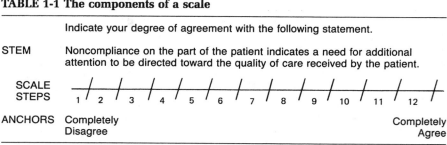

	Indicate your degree of agreement with the following statement.
STEM	Noncompliance on the part of the patient indicates a need for additional attention to be directed toward the quality of care received by the patient.
SCALE STEPS	1 2 3 4 5 6 7 8 9 10 11 12
ANCHORS	Completely Disagree Completely Agree

worthless-valuable), actual behavior, and products (e.g., samples of nursing care plans to be rated 1 to 6). Usually numerical anchors are preferred because:

1. If the meaning of each step on the scale is specified at the beginning of the rating form, as is usually the case, numbers provide an effective means of coordinating those definitions with rating scales.

2. Numbers on scales constantly remind subjects of the meanings of scale steps.

3. Numbers facilitate the analysis of data, for example, placing ratings on cards for computer analysis (Nunnally, 1967).

Summated Rating Scale. A summated rating scale contains a set of scales, all of which are considered approximately equal in attitude or value loading. The subjects respond with varying degrees of intensity on a scale ranging between extremes such as agree/disagree, like/dislike, or accept/reject. The scores for all scales in the set are summed or summed and averaged to yield an individual's attitude score. An example of a summated rating scale is given in Table 1-2.

Summated rating scales are easy to construct, usually reliable, and flexible in that they may be adapted for the measurement of many different kinds of attitudes. Nunnally (1967) suggests the reliability of summated scales is a direct function of the number of items. When there are a reasonable number (e.g., 20) of items on the scale, fewer scale steps for individual scales are required for a high degree of reliability. When there are fewer items, more scale steps for individual scales are required for reliability. In most cases, 10 to 15 items using 5 or 6 steps are sufficient. Individual scales on summated attitude scales tend to correlate substantially with each other, because it is fairly easy for the constructor to devise items that obviously relate to each other and for subjects to see the common core of meaning in the items. Additional information regarding summated attitude scales can be found in Nunnally (1967), Edwards (1957), or Shaw and Wright (1967).

Semantic Differential Scales. The semantic differential is a method for measuring the meaning of concepts that was developed by Osgood and associates (1957). The semantic differential has three components: (1) the concept to be rated in terms of its attitudinal properties, (2) bipolar adjectives that anchor the scale, and (3) a series of 5 to 9 scale steps (7 is the optimal number of steps suggested by Osgood). Table 1-3 presents an example of a semantic differential scale. The concept to be rated in Table 1-3 is noncomplying patient. Respondents are instructed to rate the concept according to how they perceive it or feel about it by placing an X along the seven-point scale anchored by the bipolar adjective pairs. The resulting scale responses can then be converted to numerical values and treated statistically.

Nunnally (1967) explains that the logic underlying the semantic differential stems from the recognition that, in spoken and written language, characteristics of ideas and objects are communicated largely by adjectives. If it is reasonable on this basis to assume that much of meaning can be and usually is communicated by adjectives, it is also reasonable to assume that adjectives can be used to measure various facets of meaning. The semantic

TABLE 1-2 Example of a summated rating scale*

Indicate your degree of agreement with each of the following statements.

a. Antagonistic behavior on the part of the patient indicates a need for additional attention and time from the nurse.

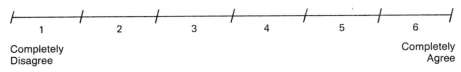

Completely
Disagree

Completely
Agree

b. Antagonistic patients receive more than their share of time and attention from the nursing staff.

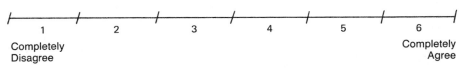

Completely
Disagree

Completely
Agree

c. The nurse should avoid reinforcing the undesirable behavior of antagonistic patients by placing limits on the time and attention given to them.

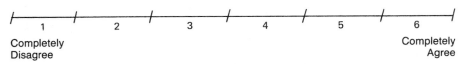

Completely
Disagree

Completely
Agree

d. The nurse should spend more time with antagonistic patients in an attempt to allay their fears.

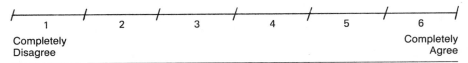

Completely
Disagree

Completely
Agree

*Adapted from Staropoli and Waltz (1978, p. 129).

differential primarily measures connotative aspects of meaning, that is, what implications the object in question has for the respondents. For example, if an individual rating the concept noncomplying patient said, "I dislike them very much," this statement would represent a connotation or sentiment for that type of patient. The semantic differential is one of the most valid measures available for assessing the connotative aspects of meaning, particularly the evaluative connotations of objects.

Factor analytic studies of semantic differential scales have suggested there are three major factors of meaning assessed by such scales: (1) evaluation, (2) potency, and (3) activity. Table 1-4 presents the pairs of adjectives most frequently used to define each of these factors. Additional information regarding semantic differential scales can be obtained from Osgood, Suci, and Tannenbaum (1957) and Snider and Osgood (1969).

Psychomotor measures seek to assess subjects' skill, that is, their ability to perform specific tasks or carry out specific procedures, techniques, and

TABLE 1-3 Example of a semantic differential scale

Rate the following concept in terms of how you feel about it at this point in time.

Noncomplying Patient

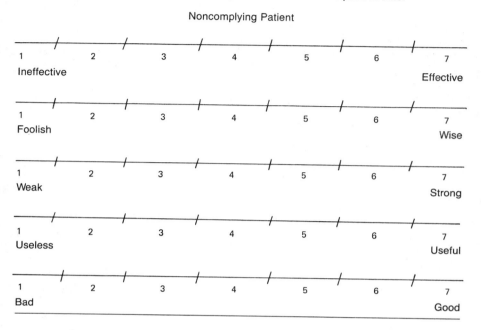

the like. An important consideration in the measurement of psychomotor objectives involves the manner in which the skills and materials or objects to be manipulated or coordinated are specified. Specificially, criteria for the successful manipulation of an object must be clearly and unambiguously stated at the time when objectives are made explicit. Task analysis procedures (Gagne, 1962) are often used to accomplish this.

The most viable approach to the measurement of psychomotor skills at this time is the observation method combined with a performance checklist or rating scale. The observation method always involves some interaction between subject and observer in which the observer has an opportunity to watch the subject perform. Although in some cases free and unstructured observation is desirable, it is more often necessary that the nurse prepare an

TABLE 1-4 Frequently employed anchors for semantic differential factors

	Factor		
	Evaluation	**Potency**	**Activity**
BIPOLAR ADJECTIVES	good . . . . bad	strong . . weak	active . . . passive
	fair . . . . unfair	large . . . small	quick . . . slow
	positive . . . . . negative	severe . . lenient	tense . . . relaxed
	honest . . . . . . dishonest	hard . . . . soft	sharp . . . dull
	successful . . . unsuccessful		
	valuable . . . . . worthless		

observation guide to structure the observations and train the observer in its use. This guide increases the probability that the crucial behaviors of concern will be considered and hence increases the reliability and validity of the method. When possible, the guide should specify when an observation begins and ends as well as what behaviors are to be observed. Frequently, time is the vehicle for accomplishing this purpose. For example, it might be specified that observation of the nurse's history taking begins when the nurse enters the room and continues for the first five minutes of the nurse-patient interaction, or, using a more elaborate scheme, that observations will begin when the nurse enters the room, continue for two minutes, and then observers will rest for the next two minutes, rate for two minutes, rest for two minutes, and so forth, until the nurse leaves the room and the encounter ends.

No matter how structured the observation or how well trained or competent the observer, observation techniques to be sound require more than one observer. This provides an estimate of the accuracy or reliability of the observations and provides a basis for determining the degree of confidence to be placed in the data.

Three factors must be considered in the discussion of observational techniques: (1) interaction between respondents and observers, (2) whether or not respondents know they are being observed, and (3) whether or not respondents know when they will be observed. Observation is difficult because watching a situation often changes it so that the observers are no longer certain of what they are observing. This implies that a basic criterion for evaluating studies in which observation is used is the extent to which the situation observed was natural. Observations of a subject's psychomotor skills should be accomplished with as little effect as possible on the natural situation in which the skills are normally performed. Webb and associates (1966) have published a useful book full of suggestions for how measures can be collected as unobtrusively as possible.

It is necessary to weigh the value of collecting observational data over time as opposed to collecting information at one isolated point in time. Observational data collected at one point in time are subject to more errors of measurement and, hence, lower reliability and validity than observational data collected at multiple points in time. When subjects' psychomotor performance is of interest, the concern is usually with how they perform most of the time or typically, that is, patterns of performance or consistency in their performance over time becomes of importance. When observational data are collected at one point in time there is greater probability that results of the measure will reflect more of the conditions surrounding that isolated point in time than the true abilities of the subject to perform the tasks or behaviors. Hence, whenever possible, measures of performance should occur at more than one point in time.

Observational techniques may be direct or indirect. In *direct observation* the observer evaluates psychomotor performance by simply watching the subject perform. A limitation of this approach stems from the fact that it is both time consuming and expensive. It is, however, an excellent technique for the assessment of behavior in conjunction with clinical performance in nursing, especially when the concern is with dynamic or process variables. Similarly, a unique strength of the observation method results from the fact that if the observer wishes to learn how a subject functions under the pressure of supervision, there is no substitute for direct observation that is known and scheduled.

Indirect methods of observation include motion picture, television, videotaping, and other devices for recording subjects' activities. The value of indirect techniques results from the opportunities they afford for subjects to become involved in the evaluation of their performance as the recording is viewed jointly by the observer and respondents. Indirect observations are limited in that they are not sensitive to the tone, mood, or affect of the situation. Another limitation is that mechanical devices selectively record depending upon their placement—where they are aimed by the operator—and hence, the total situation may be missed. This limitation can be turned into an advantage, however, if multiple devices are used so that recordings are made of all that happens before them.

Physiologic measures seek to quantify the level of functioning of living beings. Indicators of physiologic functioning include but are not limited to:
1. Blood pressure readings.
2. Temperature readings.
3. Respiratory measures.
4. Metabolic readings.
5. Diabetic and other screening devices.
6. Readings from cardiac and other monitoring instruments.
7. ECG and EEG readings.
8. Results of blood tests and analyses.
9. Measures of height and weight.

Physical functioning can often be measured by a scientific instrument, and the results of physiologic measures usually are expressed as a quantitative scale that can be graded into finely distinguished numerical values. For example, the variable diastolic blood pressure is measured using a scientific instrument referred to as a sphygmomanometer. Its scale is in a quantitative form ranging from 0 to 300, providing a total of 300 different continuous scale points or values to which a subject can be assigned and with which to differentiate among the various degrees of the variable possessed by the subjects measured. Thus, on the basis of blood pressure readings, one can state that a subject with a diastolic pressure of 100 is 20 points higher than one with a diastolic pressure of 80. This 20-point difference is of significance in comparing the physical status of two patients.

Physiologic measures are among the most precise methods one can employ; they yield data measured at the interval or ratio level of measurement, allow a wide range of statistical procedures to be employed in their analysis, and tend to produce results that demonstrate a high degree of reliability and validity.

HOW RESPONSES ARE OBTAINED AND SCORED

The distinction to be considered here is whether a measure is objective or subjective. It should be noted that a given method or technique is generally viewed as more or less objective or subjective; that is, one may think in terms of a continuum anchored by the terms objective and subjective and then place a given method on the continuum, depending upon whether it possesses characteristics more like those of an objective or subjective measure.

Objective measures contain items that allow subjects little if any latitude in constructing their responses and that spell out criteria for scoring so clearly that scores can be assigned either by individuals who know nothing of the content or by mechanical means. Multiple choice questions and physiologic measures are examples of the most objective devices that can be employed.

Subjective measures allow respondents considerable latitude in constructing their responses. In addition, the probability that different scorers may apply different criteria is greater. Examples of subjective measures are the essay test, open-ended interview questions, case studies, and nursing care plans. The *essay* question is a method requiring a response constructed by the subject, usually in the form of one or more sentences. The nature of the response is such that (1) no single answer or pattern of answers can be listed as correct and (2) the quality of the response can be judged only subjectively by one skilled or informed in the subject (Stalnaker, 1951). Thus, significant features of the essay method are (1) the freedom of response allowed the respondents, (2) the fact that no single answer can be identified as correct or complete, and (3) responses must be scored by experts who themselves usually cannot classify a response as categorically right or wrong. Essay questions may require subjects to express their own thoughts on an issue of interest to the profession of nursing, outline a research design for investigating a research question, derive a mathematical proof, or explain the nature of some nursing phenomenon. Items may require only a brief response or may demand an extensive exposition.

Advocates of the essay approach argue that an important characteristic of individuals is their ability to interact effectively with other individuals in the realm of ideas. The basic tool of interaction is language, and successful individuals are those who can react appropriately to questions or problems in their field as they encounter them. It is not enough, they contend, to be able to recognize a correct fact when it is presented or to discriminate among alternatives posed by others. Successful individuals are the masters of their collection of ideas, are able to cite evidence to support a position, to extend their range of understanding, and to contribute to the advancement of ideas and constructs within their field. The only way to assess the extent to which individuals have mastered a field is to present them with questions or problems in the field and assess how they perform. Hence, they argue, the essay format provides an avenue for assessing scholarly and/or professional performances better than other available methods (Coffman, 1971).

Even so, because of their subjective nature, essay questions have inherent limitations that must be recognized and minimized if sound measurement is to result from their use. Limitations of essays and other subjective measures as well fall into two general categories: (1) problems related to the difficulty in achieving consistency in scoring responses, and (2) problems associated with the sampling of content. Empirical evidence regarding the reliability of subjective measures suggests that different raters tend to assign different scores to the same response; a single rater tends to assign different scores to the same response on different occasions; and the differences tend to increase as the measure permits greater freedom of response (Finlayson, 1951; Hartog and Rhodes, 1933; Noyes, 1963; Pearson, 1955; Vernon and Millican, 1954). Different raters may differ as a result of a number of factors including the severity of their standards, the extent to which they distribute scores throughout the score scale, and real differences in the criteria they are applying.

Basic to problems associated with the sampling of content is the notion that each sample unit should be independent and equally likely to be chosen in the sample. In general, the greater the number of different questions, the higher the reliability of the score. The compromise to be made, however, is between the desire to increase the adequacy of the sample of content by asking many different questions and the desire to ask questions that probe deeply the subjects' understanding. Additional information regarding essay items is presented in Stalnaker (1951) and Coffman (1971). Other subjective measures are described in more detail in Chapter 9.

TYPE OF PERFORMANCE MEASURED

A nurse may seek to measure typical performance or maximum performance. If the interest is in assessing subjects as they do their best (produce their highest quality work), then a *maximum performance* measure is appropriate. Such measures are indices of cognition which generally measure a set of skills a subject possesses, but which differ among themselves in the specificity of their focus and the use to which scores are put. Maximum performance measures of particular interest include aptitude measures, achievement measures, and diagnostic measures.

Aptitude tests are specific measures of capacity for success and tend to focus on various general aspects of human ability (e.g., mechanical aptitude, artistic aptitude). They are often used as predictors of performance in special fields.

Achievement measures are tests of particular skills and knowledge and are more specific than aptitude tests. They usually sample a wide range of skills and are constructed by nurses for their own use. Commercially produced achievement measures also are available in many different content areas.

Diagnostic tests are even more specific in their focus than achievement measures, although this need not always be the case. They focus on specific skills and often employ multiple measures of particular skills. Their intent is to pinpoint specific weaknesses that might not be apparent otherwise. Once specific deficiencies are identified and remediation has taken place, one might predict that achievement, which is assumed to be dependent on these more specific skills, will improve.

If information about subjects' typical behavior (i.e., what they usually do or would do) is of interest, it is appropriate to use a *typical performance* measure. These are measures of affective behavior and usually attempt to have respondents describe the way they typically perceive themselves or their behavior. Typical performance measures usually ask the subjects for scaled responses, forced choice responses, or criterion-keyed responses. Table 1-5 presents examples of each of these types of responses.

15

TABLE 1-5 Sample responses of typical performance measures

Scaled response:
In a scaled response situation, the respondent indicates on a scale what his rating or answer is to the question posed. An example is the item:
Did this course provide information that will be meaningful to you in your clinical work? Please rate.

not at all	very little	somewhat	enough	very much
1	2	3	4	5

Forced choice response:
With a forced choice response item, the respondent is asked to choose between two or three different alternatives, all of which may be appealing responses. The point is that one particular response is most appealing to the subject. An example of this type of item is:
A program of ongoing evaluation of patient care does not exist in the agency with which you are affiliated. You are aware of a need to evaluate the various approaches to patient care management. You would prefer to have this need met by:
1. Referring the task to someone else.
2. Supporting the activities of the professional nursing organizations that are seeking to stimulate interest and involvement in evaluation of patient care.
3. Supporting a policy change in the agency responsible for care.
4. Acting as a resource person to staff by providing them with knowledge and materials to enable them to develop such a program.
5. Becoming a member of a committee of practitioners who are developing and testing a pilot program of evaluation in conjunction with the patients for whom they deliver care.
6. Initiating the idea of such a program by providing care to a small group of clients and sharing with staff your evaluation of the various approaches you use.

Criterion-keyed response:
Criterion-keyed responses depend on information previously obtained about how certain groups answered the items. If a present respondent's score looks like those from members of a certain predefined group, then he is classified as a member of that group. Criterion keying assumes that the criterion for membership in a particular group is having a set of responses on the measurement instrument that looks like those from the predefined group.
Example: The Minnesota Multiphasic Personality Inventory (MMPI) was originally used with hospitalized psychiatric patients and normal (i.e., nonhospitalized respondents) to construct a criterion-keyed set of questions which had some value as predictors of mental stability, that is, if a particular item was responded to differently by the two groups, it was included in the test.

From Staropoli and Waltz (1978, p. 116), with permission.

WHO CONSTRUCTS MEASURES

Standardized measures are developed by specialists for wide use. Their content is set, the directions for administration (often including time limits) are clearly described, and the scoring procedure to be used is completely prescribed. Norms information concerning scores is generally available.

Informal devices are typically constructed by nurses for their own use. They are not content constrained, that is, the user is free to define the content as well as administration procedures and scoring. Norms may be available for local groups but usually are not available on any group.

In summary, the measurement framework employed in a given situation will have important implications for instrument development and for what can be done with and on the basis of the resulting information. Thus, nurses must clarify at the outset the type of measurement that will yield data appropriate for the types of questions and/or hypotheses they seek to answer. In Chapters 2 through 7 attention focuses on tool development and testing in both the norm-referenced and criterion-referenced cases. In Chapters 8 through 10 and the Appendix characteristics and important considerations to be made in using the types of measures presented in this section are addressed.

RELIABILITY AND VALIDITY OF MEASURES

As indicated in the foregoing sections reliability and validity are essential characteristics of any measuring device or method. Factors that may affect the degree of consistency obtained for a given measure (reliability) are (1) the manner in which the measure is scored, (2) characteristics of the measure itself, (3) the physical and/or emotional state of the individual at measurement time, and (4) properties of the situation in which the measure is administered (e.g., the amount of noise, lighting conditions, temperature of the room).

Strictly speaking, one validates not the measuring device but rather some use to which the measure is put. For example, an instrument designed to select participants who would benefit from a primary care fellowship experience must be valid for that purpose, but it would not necessarily be valid for other purposes, such as measuring how well participants master objectives at the completion of the fellowship experience.

Both reliability and validity are matters of degree rather than all or none properties. Measures should be assessed each time they are used to see if they are behaving as planned. New evidence may suggest modifications in an existing measure or the development of a new and better approach to measuring the attribute in question. Reliability is a necessary prerequisite for validity, that is, if a measure does not assign scores consistently it cannot be useful for the purposes for which it is intended. Reliability is not, however, a sufficient condition for validity, that is, because a measure consistently measures a phenomenon does not ensure that it measures the phenomenon of interest.

As stated earlier, the determination of the reliability and validity of a specific device or method will differ depending upon whether it is norm-referenced or criterion-referenced. Specific techniques for determining reliability and validity in each case are discussed in Chapter 4 (norm-referenced) and in Chapter 7 (criterion-referenced). In either case, the reliability and validity of the measurement process itself is increased when multiple measures of the same thing are employed, that is, more than one type of instrumentation is used to answer a given question. Similarly, reliability and validity increase when the answer to a given measurement concern is elicited by collecting data from a number of different sources using the same measure or device.

REFERENCES

ANGOFF, WH: "Scales, Norms, and Equivalent Scores." In THORNDIKE, RL (ed.): *Educational Measurement*, ed. 2. American Council on Education, Washington, D.C., 1971, p. 508–600.

BORLICK, M, et al: *Nursing Examination Review Book*, Vol. 9. *Community Health Nursing*, ed. 2. New York, Medical Examination Publishing Co., Inc., 1974.

CAMPBELL, DT: "Social Attitudes and Other Acquired Behavioral Dispositions." In KOCH, S (ed): *Psychology: A Study of a Science*, Vol. 6. New York, McGraw-Hill Book Co., 1963.

COFFMAN, WE: "Essay Examinations." In THORNDIKE, RL (ed): *Educational Measurement.* American Council on Education, Washington, D.C., 1971, pp. 271–302.

EDWARDS, A: *Techniques of Attitude Scale Construction.* New York, Appleton-Century-Crofts, 1957.

FINLAYSON, DS: "The Reliability of the Marking of Essays." *British Journal of Educational Psychology* 21:126–134, 1951.

GAGNE, RM: "The Acquisition of Knowledge." *Psychological Review* 69:355, 1962.

HARTOG, P AND RHODES, EC: *The Marks of Examiners.* Macmillan, New York, 1936.

MARTUZA, VR: *Applying Norm-Referenced and Criterion-Referenced Measurement in Education.* Allyn and Bacon, Inc., Boston, 1977.

MARTUZA, VR: et al: "EDF660 Tests and Measurements Course Manual," 4th revision. University of Delaware, College of Education, 1975, p. 1.

NOYES, ES: "Essay and Objective Tests in English." *College Board Review*, 49:7–10, 1963.

NUNNALLY, JC: *Psychometric Theory.* McGraw-Hill Book Co., New York, 1967.

OSGOOD, CE, SUCI, GJ, AND TANNENBAUM, PH: *The Measurement of Meaning.* University of Illinois Press, Chicago, 1957.

PEARSON, R: "The Test Fails as An Entrance Examination." In Should the General Composition Test be Continued? *College Board Review*, 25, 209, 1955.

SHAW, RE, AND WRIGHT, JM: *Scales for the Measurement of Attitudes.* McGraw-Hill Book Co., New York, 1967.

SNIDER, JG AND OSGOOD, CE (eds): *Semantic Differential Technique.* Aldine Publishing Co., Chicago, 1969.

STALNAKER, JM: "The Essay Type of Examination." In LINDQUIST, EF (ed): *Educational Measurement.* American Council on Education, Washington, DC, 1951, pp. 495–530.

STAROPOLI, CJ AND WALTZ, CF: *Developing and Evaluating Educational Programs for Health Care Providers.* F.A. Davis Co., Philadelphia, 1978.

VERNON, PE AND MILLICAN, GD: "A Further Study of the Reliability of English Essays." *British Journal of Statistical Psychology* 7:65–74, 1954.

WALTZ, CF AND BAUSELL, RB: *Nursing Research: Design, Statistics, and Computer Analysis.* F.A. Davis Co., Philadelphia, 1981.

WEBB, EE, et al: *Unobtrusive Measures: Nonreactive Research in the Social Sciences.* Rand McNally and Co., Chicago, 1966.

2

OPERATIONALIZATION
OF NURSING CONCEPTS

Within a scientific discipline such as nursing, concepts provide the means for communicating essential subject matter. They are the building blocks of thought and communication. As such, they constitute the logical starting point for nursing measurement. The conceptual approach to measurement advocated in this book highlights the importance of linking observations and experience to accumulated knowledge, thereby increasing the relevance and utility of any measurement activity. The purpose of this chapter is to provide an orientation to concepts as a basis for measurement and to present strategies for defining and operationalizing them.

DEFINITION OF TERMS

A *concept* is a term that symbolizes aspects of reality that can be thought about and communicated to others. It denotes an idea, often one formed from particular observations or sensory experiences (Burr, 1973, p. 5; King, 1975, p. 29; Newman, 1979, p. 5). The concept name is used to denote phenomena (objects, attributes, or events) that share a combination of essential properties that set them apart from other phenomena. Because a concept is a symbol, it is an *abstraction* from reality, a kind of shorthand device for labeling ideas; thus, it may serve as a language link between abstract thought and sensory experience.

Concepts are often considered the basic elements of scientific theories. In order to clarify this statement, it is necessary to define related terms encountered in the nursing literature. A *proposition* is a statement that includes and specifies a relationship between two or more concepts. The statement "Time is a function of movement" (Newman, 1979, p. 60) is an example of a proposition. The key concepts in this proposition are time and movement. A *theory* is an interrelated set of propositions or statements that provides the basis for describing, explaining, predicting, and/or controlling phenomena. The proposition above is one of several included in Newman's (1979) theory of health. A given theory may include many concepts. A *conceptual framework* (or conceptual model) also includes a number of concepts. In a conceptual framework concepts are identified, defined, and linked by broad generalizations. A conceptual framework provides an orienting scheme or world view that helps to focus thinking and provides direction for the development of specific theories. A number of theories may be developed under the rubric or perspective of one conceptual framework. Newman's theory of health has been guided by Rogers' (1970) conceptual framework. Usually a conceptual framework is more abstract and general than a theory, the latter including concepts that are more specific, precisely defined, and explicitly interrelated (Fawcett, 1978). The important point is that concepts provide the basis for building the complex statements and theories that form the subject matter of a discipline.

A distinction is generally made between concepts and *observables*. The former are abstractions from the latter. The term observable is used to include objects, behaviors, or properties that can be perceived through any of the senses either directly or indirectly. The color of a patient's skin or the size of his wound can be observed directly, as can behaviors that he carries out before an observer. Some behaviors and characteristics are observed indirectly via responses to questions; for example, behaviors that the patient performed in the past, his or her attitude toward illness, or his or her level of educational achievement. Some properties of individuals require amplification or transformation devices to be made observable. For example, cardiac arrhythmias are observed indirectly through an electrocardiograph which records electrical impulses.

Observables associated with a given concept are often termed *indicators* of the concept. In the examples cited above, number of years of schooling is an indicator of educational achievement; another indicator might be the highest degree earned. An abnormal P wave, as reflected in an electrocardiogram recording, is an indicator of a cardiac arrhythmia; other indicators might be palpitation, shortness of breath, or an irregular pulse. A given observable may be an indicator for more than one concept. For example, shortness of breath may be an indicator of anxiety or of pulmonary edema.

Operationalization is the process of delineating how a concept will be measured; that is, making a concept explicit in terms of the observables associated with it and/or the operations that must be carried out in order to measure it. To operationalize a concept is to specify the empirical indicators that will be used to signify its meaning and the procedures that will be used to measure it. The process of operationalization involves a mode of thinking that proceeds from the abstract to the concrete, in that one moves from an abstract idea (the concept) to identifying the concrete observables associated with it and the way in which those observables will be measured. The process of operationalization will be described in later sections of this chapter.

Operationalization is inherent in virtually every aspect of nursing practice. Consider the following discussion between Ms. X, the night charge nurse, and Ms. Y, the day charge nurse, during morning report on a surgical unit.

Ms. X: Mr. Jones, in Room 305, seemed very anxious about his surgery, which is scheduled for this morning.

Ms. Y: Why do you say that?

Ms. X: Well, he didn't sleep all night, even though I repeated his medication. I suggested that he try to read or watch TV but he couldn't concentrate. He paced around the halls most of the night and complained of diarrhea and stomach cramps.

In the above scenario, Ms. X has operationalized the concept anxiety (or anxious) by suggesting several observable indicators of the term: inability to sleep, inability to concentrate, pacing, diarrhea, and stomach pain.

Many nursing activities require that concepts be operationalized in writing and with as much precision as possible. Careful operationalization of concepts is an essential step in nursing research. Given a research problem or question to be investigated or a theory to be tested, the researcher must identify the key ideas or concepts and must define and operationalize each of them before a study can be carried out. Other nursing activities require precise operationalization of concepts as well. For example, in order to develop a nursing care plan the nurse must decide what needs to be known about the patient and which observations must be made to yield the information. Specifying the observations that must be made in order to assess a patient's nutritional status is an example of operationalizing that concept. To render nursing assessment precise and to assure that other nurses will base their judgments on the same kinds of observations, checklists, protocols, or guides may be developed. All such devices incorporate the operationalization of concepts. Other examples of activities that require precise operationalization of relatively complex concepts include evaluating the quality of nursing care, appraising patient responses to specific nursing interventions, and assessing student performance in the classroom or clinical setting.

In summary, concepts are the basic elements of language that convey ideas. As such they comprise the building blocks of more complex statements and theories. Because they also summarize and categorize concrete observations, they serve to link abstract thought and sensory experience. The process of operationalizing a concept makes explicit the inherent linkages between thought and experience by delineating how it can be identified and measured in concrete terms.

EXAMPLES OF NURSING CONCEPTS AND THEIR OPERATIONALIZATION

Nursing, like other disciplines, has key concepts that designate its essential subject matter. Some represent ideas that are vital to the thought and language of all nurses, regardless of the settings and specialty areas in which they practice. Others represent narrower domains of knowledge because they are of primary concern to certain subgroups within the profession.

Health, care, and interaction are examples of generic concepts that are essential building blocks of knowledge employed by all nurses. Examples of concepts that are more specific to subspecialty areas within nursing would include sibling rivalry (of primary interest to nurses working with children and young families) and dyspnea (of primary interest to nurses working with patients who have pulmonary or cardiac problems).

Because nursing is practiced in diverse settings and takes into account a wide variety of concerns, it is virtually impossible to generate a list of concepts that all nurses would agree are essential or central to the knowledge of the discipline. Individual nurse theorists who have developed conceptual frameworks to guide nursing knowledge and practice have identified different key nursing concepts (see the Appendix). Likewise, nursing curricula differ in the concepts that are highlighted. Choice of particular concepts for emphasis reflects one's background, perspective, and philosophy. It is not necessary that there be universal agreement that a given concept is important to nursing knowledge. In fact, it may be argued that inability to agree on a specific set of concepts reflects the diversity of the discipline and encourages thought and dialogue. It can be expected that over time certain concepts will emerge as more important than others for building nursing knowledge.

Nursing concepts represent a wide variety of phenomena that are of concern to the profession. Some represent objects (e.g., syringe, bed, patient), while others represent attributes or characteristics of objects or people (e.g., anxiety, attitude, intelligence). Some nursing concepts represent static entities or states occurring at a given point in time (e.g., asepsis, health status), while others represent dynamic processes that occur over time intervals (e.g., socialization, interaction, transaction). Whereas some concepts refer to individuals or properties thereof, others represent relations between individuals (e.g., subordination) or properties of collective units such as families, groups, or communities.

Table 2-1 contains examples of some concepts used in nursing research projects and specifies the ways in which each was operationalized. Inspection of this table reveals that nursing concepts differ in several respects. First, they differ in their complexity or the number of observable properties, characteristics, or behaviors designated by the concept name. Concepts such as identity and functionality are highly complex, in that they encompass a large number of characteristics and behaviors and their meanings have many dimensions. In general, the more complex the concept, the more difficult it is to specify its meaning, the less likely it is to be defined identically by all using it, and the more complex its operationalization. The relatively complex concepts in Table 2-1 are either operationalized in terms of several discrete observables (e.g., functionality, attachment behavior) or by means of indices that combine several discrete observables into one score (e.g., socioeconomic class, functional health, sex role identity).

Nursing concepts also differ in their level of abstraction, that is, in the number of inferential steps required to translate observation into meaning. The concept table is relatively concrete, in that most of its properties are directly observable. The concepts in Table 2-1 are more abstract, since they cannot be observed directly and occurrence must be inferred. For example, attachment behavior and defensiveness are inferred through observation of

TABLE 2-1 Concepts and indicators from reports of nursing research

Concept	Operationalization
Socioeconomic class	Score on Hollinghead's Two-Factor Index of Social Position (categorizes class on the basis of reported occupation and education)[1]
Gastric motility	Changes in intragastric pressure as measured by a pressure transducer and recorded on a dynograph recorder[2]
Functionality (of the hand)	Grip strength; palmar pinch strength; three-point pinch strength; lateral pinch strength[3]
Sex role identity	Score on the Bem Sex Role Inventory (a 60-item scale of Likert-like items which yields a masculinity score, a femininity score, and a social desirability score)[4]
Attachment behavior	Inspection; verbalization; smiling; touching; en face position; holding (Behaviors were observed at 30-second intervals over a 15-minute time period.)[5]
Defensiveness	Crossed arms; crossed legs[6]
Functional health	Score on the Guttman Health Scale for the Aged (a scale of 6 items that refer to the person's subjective evaluation of his capacity for functional activity)[7]

1. Ford, A.H. "Use of automobile restraining devices for infants." *Nursing Research* 29:281–284, 1980.
2. Kagawa-Busby, K., et al. "Effects of diet temperature on tolerance of enteral feedings." *Nursing Research* 29:276–280, 1980.
3. Jamison, S.L. and Dayhoff, N.E. "A hand-positioning device to decrease wrist and finger hypertoncity." *Nursing Research* 29:285–288, 1980.
4. Till, T.S. "Sex role identity and image of nursing of females at two levels of baccalaureate nursing education." *Nursing Research* 29:295–300, 1980.
5. Bowen, S.M. and Miller, B.C. "Paternal attachment behavior as related to presence at delivery and preparenthood classes: A pilot study." *Nursing Research* 29:307–311, 1980.
6. Hardin, S.B. "Comparative analysis of nonverbal interpersonal communication of schizophrenics and normals." *Research in Nursing and Health* 3:59, 1980.
7. Fuller, S.S. and Larson, S.B. "Life events, emotional support and health of older people." *Research in Nursing and Health* 3:83, 1980.

behavior. Concepts such as sex role identity and functionality require the use of special devices or instruments. The more abstract the concept, the more difficult it is to operationalize and to achieve consensus about its meaning. Most nursing concepts are relatively abstract; thus, careful attention must be directed toward specifying the multiple dimensions and characteristics included in their meaning.

Concepts representing ideas that are important in nursing may be used by other disciplines as well. The concept health, for example, is an idea that is central to nursing. Other disciplines (e.g., medicine, dentistry, social work, medical sociology, and medical economics) certainly would also claim the concept to be central. Because nursing incorporates and builds on related sciences and the humanities, its concepts, for the most part, are not isolated or unique. Its perspective does, however, guide the selection of concepts from other disciplines and influences the way in which those concepts are defined, operationalized, and reformulated.

In order to designate a particular idea as unique and different from what has gone before, new terms or neologisms are sometimes invented to name these ideas. Rogers' (1970) work contains several neologisms which she developed to avoid confusion between the unique meaning she assigned to an idea and meanings that may be conveyed by the use of other, more conventional terms. While neologisms may serve to highlight subtle differences, they sometimes result in terminological confusion and should be used and interpreted carefully. It is important to note that merely assigning a new or invented name to an idea does not necessarily result in a unique concept. As nursing progresses and new discoveries are made, new concepts and operations may be formulated to represent this new information. It is hoped that these new concepts and operations will be useful to other disciplines as well.

THEORETICAL AND OPERATIONAL DEFINITIONS

A *theoretical definition* provides meaning by defining a concept in terms of other concepts; it involves substituting one or several words for another. An *operational definition* provides meaning by defining a concept in terms of the observations and/or activities necessary to measure it.

The theoretical definition of a concept generally consists of a word, phrase, or sentence that is selected from among several alternative or possible meanings. Sometimes several meanings, each equally plausible, are included. The operational definition is stated in terms of the empirical indicators of the concept and represents the outcome of the process of operationalization. For example, the concept self esteem has been defined as follows by Goldberg and Fitzpatrick (1980):

Theoretical definition: "Self esteem is an individual's self-evaluation which expresses an attitude of self-approval or disapproval, and indicates the extent to which individuals believe themselves capable, significant, successful and worthy" (p. 341).

Operational definition: Self esteem of an individual is "the sum of the scores on the six scale items of the adapted Rosenberg (1965) Self-Esteem Scale" (p. 342).

Generally, the operational definition for a concept refers to the way in which that concept is measured within the context of a particular study or activity. It is frequently acknowledged that a given operationalization does not completely reflect the theoretical meaning of a concept. Thus, the operational definition usually is more restrictive and situationally specific than the theoretical definition. Examples of theoretical and operational definitions of some other nursing concepts are included in Table 2-2.

Both theoretical and operational definitions are important and useful and should be employed in nursing. To define nursing concepts either exclusively in terms of their observable indicators and operations or exclusively in terms of other concepts would preclude essential links between theory and research. Hage (1972) states:

It is much easier to decide if the indicators are valid with the presence of a theoretical definition, while indicators are a check on the utility of the definition. A concept can be measurable but not relevant because it bears little relationship to any other theoretical idea. . . . Similarly, a grand idea that is unmeasurable remains largely useless. Without a theoretical definition, the indicators can remain too specific. Without an operational definition the meaning can remain too diffuse (p. 67).

Thus, communicating the meaning of a concept by using both theoretical and operational definitions provides the links between theory and empirical reality that are essential for knowledge and practice.

OPERATIONALIZING NURSING CONCEPTS

The process of operationalizing a concept is an ongoing and cumulative process that involves several interrelated steps: (1) developing the theoretical definition; (2) specifying variables derived from the theoretical definition; (3) identifying observable indicators; and (4) developing means for measuring the indicators. Each of the steps represents progression from the abstract to the concrete; however, in actuality, there is considerable interplay between steps and one is rarely completed before the next is begun.

Although there is no specific way to go about operationalizing a concept, the following is a description of the approach that the authors have found to be useful. Each of the four major steps is considered in detail with specific strategies included.

DEVELOPING THE THEORETICAL DEFINITION

The purpose of defining a concept is to convey as clearly as possible the idea that is represented when a given term is used. Generally, when a concept is used in conversation or encountered in the literature, the user/reader has some idea, more or less precise, of the meaning assigned to the term. In order to formulate a theoretical definition for a concept that is to be used in nursing theory, research, or practice, it is necessary to translate one's informal, personal, working definition of the concept into a theoretical definition that is precise, understandable to others, and appropriate for the context in which the term will be used. A series of activities are involved: (1) developing a preliminary definition, (2) reviewing literature, (3) mapping the concept's meaning, and (4) stating the theoretical definition. As a means of shortcutting the process the nurse may be tempted to turn to the dictionary or to a frequently cited reference and simply borrow the definition supplied therein. These shortcuts to concept definition present potential problems. Dictionary definitions reflect the meanings of terms as they are used in everyday language. These common sense meanings may differ from and are much less precise than scientific meanings, which reflect the result of systematic study and have been validated by consensus among the members of a scientific community. For example, a dictionary definition of the concept care (painstaking or watchful attention from *Webster's Seventh New Collegiate Dictionary*, 1965, p. 126) does not ade-

TABLE 2-2 Examples of theoretical and operational definitions

Concept	Theoretical Definition	Operational Definition
Anxiety	A transitory emotional state characterized by subjective feelings of apprehension and autonomic nervous system arousal.[1]	Score on the State-Trait Anxiety Inventory State Scale.[2]
	A normal mental process in reaction to a real or perceived-as-real threat to an individual which is accompanied by specific physiological responses.[3]	Anxiety was operationally defined as total generalized free or total anxiety as measured by the IPAT Anxiety Scale Questionnaire.[3]
		Physiological responses to anxiety were measured by mean systolic blood pressures and mean heart rates.[3]
Autonomy	Perceived independence or control over work activities.[4]	Score on a "four-item scale from the Quality of Employment Surveys, tapping workers' perception of their decision-making power relative to the conduct of their jobs." Each item is scored on a 4-point scale and scores are summed.[5]
Maternal-fetal attachment	The extent to which women engage in behaviors that represent an affiliation and interaction with their unborn child.[6]	Scores on each of six subscales of the 37-item Maternal-Fetal Attachment Scale. The subscales are (1) differentiation of self from fetus, (2) interaction with the fetus, (3) attributing characteristics and intentions to the fetus, (4) giving of self, (5) role-taking, and (6) nesting. Items are statements followed by five response options designating frequency of behavior.[6]

quately reflect the richness of its meaning as used in nursing. Use of a preexisting theoretical definition may be necessary in some instances, for example, if one is testing a particular theory in which clear theoretical definitions have been stated. Borrowing another's theoretical definition may also be acceptable if it clearly represents the meaning to be conveyed. Usually, however, its appropriateness cannot be determined until a variety of possible definitions have been explored. The activities required to develop a theoretical definition are detailed below.

THE PRELIMINARY DEFINITION. Writing one's own definition of a concept, including key ideas and synonyms, is frequently a useful starting point for developing a theoretical definition. If examples of the concept can be provided, or if questions about whether certain ideas fit within the boundaries of the concept can be posed, these also should be jotted down for future reference and clarification. In addition, it is helpful to indicate the purpose for which the concept is being defined and operationalized. Possible purposes might include testing a particular theory, conducting

TABLE 2-2 Continued

Concept	Theoretical Definition	Operational Definition
Unstructured teaching	The imparting of knowledge to another in a random and unorganized manner.[3]	Unstructured pretransfer teaching . . . was operationally defined to include any teaching conducted by CCU nurses for any of the study subjects while the subjects were patients in the CCU.[3]
Morale	Outlook on life or one's assessment of the quality of life.[7]	Sum of the three factor scores on the Philadelphia Geriatric Center Morale Scale. The three themes that are components of the scale include the agitation factor (6 items), the attitude toward own aging factor (5 items), and the lonely dissatisfaction factor (6 items).[8]

1. Barsevick, A. and Llewellyn, J. "A comparison of the anxiety-reducing potential of two techniques of bathing." *Nursing Research* 31(1):22–27, January-February, 1982, (p. 22).
2. Ibid, p. 24.
3. Toth, J.C. "Effects of structured preparation for transfer on patient anxiety on leaving coronary care unit." *Nursing Research* 29(1):28–34, January-February, 1980, (p. 30).
4. Alexander, C.S., Weisman, C.S., and Chase, G.A. "Determinants of staff nurses' perceptions of autonomy within different clinical contexts." *Nursing Research* 31(1):48–52, January-February, 1982, (p. 48).
5. Ibid, p. 50.
6. Cranley, M.S. "Development of a tool for the measurement of maternal attachment during pregnancy." *Nursing Research* 30(5):281–284 (p. 282).
7. Goldberg, W.G. and Fitzpatrick, J.J. "Movement therapy with the aged." *Nursing Research* 29(6):339–346, November-December, 1980, (p. 340).
8. Ibid, p. 342.

research to describe a nursing phenomenon, developing and testing patient assessment tools, or documenting the outcomes of nursing interventions. By way of example, assume that the concept to be operationalized for research purposes is help-seeking. A preliminary definition might be stated as follows: help-seeking is the process of looking for assistance to solve a problem. This preliminary definition suggests that the concept involves a sequence of behaviors purposely undertaken by the searcher in order to achieve a goal.

These preliminary activities help to set the stage for concept definition in several ways. First, they force translation of a mental image into words and call attention to aspects of the image that are crucial to include in a later, more precise formulation of the definition. Second, they help to place limits or boundaries around the concept and eliminate meanings that are irrelevant to the purpose at hand. Many concepts have a wide range of possible meanings depending on the context in which they are used. For example, the concept interaction conveys a different sense when used in the context of pharmacology (e.g., drug interaction) than when used in the context of human communication (e.g., nurse-patient interaction). Third, the preliminary definition helps to identify the perspective or world view that will be used and the assumptions that will be made in defining the concept. One's own orientation should be recognized and compared with others' orientations in order to reveal biases or inconsistencies which should be rectified as the definition is refined.

LITERATURE REVIEW. Once the preliminary working definition has been written, an essential next step is to examine the current knowledge about the concept by means of a review of relevant literature. The review should be carried out carefully and critically (Batey, 1977, p. 327), with attention to inconsistencies in use of the concept, incompleteness of meanings, and subtle differences between the concept being defined and others related to it. Regarding the conduct of the review, several points should be considered. First, given the overlap among scientific disciplines in the use of a given concept, the review should include but not be limited to nursing literature. Frequently, literature in related disciplines is very helpful in defining a concept. Caution should be used, however, to scrutinize the relevance of the information for application to nursing situations and to interpret the information carefully, recognizing possible limitations in one's ability to understand what is written. Second, choice of literature to review should be guided by the purpose for which the concept is being developed and the conceptual or theoretical framework that is being used. While the review should not be overlimited in scope, choice of literature should not be random. Third, the review should include, but not be limited to, recent publications. Frequently tracing the historical evolution of a concept in the literature reveals important advances that have been made in reformulating the concept or adding new dimensions to its meaning.

A number of techniques that can be used to help construct theoretical definitions using information gleaned from the literature review are listed below. Usually a combination of techniques is required.

1. List all definitions from the literature that are potentially relevant, including both explicit and implicit (suggested but not stated as such) definitions. Then identify commonalities and differences. Elements common to all definitions of a concept are considered *critical attributes* which should be included in the theoretical definition.

2. List synonyms and their definitions. This activity is useful in differentiating terms and identifying subtle differences in meaning.

3. List examples or instances of the concept recorded in the literature. Then, using the examples as a starting point, perform the following mental exercises described by Wilson (1963) and Forsyth (1980), to clarify concept meaning:

   a. Select model cases that clearly exemplify the concept. Features present in all model cases represent critical attributes of the concept; features not present in all model cases can be eliminated.

   b. Select contrary cases that clearly are not instances of the concept and reflect an opposite meaning. Essential features of the concept should not be present in contrary cases.

   c. Select and describe borderline cases, those which one is not sure would be instances of the concept. Borderline cases generally share some features with model cases but are somehow different. By examining these cases to determine what makes them different, it becomes easier to identify the central features of the concept.

d. Select and describe related cases, instances of concepts that are similar or related to the focal concept. This helps increase understanding of how the concept fits into a larger network of ideas of which it is a part and may also help to differentiate concepts that are similar, but not identical, in meaning.

The literature review and the above techniques serve several useful purposes. They set limits and boundaries around the meaning of a concept, help differentiate the concept from others related to it, and indicate the aspects of meaning that should be included in the theoretical definition.

MAPPING. After having determined the critical attributes of a concept and the aspects of its meaning, it is necessary to develop a scheme for logically organizing the meaning of the concept (often termed its meaning space). Although the mapping process can be difficult, the purpose and context for use of the concept, the theoretical framework (orienting perspective), and the literature provide helpful cues. For example, the literature reveals that the concept health includes both objective (perceivable by others) and subjective (perceivable only by the individual experiencing it) aspects. Although both aspects might make up the meaning in the larger sense, one aspect might be eliminated as irrelevant for a given purpose. For example, if the purpose of an inquiry were to determine whether an individual's perception of health had an influence on behavior, objective aspects of the meaning might be eliminated and attention directed toward specifying subjective aspects of health. Another example of how the literature may suggest ways to organize the meaning of a concept is reflected in a study of fathering by Eversoll (1979). The author organized the meaning of the concept fathering into five separate aspects: nurturing, problem solving, providing, serving as a societal model, and recreational.

In order to construct or select a mapping that is appropriate, it is necessary to take into account the guiding conceptual or theoretical framework. For example, if the nursing conceptual framework that is guiding the development of a concept includes the assumption that man is a biopsychosocial being, then it is necessary to include biophysical, psychological, and social aspects in mapping the meaning. This assumption would result in a very different map than would a framework that addresses man as a solely physiologic entity.

Strategies that may be helpful in mapping the meaning space of a concept include the following:

1. List major elements in each author's organizing scheme and identify similarities and differences. Determine whether one set of organizing elements or categories can be subsumed under another. Eliminate schemes that do not apply to the purpose at hand.

2. Construct an outline or table with major headings representing key aspects of meaning. Include under each heading elements that are subsumed or summarized. Figure 2-1 is an example of an outline depicting the process of help-seeking.

Key Steps	Type of Process
I. Stimulus: Perception of need for help	(Cognitive)
II. Preliminary Activities	
A. Defining the goal	(Cognitive)
B. Deciding whether to seek help	(Cognitive)
III. Information Seeking	
A. Searching for information about possible resource options	(Behavioral)
B. Acquiring information about possible resource options	(Cognitive)
IV. Resource Selection	(Cognitive)
A. Evaluating possible options	
B. Selecting the desired resource from those available	
V. Resource Contact	(Behavioral)
Contacting the selected resource	
VI. Outcomes	
A. Receipt of help or nonreceipt of help	(Behavioral)
B. Evaluation of goal achievement	(Cognitive)
C. Termination or continuation of search	(Behavioral)

FIGURE 2-1. Preliminary outline of steps in the help-seeking process.

3. Pose questions about the concept that derive from the theoretical framework and/or purpose. Regarding the help-seeking concept, possible questions might include: what is being sought, from whom is it being sought, how is it being sought, for what purpose is it being sought, and to what extent is the purpose achieved?

4. Construct diagrams to represent the concept meaning. Venn diagrams that depict meanings in terms of discrete, overlapping, and/or inclusive sets are particularly useful (Thigpen and Drane, 1967). Flow diagrams are often used for mapping concepts that denote processes. Figure 2-2 provides examples of these two types of diagrams.

Depending on the nature of the concept, the mapping may be simple, consisting of one or two words that designate aspects of the meaning, or may be highly complex. The map is essentially a tool that organizes the meaning of the concept into a usable framework and helps to assure that critical elements are included in the definition. A preliminary map which provides the basis for the theoretical definition generally becomes more precise as the concept is operationalized. For a more detailed discussion of strategies that can be used for mapping the meaning of concepts, the reader is referred to Norris (1982) and Walker and Avant (1983).

STATING THE THEORETICAL DEFINITION. Having carried out preliminary procedures to identify and organize essential elements and dimensions of meaning denoted by a concept, selecting or constructing a theoretical definition is a relatively straightforward, logical exercise. The definition should include critical attributes of the concept's meaning that differentiate it from other terms and should reflect the way in which these attributes are organized in the mind of the definer. The theoretical definition should orient the reader to the definer's frame of reference and help assure that the concept will be interpreted similarly by all who read it.

Consider the following theoretical definition: help-seeking is defined as a multistage cognitive and behavioral process which an individual undertakes for the purpose of securing needed assistance from another. This defi-

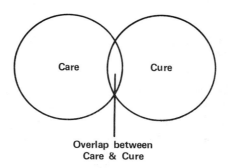

Overlap between
Care & Cure

Venn Diagram Representing Aspects of Nursing

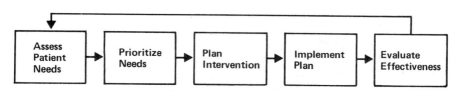

| Assess Patient Needs | → | Prioritize Needs | → | Plan Intervention | → | Implement Plan | → | Evaluate Effectiveness |

Flow Diagram of the Nursing Process

FIGURE 2-2. Examples of diagrams that represent the meaning of a concept.

nition denotes several essential aspects of the meaning intended by the definer: that help-seeking (the concept) represents both cognition and behavior, that it involves a sequence of several activities carried out over time, that the sequence is carried out for a purpose and with a perceived need and goal in mind, that the goal involves at least one other individual, and that the goal need not be achieved. This definition also serves to orient the reader to the way in which the definer has mapped the meaning of the concept: as a sequence of cognitive and behavioral steps initiated by a mental process (perception of need). This definition helps the reader to eliminate certain phenomena that do not meet the definitional criteria for consideration. For example, random behaviors are eliminated, as are actions such as seeking help from books. The former are not purposeful or goal-directed; the latter does not involve help from other individuals but from inanimate sources. On the basis of the definition, the reader is able to differentiate help-seeking from related concepts that denote different phenomena, for example, help-finding, helping, acquisition of help. Help-finding suggests that help has been secured; helping denotes behaviors that are undertaken in order to provide rather than to look for assistance; acquisition of help denotes a passive rather than an active stance. This example underscores the importance of precision and care in translating the map of meaning into the theoretical definition.

Theoretical definitions of relatively abstract and complex concepts are frequently supplemented with definitions for included terms and/or with statements that clarify the definition. For example, the abstract concept social dependence has been defined as ". . . the state in which patients require help or assistance from others in performing activities or roles that under ordinary circumstances adults can perform by themselves" (Benoliel, *et al.*, 1980, p. 4). The authors go on to specify that social dependence involves the absence of, or at least diminished capacity for, three basic competencies (everyday self-care competence, mobility competence, and social competence) that are necessary for normal and expected role performance. They then provide explicit definitions for each of the three competencies, which are the subconcepts included in the meaning of the more inclusive concept. The clarifying statements that supplement the definition help the reader to reconstruct the authors' mental image of the concept and provide the groundwork for the subsequent steps in operationalization.

There are no rules that specify the level of generality or abstraction that a theoretical definition should reflect. Abstract theoretical definitions generally require supplementary definitions of their major components or subconcepts in order to clarify meaning and bridge the gap between language and experience. Regardless of the level of abstraction, theoretical definitions should be stated with sufficient generality to allow application across a variety of real-world situations. In the example cited above, the concept social dependence was used in a study of chronic illness. However, the theoretical definition was stated in general terms that would allow its applicability to all adult patients. An even more general statement of the definition, substituting the term person for patient, would signify that the concept represented a potential characteristic of all adults. Generic theoretical definitions that are precise, yet have not been unnecessarily qualified by terms that restrict their use, facilitate knowledge-building.

It is not always necessary to develop a theoretical definition from scratch. Having determined critical attributes which define a concept and having constructed a map of the concept's meaning, one may find that a theoretical definition already exists in the literature which accurately conveys the intended meaning and is appropriate for the current purpose and context. In this case it is preferable to use the existing theoretical definition, in order to provide for accumulation of evidence about the concept as defined. Use of an existing definition is *not* appropriate if it does not represent the desired meaning accurately or cannot legitimately be applied to nursing situations without changing the meaning intended by the originator of the definition.

SPECIFYING VARIABLES
DERIVED FROM THE THEORETICAL DEFINITION

Generally speaking, variable concepts are more useful than nonvariable concepts. For example, the concept needle is a nonvariable concept. What is most useful to nurses, however, is not whether a particular object can be classified as a needle, but how sharp it is, how long it is, and whether a given substance can flow through it. Length, diameter, sharpness, curvature, and composition are variable dimensions of the meaning of the concept needle. To make concepts most useful for nursing, a necessary step in the operationalization process is to specify the dimensions of the concept's meaning with respect to which variation can occur, that is, the variables associated with it. This activity is closely related to the mapping procedure but carries it a step further in that essential aspects (or parts) of the meaning are expressed in terms of characteristics that can assume different values. The identification of variable dimensions of meaning may range from simple to difficult, depending on the existence of relevant supporting literature and the precision with which the meaning space was mapped prior to developing the theoretical definition of the concept.

A well-developed theoretical definition generally provides important clues to salient dimensions of the concept. This may be true even when the concept is theoretically defined as a nonvariable concept. For example, the concept social dependency, as described above, was defined theoretically as a "state in which patients require assistance . . ." (Benoliel, et al., 1980). Although this definition reflects a nonvariable concept, the authors specified that the described state represented one end of a continuum ranging from total dependence to total independence in carrying out activities related to self-care, mobility, and social interaction. Thus, dependency was actually envisioned as variable. Variable dimensions of this concept included the degree to which assistance is required for carrying out activities necessary for (1) everyday self-care (self-care competency), (2) physical movement (mobility competency), and (3) communication and interaction with others (social competency). In cases such as this, wherein a theoretical definition reflects several aspects of meaning, the identification of variables may be simply a matter of thinking of them as varying in the degree to which they are present.

Sometimes variable dimensions of a concept are not easily derived from the theoretical definition and require a return to the literature. Research reports frequently suggest variables that are applicable to many concepts. For example, most studies of expectations or beliefs (e.g., expectation or belief that one should have a yearly physical examination) reveal differences among people in the strength with which they hold the expectation or belief. Therefore, strength of belief would represent a potentially salient variable if one were attempting to operationalize a concept in which expectation or belief was a major component. Studies of behavior often report differences in the frequency with which a particular behavior occurs, indicating that frequency may represent an important variable dimension for behavioral concepts. To apply these ideas to a previous example, one might want to identify the variables of frequency and strength in operationalizing the concept fathering, which was mapped as having five major aspects of meaning and has behavioral and expectation components. Knowing the frequency with which a father performs specific behaviors and the strength with which he holds the belief that a particular behavior is expected tells us more about him than a statement about whether or not he has ever carried out a particular behavior or holds a given belief.

Literature about a given concept often yields clues about relevant variables. For example, literature related to the concept collegial relationships shows that these relationships vary in several respects; for example, degree to which functions overlap, degree to which philosophies are compatible, degree to which prestige is equal, degree of shared accountability, degree of mutual respect, and degree of mutual involvement in decisions. To continue the example of the help-seeking concept, descriptions of the ways in which people go about seeking help suggest differences in the nature of the stimulus, the number of activities carried out, the length of time spent looking, the degree to which other persons are consulted for information, the number of consultants used, the amount and type of information acquired, the number of resources contacted, and the outcomes. These descriptions suggest variable dimensions of help-seeking, which are shown in Figure 2-3.

In addition to reviewing literature, it may be helpful to cite examples of the concept and then determine the ways in which the examples differ or vary. Asking oneself about possible differences among hospital rules can reveal several inherent variable dimensions of the concept rule, such as explicitness, clarity, enforcibility, and conformity.

Once possible variables are identified, the selection of those that ultimately will be included in the operationalization of the concept is determined by the purpose for which the concept is being developed and the context in which it will be used. Given several possible variables, a decision often must be made to include some and exclude others. Possible questions to ask oneself to aid in selecting variables include the following:

1. Which variables will provide the most useful information to nurses?

2. Which variables have others found to be most important in understanding the phenomenon?

3. Which variables have others found to be related to other concepts of interest or to help explain or predict occurrences of interest to nurses?

4. Which variables can be rendered observable and measurable, given our present state of knowledge?

I. Stimulus
   A. Type of problem
   B. Specificity
   C. Immediacy
II. Preliminary Activities
   A. Feasibility of goal
   B. Specificity of goal
III. Decision to Seek Help
   A. Immediacy
   B. Active vs. passive
   C. Amount of input from others
IV. Information Search
   A. Extent
   B. Duration
   C. Type of method
   D. Number of consultants
   E. Expertise of consultants
V. Information Acquisition
   A. Extent
   B. Specificity
   C. Degree of fit with goal
VI. Resource Selection
   A. Relevance of criteria to goal
   B. Specificity of criteria
   C. Number of options considered
VII. Resource Contact
   A. Success
   B. Type of resource contacted
VIII. Outcomes
   A. Success (receipt of help)
   B. Level of satisfaction with help received
   C. Continuation of search/termination of search

FIGURE 2-3. Outline of several variable dimensions of the help-seeking process.

IDENTIFYING OBSERVABLE INDICATORS

The selection of observable indicators for the concept is guided by the theoretical definition, the map of the concept's meaning, and the variable dimensions that have been identified. Three examples are provided to demonstrate the way in which the selection of indicators flows directly from the previous steps.

Example 1. Continuing the example of help-seeking, specific indicators can be identified for each of the variable dimensions listed in Figure 2-3. Examples of possible indicators for the information search stage and outcomes are provided in Table 2-3.

Example 2. Assume that the meaning of the concept fathering is determined to involve both behaviors and expectations about the behaviors which should be

TABLE 2-3 Variables and indicators for selected aspects of help-seeking*

Variable	Indicator
Extent of search	Number of search activities reported by the individual, calculated as the sum of separate activities undertaken by the individual for the purpose of acquiring information about potential sources of help.
Duration of search	Number of days during which the individual reportedly engaged in information-seeking activities, i.e., interval between deciding to seek help and contacting a potential source of help.
Method of search	Designation of reported search activities as personal or impersonal, with the categories defined as follows: personal method involves use of an individual known personally to the searcher as a source of information; impersonal method involves using a nonhuman source of information or an individual not known personally to the searcher.
Number of consultants	Number of persons whom the searcher reportedly contacted for information about sources of help, calculated as the sum of individuals from whom information was sought and/or received.
Expertise of consultants	Median level of expertise of persons consulted for information, with level of expertise being designated as lay or professional with respect to the health-care system.
Receipt of help	Reported occurrence of receipt of assistance from a local resource contacted voluntarily for such help.
Level of satisfaction with help received	Expressed level of satisfaction with each resource from which help was received, as measured on a five-point Likert-type scale ranging from very dissatisfied to very satisfied.
Continuation/termination of search	Reported occurrence (continuation) or nonoccurrence (termination) of any additional help-seeking activity carried out following receipt of service from a local resource.

*Adapted from Lenz (1976).

carried out. This would suggest that indicators for the concept should include both observable behaviors (or reports that an individual performed the behaviors) and responses that reflect the individual's expectations. A mapping scheme previously described (Eversoll, 1979) subdivided the father role into five parts. On this basis a grid (Table 2-4) could be constructed to guide the selection of indicators. One possible indicator has been inserted into each space; ideally several indicators would be selected for each space.

Example 3. The meaning of the concept infant development is frequently mapped as progressive change in several different aspects of functioning such as gross motor ability, fine motor coordination, language ability, and social ability. Within these broad categories of functioning, specific behaviors have been found to emerge at different ages. Indicators of infant development would therefore have to be specific to a given age and should represent each major category of functioning. Figure 2-4 exemplifies the mapping of this concept into separate aspects of meaning and includes some observable indicators which might be used to measure the level of development of a six-month-old infant. Indicators for a 12-month-old infant would be different.

When selecting indicators it is crucial to determine whether the concept represents an either-or phenomenon (i.e., a state or object) or a phenomenon that varies. One could define pain, for example, in terms of presence or absence or in terms of its degree of severity. The indicators for the two ideas of pain would differ. If pain were defined as an either-or phenomenon, possible indicators might include a patient's positive response to the ques-

TABLE 2-4 Meaning categories and indicators for the concept fathering

Fathering Sub-Roles*	Behavior	Expectation
Nurturing Role	Frequency with which the individual speaks softly to crying child during the observation period.	Extent of agreement[†] with statement that a father should rock a crying baby.
Problem-Solving Role	Number of times per week the individual asks child to tell him about problems encountered in school (self report).	Extent of agreement with statement that a father should decide the outcome of disagreements among family members.
Provider Role	Percentage of time within last five years that the individual held a full-time job (self report).	Extent of agreement with statement that a father should be a wage earner.
Societal Model Role	Number of times within past five years that the individual has voted in local, state, and national elections (self report).	Extent of agreement with statement that a father should set an example for his family by attending church regularly.
Recreational Role	Number of times per week the individual plays ball with child (self report).	Extent of agreement with statement that a father should take his child to ball games.

*Categories were derived from Eversoll (1979).
[†]Extent of agreement is measured as response on a five-point Likert-type scale.

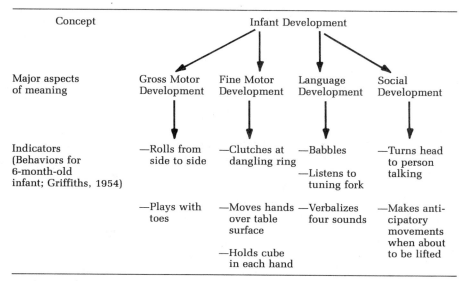

Concept	Infant Development			
Major aspects of meaning	Gross Motor Development	Fine Motor Development	Language Development	Social Development
Indicators (Behaviors for 6-month-old infant; Griffiths, 1954)	—Rolls from side to side	—Clutches at dangling ring	—Babbles —Listens to tuning fork	—Turns head to person talking
	—Plays with toes	—Moves hands over table surface —Holds cube in each hand	—Verbalizes four sounds	—Makes anticipatory movements when about to be lifted

FIGURE 2-4. Meaning categories and indicators for the concept normal infant development as measured at six months of age.

tion "Are you in pain?" or whether or not a patient requests pain medication. On the other hand, defining pain as variable in intensity would require indicators of the degree of severity. Possible indicators might include a patient's rating of the severity of pain on a scale from 1 (no pain) to 10 (unbearably severe pain), the frequency of requests for pain medication in a specified period of time, or the dosage of medication required to alleviate the pain.

In Example 1, some dimensions of help-seeking were conceptualized as varying in number or degree (e.g., number of activities carried out, level of satisfaction) and others were conceptualized as either-or phenomena (e.g., receipt of help, continuation of search); in Example 2, fathering was conceptualized as a variable phenomenon throughout. In Example 3, infant development was conceptualized as variable; however, the indicators were stated as behaviors that the infant would or would not perform (either-or). In order to determine an infant's *level* of development it would be necessary to sum the number of behaviors that the infant performed.

The literature related to a concept is a rich source of possible indicators. A good strategy is to list indicators from the literature, then examine each to determine its degree of fit with the theoretical definition and purpose. For example, assume that a nurse is interested in operationalizing the concept hospital size for the purpose of studying nursing staff turnover patterns. Various indicators that may be found in the literature include number of square feet, number of beds, number of departments or units, number of employees, number of patients served per year, and annual budget. Indicators such as number of beds and number of employees would be more relevant for most nursing purposes than those reflecting spatial or economic aspects of hospital size. Because there are several ways in which numbers of beds and employees may be counted, additional decisions about appropriate indicators would have to be made in relation to the purpose of the investigation and the meaning to be conveyed.

The nursing literature often refers to instruments (e.g., questionnaires, checklists, attitude scales, or machines) that have been developed to measure a particular concept. Such instruments should not automatically be assumed to generate appropriate indicators. Considerations to be employed in selecting instruments are addressed in Chapters 8 and the Appendix, and issues related to the use of borrowed instruments are addressed in Chapter 10. The prime criterion for evaluating the appropriateness of any instrument or indicator suggested in the literature is congruence with the theoretical definition. Also important are evaluative statements in the literature. Evidence about specific indicators accrues over time through research and should be carefully sought and examined.

In addition to the literature there are other sources of potential indicators. One's past experience can be used to generate instances or examples of the concept. These examples can then be studied using Wilson's (1963) techniques described above to determine observable characteristics or properties that are universally present and represent potential indicators. Other nurses can be a valuable resource for suggesting indicators, particularly when they are in daily contact with patients. They may also help evaluate the relevance and potential observability of indicators derived from the literature in the light of practical experience. It is important that the selection of indicators not be isolated from reality and common sense.

DEVELOPING MEANS FOR MEASUREMENT

The final step in the operationalization process is to develop means by which the indicators can be observed and measured. This step constitutes the focus for the remainder of the book. Suffice it to say at this point that the operations by which a particular indicator can be rendered observable and the rules by which numbers will be assigned to various states or degrees of the indicator must be specified. Operations that are required to measure indicators of nursing concepts range in complexity from unassisted sensory observation to the construction of written instruments and machinery that augment the senses. Having determined the way in which the concept is to be measured, it is possible to state the *operational definition*, which expresses the meaning of the concept in terms of the way in which it will be measured in a particular context. Although operational definitions can take a variety of forms, their purpose is to make clear to the reader the way in which the concept has been operationalized. The theoretical and operational definitions, therefore, can be viewed as the two products of the operationalization process.

EVALUATING THEORETICAL AND OPERATIONAL DEFINITIONS

Judgment about the adequacy with which a concept has been defined and operationalized ultimately should be made on the basis of accumulated evidence from empirical investigation. Unfortunately, very few key nursing concepts have yet received sufficient attention to allow such evidence to accrue. There are, however, a number of criteria that one might apply to evaluate how well a concept has been defined and operationalized. Before listing these criteria, it is important to note that an operationalization cannot be judged in terms of truth or falsity. One theoretical or operational definition can be judged to be better or worse than another when compared according to the following criteria. However, truth value is not a criterion that can legitimately be applied in evaluating concepts and their operationalization.

Criteria that can help guide the nurse in evaluating the adequacy of an operationalization include the following:

1. Clarity. This criterion requires that the definition, indicators, and operations for the concept be presented in a way that can be easily understood.

2. Precision. This criterion reflects the desirability of describing observations and operations in explicit and specific terms. Mathematical formulae exemplify precise operationalizations of concepts. Although this degree of precision is difficult to achieve in nursing, verbal operationalizations can also be very precise. For example, instructions about how to make a given observation or how to carry out an operation can and should be stated explicitly.

3. Reliability. This criterion refers to the replicability or reproducibility of observations and operations and is described in detail in Chapters 5 and 7.

4. Consistency. The criterion of consistency includes not only use of terms in a consistent manner but also logical consistency; that is, use of logical reasoning to guide selection of indicators and explication of the linkages between the language meaning of the concept and observable reality.

5. Meaning Adequacy. This criterion addresses the congruence that must exist between the meaning designated by a concept and the indicators selected to represent that meaning. An adequate operationalization is one which (as fully as possible) accounts for the various dimensions of meaning designated by a concept.

6. Feasibility. Indicators and operations should be capable of being executed, at least theoretically. This criterion represents a utilitarian view. Concepts are sometimes operationalized in terms of hypothetical or imaginary observations that are impossible to make because either the required technology or the condition or state to be observed does not exist. While such efforts may be intellectually interesting, they are useful only in the sense that they suggest the need for new technology. A potential danger exists in that suggested indicators that cannot be observed also cannot be evaluated empirically as to the adequacy with which they relate to a concept.

7. Utility. This criterion requires that an operationalization must be useful (1) within the content of the specific investigation or other activity and (2) to the discipline of nursing. An operationalization that includes observations that could be made by the practicing nurse caring for patients in a clinical setting would be potentially more useful to the discipline than

one that required the use of highly complex electronic equipment available only in a laboratory. Furthermore, concepts that are operationalized with variable indicators are more useful than those that are operationalized in terms of nonvariable observations.

8. Validity. This criterion refers to the requirement that the observations selected to represent or indicate a concept in fact do so. Assessment of the validity of an operationalization is an on-going process that requires empirical investigation and will be discussed in Chapters 5 and 7.

9. Consensus. The ultimate test of an operationalization is that it is accepted by consensus of the scientific community on the basis of empirical evidence.

SUMMARY

Concepts are abstract verbal symbols which help to summarize and categorize observations. They are the basic elements of the complex statements and theories that make up the language of any scientific discipline; thus, they link thought and experience. Nursing concepts designate the subject matter of the discipline but are not necessarily unique to nursing. Because key nursing concepts tend to be complex and relatively abstract, they must be defined and operationalized carefully if they are to be useful in knowledge-building.

To operationalize a concept is to delineate how it will be measured. A multistep procedure is required. The first step is to formulate a theoretical definition that supplies meaning through the use of other concepts. The theoretical definition is developed following a careful review of the literature in which essential elements of the concept's meaning are delimited and logically organized. Subsequent steps are to specify variable dimensions of the concept's meaning, identify observable indicators of the concept, and develop means to measure the indicators. The steps are interrelated, such that each logically flows from and builds upon those that precede it. The product of the operationalization process is the operational definition, which provides meaning in terms of the observations or operations necessary to measure the concept. Operationalization is an ongoing and cumulative process.

Criteria for evaluating the operationalization of a concept include clarity, precision, reliability, validity, adequacy of meaning, feasibility, and utility. The ultimate test of the adequacy with which a concept is defined and operationalized is consensus of the scientific community based on accumulated empirical evidence.

REFERENCES

BATEY, MV: "Conceptualization: Knowledge and logic guiding empirical research." *Nursing Research* 26(5), 324–329, 1977.

BENOLIEL, JQ, McCORKLE, R, AND YOUNG, K: "Development of a social dependency scale." *Research in Nursing and Health* 3(1), 3–10, 1980.

BURR, WR: *Theory Construction and the Sociology of the Family.* Wiley, New York, 1973.

EVERSOLL, D: "A two-generational view of fathering." *The Family Coordinator* 28(4), 503–508, 1979.

FAWCETT, J: "The relationship between theory and research: A double helix." *Advances in Nursing Science* 1(1), 49–62, 1978.

FORSYTH, GL: "Analysis of the concept of empathy: Illustration of one approach." *Advances in Nursing Science* 2(2), 33–42, 1980.

GOLDBERG, WG AND FITZPATRICK, JJ: "Movement therapy with the aged." *Nursing Research* 29(6), 339–346, 1980.

GRIFFITHS, R: *The Abilities of Babies: A Study in Mental Measurement.* Association for Research in Infant and Child Development, Amersham, Bucks, England, 1954.

HAGE, J: *Techniques and Problems of Theory Construction in Sociology.* Wiley, New York, 1972.

LENZ, ER: *The Search for Health-Service Information by Newcomers to a Community.* Unpublished doctoral dissertation, University of Delaware, Newark, Delaware, 1976.

KING, I: "A process for developing concepts for nursing through research." In VERHONICK, PA (ed.): *Nursing Research I.* Little, Brown, Boston, 1975.

NEWMAN, M: *Nursing Theory.* F.A. Davis, Philadelphia, 1979.

NORRIS, CM: *Concepts Clarification in Nursing.* Aspen, Rockville, Md., 1982.

ROGERS, ME: *An Introduction to the Theoretical Basis for Nursing.* F.A. Davis, Philadelphia, 1970.

THIGPEN, LW AND DRANE, JW: "The Venn diagram: A tool for conceptualization in nursing." *Nursing Research* 16(3), 252–260, 1967.

Webster's Seventh New Collegiate Dictionary. G & C Merriam, Philadelphia, 1965.

WILSON, J: *Thinking With Concepts.* Cambridge University Press, New York, 1963.

WALKER, LO AND AVANT, KC: *Strategies for Theory Construction in Nursing.* Appleton-Century-Crofts, 1983.

3

MEASUREMENT THEORY: PRINCIPLES AND PRACTICES

The purpose of this chapter is to present basic principles of statistics and measurement theory which are requisite for understanding the process of measurement.

How to measure phenomena of interest is a common concern for nurses who work in all types of settings. Measurement problems may range from determining the best method for obtaining the accurate length, weight, and body temperature of a newborn infant to trying to ascertain the quality of patient care provided on a clinical unit. In each of these situations the goal is to describe the kind and/or amount of an attribute possessed by some object.

What is measured is not the object but a characteristic or attribute of the object. In the previous examples, the nurse is not concerned with measuring the infant, but its length, weight, and body temperature. In the latter situation, the clinical supervisor is not concerned with measuring the clinical unit but the quality of patient care administered on the unit. When a nursing instructor evaluates the level of clinical performance of nursing students, the objective is to measure students' ability to perform within the clinical setting, not to measure the students themselves. The attribute to be measured varies in amount and/or kind and different objects may be assigned to different categories that represent the amount or kind of the attribute possessed. For example, various infants in a nursery have different weights. Similarly, different nursing students in a class will have different levels of ability. Therefore, attributes that are measured are variable and take on different values for different objects. Measurable attributes are often termed variables in scientific language. An attribute must be variable in order for it to be measured. Measurement provides for meaningful interpretation of the nature of an attribute possessed by an object or event. The results of measurement are usually expressed in the form of numbers.

In nursing, as in other disciplines, there are many attributes of objects that are not easily measured. In such cases, the attribute of concern may be defined in a manner whereby it can be made measurable, that is, the attribute or concept is operationalized. Whenever an attempt is made to measure an attribute it is necessary to define it in qualitative or quantitative terms. A unit of measurement for categorizing the kind and/or amount of the attribute must be established and a measurement procedure or rule must be derived which is in concert with the established unit of measurement. The unit may be a score, a centimeter, a milliliter, a second, a degree Centigrade, or any appropriate unit or category of measurement. The need for the establishment of a suitable unit of measurement and for precision in measurement has fostered the development and use of tools such as tests, thermometers, rulers, and balance scales.

Measurement is the process of using a rule to assign numbers to objects or events which represent the amount and/or kind of the specified attribute possessed. The measurement rule is the precise procedure used to assign numbers to phenomena, for example, procedures for administering and scoring tests or using a balance scale to measure weight.

Stevens (1946) has classified the rules used for assigning numbers to objects to represent the amount and/or kind of a specified attribute possessed by them in a hierarchical manner. From lower to higher levels, the scales of measurement are *nominal, ordinal, interval,* and *ratio.*

In *nominal-scale measurement* objects are placed into categories according to a defined property. Numbers assigned represent an object's membership in one of a set of mutually exclusive, exhaustive, and unorderable categories. Numbers are used for labeling purposes only and have no quantitative significance. Categories used in nominal-level measurement differ in quality rather than quantity; hence, no statement can be made about the amount of the attribute possessed. All members of a category are regarded as similar or equal in some respect. For example, a group of registered nurses may be assigned to categories based on their sex, that is, 1 = male and 2 = female. The basis for classifying is the definition of the class. The basic distinguishing signs for determining inclusion within the class are specified by the definition. Regardless of the number of categories used, two essential conditions should be met. First, a set of categories should be *exhaustive,* that is, every object that is to be classified should belong to at least one category. Second, the designated categories should be *mutually exclusive,* that is, the definition of the categories should be such that no object could be placed in more than one category.

In *ordinal-scale measurement* numbers are assigned to objects according to rank order on a particular attribute. Numbers assigned represent an object's membership in one of a set of mutually exclusive and exhaustive categories that can be ordered according to the amount of the attribute possessed. Ordinal-scale measurement may be regarded as the rank ordering of objects into quantitative categories according to relative amounts of the specified attribute. The rankings do not imply that the ranked categories are equally spaced on a scale nor that the intervals between the scale categories are equal. Ordinal assignment of numbers merely means that the ranking of 1 (for first) has ranked higher than 2 (for second), and since 2 has a higher ranking than 3, then 1 also must rank higher than 3. If, for example, a group of clients are ranked according to their ability to provide self care such that 1 would represent the highest level of ability, then a client ranked as 3 would possess less self-care ability than one ranked 2 and would possess more ability for self care than one ranked 4.

An *interval scale* is one for which equal numerical distances on the scale represent equal amounts with respect to the attribute or the object that is the focus of measurement. Numbers assigned in interval-scale measurement represent an object's membership in one of a set of mutually exclusive, exhaustive categories that can be ordered and are equally spaced in terms of the magnitude of the attribute under consideration. However, the absolute amount of the attribute is not known for any particular object, because the zero point in an interval scale is placed in some arbitrary position. In addition to being able to categorize and rank objects, at the interval level one can also order objects according to the size of their numerals and the relative size of the differences between two objects. The Farenheit temperature scale is an example of a commonly used interval scale. One can say that two objects having temperatures of 90° and 100° are as far apart on the scale as two other objects with temperatures of 50° and 60°. One can also say, for example, that a patient's temperature at 6:00 p.m. is 3° higher than it was at noon, or that the drop in temperature after taking an aspirin was greater than after taking a sponge bath. One cannot say, however, that an object with a temperature of 0°F does not have a temperature at all.

Ratio-level measures provide all information that is provided by interval level measures, but in addition they have absolute zero points, where zero represents an absolute absence of the relevant attribute. The category and rank-order of objects with respect to the attribute is known, the intervals on the scale are equal, and the distance or magnitude from the actual zero point is known. Volume, length, and weight are commonly measured by ratio scales and all can be assigned absolute zero values. With a ratio scale one can say that Roy is two times as heavy as John if Roy weighs 100 pounds and John weighs 50 pounds.

There is a great deal of controversy about the levels of measurement and the types of statistical operations that can be properly used with the resulting scores. Either the fundamentalist or pragmatist view of measurement rules may be taken. The fundamentalist view purports that all measures of attributes can be classified into one of the distinct levels of measurement, and that, once classified, the level of measurement specifies the type of statistical operations that can be properly used. The hierarchical nature of the scales of measurement is considered when statistical operations are applied with scores derived at different levels of measurement. The higher the level of the scale, the broader the range of statistical operations that can be applied with the numbers obtained from measurement. Only nonparametric statistics are considered appropriate with lower level data, that is, nominal or ordinal data; but parametric statistics are permissible with higher level data, that is, interval and ratio data. Frequencies, percentages, and contingency-correlation coefficients are considered permissible at the nominal-scale level of measurement. Ordinal-scale data are believed to allow the same statistical operations permissible with nominal-scale data, but in addition, it is possible to use medians, centiles, and rank-order coefficients of correlation. Practically all of the common statistical procedures are considered permissible with interval and ratio data.

The pragmatists point out that most measurement rules are not as clear-cut and easily classified as fundamentalists believe they are, and that it is not practical to waste effort in attempting to classify a variable into a level of measurement. For example, there is some controversy among measurement specialists as to whether scores from psychological tests represent ordinal or interval level measurement, because there is no assurance that equal differences between scores represent equal differences in the amount of the attribute of concern. Some contend that test scores simply order subjects according to the amount of the specified attribute possessed, while others purport that test scores represent the magnitude of the attribute possessed. Pragmatists minimize the emphasis on levels of measurement and suggest that the statistical techniques applied to any set of numbers should be determined by the nature of the research question addressed rather than by the level of measurement. The authors believe that the statistical treatment of any data or set of numbers should be determined by the nature of the scientific inquiry, that is, the research question one is trying to answer, rather than the level of measurement alone.

BASIC STATISTICAL PRINCIPLES AND PROCEDURES

In most instances, measurement results in a number. This number represents the amount and/or kind of some attribute or characteristic of the object or event that is measured. The number that results from measurement may be referred to as either the *observed score* or *raw score*.

In many situations a group of objects is measured on the same attribute, which results in a series or group of observed scores. One might determine, for example, the lung capacity of a group of adult smokers, the arterial pressure of a group of cardiac patients, or the scores on a nursing vocabulary test for a group of nursing students. Unfortunately, it is difficult to make much sense out of a group of numbers obtained from such situations when they are presented in this raw form. One usually would want to know what the highest and lowest scores are, if the scores are spread out or concentrated at some point along the distribution, and what score occurs most often. Statistical procedures enable one to better understand such groups of numbers and to answer these basic kinds of questions about the characteristics of the group of scores. This section presents some basic statistical principles and procedures that are important for understanding measurement.

DISTRIBUTION

One step in obtaining information about any group of measures or scores is to arrange them in order from their highest to lowest value and to note how many times a particular score occurs, or whether it occurs at all. This will indicate the *distribution* of scores, which can be represented by a table or graph in which each score is paired with its frequency of occurrence. An illustration of a frequency distribution of the hematocrit levels for 50 female patients is shown in Table 3-1. The first column includes scores, that is, the hematocrit values, which are ordered from the highest to the lowest. The second column contains the frequencies, that is, the number of patients with each hematocrit value, and clearly displays how many patients had each.

Frequency distributions also can be presented in the form of a histogram. A histogram is a bar graph representation of a frequency distribution and makes the shape of the distribution more obvious. Figure 3-1 presents the histogram for the data in Table 3-1. Further discussion of the ways to present frequency distributions is provided in Chapter 4.

DISTRIBUTION SHAPE

Frequency distributions can occur in various shapes. Because the shape of a distribution is often important information, it is necessary for one to know some of the descriptive terms used to indicate the various shapes. Several common distribution shapes are shown in Figure 3-2. The shape of a frequency distribution can be either symmetrical or asymmetrical. A symmetrical distribution is one in which both halves of the distribution are identical in shape. Normal and flat distributions are symmetrical in shape. Skewed distributions, that is, distributions in which scores trail off in one direction, are asymmetrical.

A bimodal distribution may be symmetrical or asymmetrical. The extent to which a distribution departs from symmetry is referred to as its degree of *skewness*. The direction of skewness refers to the fact that in some asymmetrical distributions most scores pile up at one end of the scale as far as frequency of occurrence is concerned, while there are fewer scores at the other end. When the frequency of scores is low on the right side of the distribution, it is positively skewed. If the frequency of scores is low on the left side of the distribution, then it is negatively skewed. Difficult tests or

TABLE 3-1 Frequency distribution of hematocrit values (scores) for 50 female patients

Hematocrit Value or Score	Frequency
48	1
47	1
46	2
45	3
44	6
43	6
42	9
41	7
40	6
39	3
38	2
37	2
36	0
35	2
	n = 50

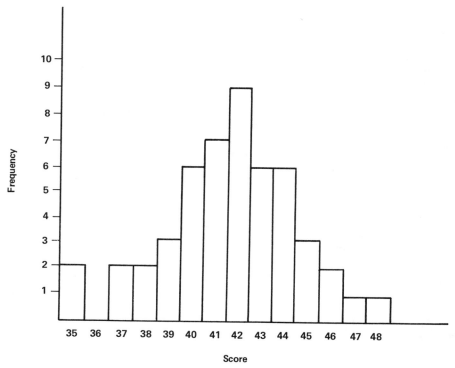

FIGURE 3-1. Histogram for data presented in Table 3-1.

situations in which scores are generally low in a group will result in distributions that are positively skewed. Easy tests or instances in which most scores tend to be high within a group will yield negatively skewed distributions. In instances in which scores occur in the middle range with few scores in the low and high levels, normal distributions will result. Bimodal distributions will often occur when two distinctly different populations are measured on a selected attribute. For example, if the hematocrit levels of a group of males and females were determined, a bimodal distribution would be likely to result, because males normally have higher hematocrit levels than females. In this case, males and females are actually two different populations, because the variable of interest, that is, hematocrit, is influenced by sex.

In the norm-referenced measurement situation a normal distribution is desirable. A skewed distribution would be expected in a criterion-referenced measurement situation following a specific intervention or treatment. The theoretical basis for the occurrence of these distributions as indicated for each measurement framework is discussed in Chapters 4 and 6.

The shape of a distribution also may vary in regard to the peakedness of the curve of the distribution as shown in Figure 3-3. *Kurtosis* refers to the peakedness of a distribution's curve.

The curve of a normal distribution, as indicated by curve A in Figure 3-3, is referred to as *mesokurtic* and is used as the standard with which the

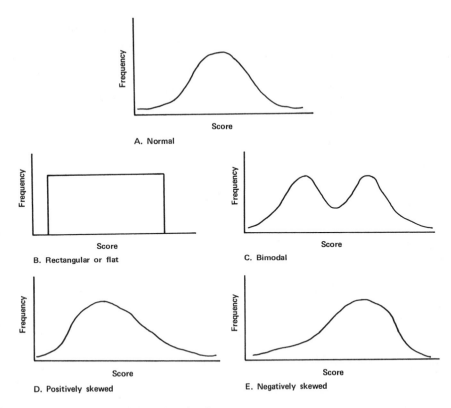

FIGURE 3-2. Common distribution shapes.

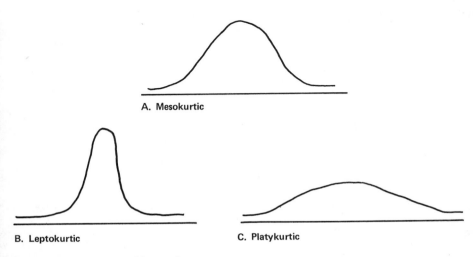

FIGURE 3-3. Types of kurtosis.

curves of other distributions are compared to determine their kurtosis. A very peaked slender curve is called *leptokurtic* and is illustrated by curve B. A *platykurtic* curve is flat or broad as shown by curve C. The scores in a leptokurtic curve are more close together, that is, have less variance, than in the normal curve. On the other hand, the scores in a platykurtic curve are more spread out, that is, have more variance, than in the normal curve. If a distribution is bimodal, the kurtosis of each curve is considered separately.

MEASURES OF CENTRAL TENDENCY

Rarely do all the individual members of a group or population have the same amount of some common attribute. Instead different objects vary on the attribute of interest. In many instances, one might be interested in the averageness of some specific attribute. For example, one might want to know the average weight and length of a group of newborn infants or the average score on a depression scale for a group of psychiatric clients. The mode, median, and mean are three statistical indices of averageness or central tendency.

The *mode* is the score in a distribution that occurs most frequently. The mode of the scores in Table 3-1 is 9. The mode is determined by inspecting the data to ascertain which score occurs most often. It is the easiest measure of central tendency to calculate.

Occasionally a frequency distribution will have two modes rather than one. In such cases two scores will have occurred at maximum frequency. This type of distribution is called bimodal and is illustrated in Figure 3-2.

The *median* is the score value in a distribution above which 50 percent of the scores fall and below which 50 percent of the scores fall. The fiftieth percentile is another label for the median. When a distribution includes an unequal number of scores the median is the middle score. For example, if a distribution included the scores 4,6,10,11,13,15, and 16, the median would be 11.

Because the median represents the middle score, it may be a value that is not included in the scores in the distribution. This may be the case when the distribution includes an even number of scores. Where there is an even number of scores, the median is calculated in the following manner.

1. The scores in the distribution are arranged from the lowest to the highest value.
2. If no score occurs more than once, the median is the midpoint between the two middle scores. For example, in the case in which the scores are 3,5,6, and 8, the median is the midpoint between 5 and 6. Thus:
$$\text{Median} = (5 + 6)/2$$
$$= 5.5$$
3. When tied scores occur, as in Figure 3-4, a frequency tabulation is required.
   A. Determine placement of the median score. In this case the median score is n/2 or 40/2. Hence, the median score will be the 20th score from the bottom of the distribution.
   B. Find the score corresponding to the 20th score.

SCORE	FREQUENCY	CUMULATIVE FREQUENCY
100	2	40
95	3	38
93	5	35
88	4	30
85	8	26
81	7	18
78	4	12
69	3	7
61	3	4
55	1	1
	n = 40	

FIGURE 3-4. Frequency distribution used for demonstrating computation of median.

(1) The 20th score is located between the score interval from 81 to 85.
(2) A cumulative frequency of 18 is found in the lower limit of this interval: Thus, 20 − 18 = 2 above 18 is required for the 20th score.
(3) The number of frequencies in the interval containing the 20th score is equal to 26 − 18 = 8 frequencies.
(4) Multiply 2/8 by the width of the interval containing the 20th score, that is, 85 − 81. Thus, 2/8 × 4 = 1.
(5) Hence, 81 + 1 = 82. This is the score equal to the median.

The median has the advantage that its value is not influenced by extreme scores. This makes it a useful measure of central tendency when small samples are used.

The *mean* is the sum of scores in a distribution divided by the number of scores entered into the computation of the sum. A shorthand way to express this definition is presented in the formula below.

Formula 3-1
$$\overline{X} = \frac{\Sigma X}{n}$$

Where: $\overline{X}$ = arithmetic mean
Σ means the sum of a series of scores
X = raw score
n = number of scores summed

Example: The mean of 2,4,8,6, and 10 is calculated as follows:

$$\overline{X} = \frac{\Sigma X}{n} = \frac{2+4+8+6+10}{5} = \frac{30}{5} = 6$$

The mean is the balancing point of a distribution. It is the point value where a linear scale would balance as illustrated in Figure 3-5. The more equal the difference between the size of the scores around the mean, the more likely is the mean to be in the center of the scale. However, when

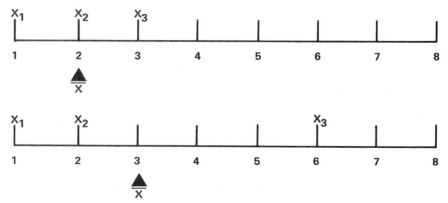

FIGURE 3-5. Representation of the shift of the mean with extreme scores away from the middle score.

extreme scores occur, the mean shifts toward the extreme score away from the middle score on the scale.

The location of the median and mean in a distribution is related to the shape of the distribution. Figure 3-6 illustrates the relationship between the measures of central tendency and the shape of a distribution of scores. The values of the mode, median, and mean are the same in a normal distribution (A). When a distribution is positively skewed (B), the mean is larger than the median and mode, and the mode is the smallest value. In a negatively skewed distribution (C), the opposite occurs; that is, the mean is the smallest value, then the median, and the mode is the largest.

The mean is usually the most preferable measure of central tendency, particularly when large samples are used or when the distribution of scores is nearly symmetrical. The mean also has the greatest stability and can be

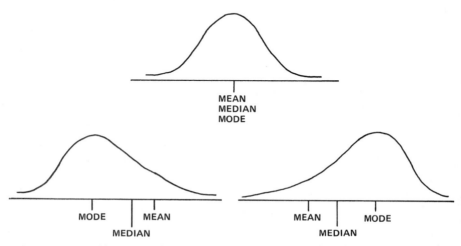

FIGURE 3-6. Relationship between the shape of a distribution and the values of its measures of central tendency. (From Waltz and Bausell, 1981, with permission.)

used for further statistical manipulations. The median is most appropriately used when the distribution shows marked skewness. The mode is best used in situations in which a rough estimate of central tendency is required quickly or where the typical case is needed. Although these rules are generally appropriate, one should consider each set of data in terms of the specific situation or particular need to determine which measure of central tendency is best to employ.

DISPERSION

An important characteristic of any distribution of scores is the amount of spread or scatter among the scores, which is referred to as dispersion. To illustrate this concept further, assume that fasting blood sugar levels are taken over a six-month period for two diabetic children. One child has diabetes that is easy to control, and the other has diabetes that is difficult to control. One might obtain distributions of blood glucose levels for the two children similar to the ones shown in Figure 3-7.

Note that the two distributions have means that are equal; however, the spread or dispersion of blood glucose levels for the two children is quite different; that is, the dispersion of the fasting blood glucose levels for the child with diabetes that is difficult to control is more spread out than that of the child with controlled diabetes. The fasting blood glucose levels for the child with easily controlled diabetes is rather consistent and more easily kept within the normal range with treatment, while the child with difficult to control diabetes has fasting blood glucose levels that are sometimes low, sometimes normal, and sometimes high. In other words, the variability of fasting blood glucose levels for the child with diabetes that is difficult to control is greater than those for the child with easily controlled diabetes.

The dispersion of a distribution of scores may be measured by three indices: (1) range, (2) variance, and (3) standard deviation.

The *range* is the distance from the lowest score in a distribution to the highest score. Hence, it is calculated by subtracting the lowest from the highest score. The range is the simplest of the three indices of dispersion and is useful for a quick gross description of a distribution's dispersion. It is limited by the fact that its value is totally dependent upon two extreme scores.

The *variance* and *standard deviation* are based on the deviation of each score in a distribution from the arithmetic mean. A deviation score represents the distance between a subject's raw score and the mean of the distribution. It is calculated by subtracting the mean from the raw score $(X - \overline{X})$. If, for example, infant A weighs 6 lb., infant B 10 lb., infant C 8 lb., and infant D 4 lb., the mean of this distribution of weights is 7 lb. The deviation score, in terms of each infant's weight, is $6 - 7$ or -1 for infant A, $10 - 7$ or $+3$ for infant B, $8 - 7$ or $+1$ for infant C, and $4 - 7$ or -3 for infant D. It should be noted that the sign of the deviation score indicates whether the raw score is above (+) or below (−) the mean. In addition, the sum of the deviation scores in a distribution should always equal zero.

The variance of a distribution of scores may be calculated by using the deviation scores or by using raw scores. Illustrations of each of these approaches using the example cited above follow.

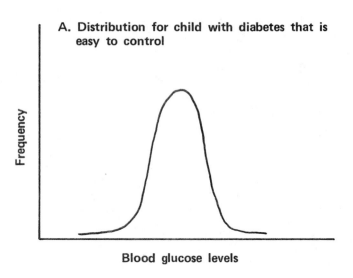

A. Distribution for child with diabetes that is easy to control

Frequency

Blood glucose levels

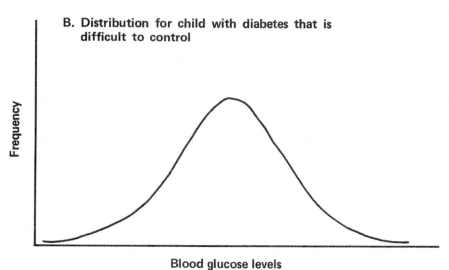

B. Distribution for child with diabetes that is difficult to control

Frequency

Blood glucose levels

FIGURE 3-7. Hypothetical distributions of fasting blood glucose levels for two children with diabetes.

Formula 3-2 Calculation of variance using deviation scores:

$$\sigma_x^2 = \frac{SSx}{n}$$

Where:
σ_x^2 = variance of the distribution of scores
SS_x = the sum of the squared deviation scores
n = the number of scores in the distribution

Example: Given the infant weights of 6 lb., 10 lb., 8 lb., and 4 lb., with $\overline{X} = 7$ lb.

$$SS_x = (6 - 7)^2 + (10 - 7)^2 + (8 - 7)^2 + (4 - 7)^2$$
$$= (-1)^2 + (+3)^2 + (-1)^2 + (-3)^2$$
$$= 1 + 9 + 1 + 9$$
$$= 20$$

$$\sigma_x^2 = \frac{20}{4}$$
$$= 5 \text{ square units}$$

It can be seen from this computational method that the variance is the average of the sum of the squared deviation scores.

Formula 3-3 Calculation of variance using raw scores:

$$\sigma_x^2 = \frac{\Sigma X^2 - \frac{(\Sigma X)^2}{n}}{n}$$

Where:
σ_x^2 = the variance of the distribution of scores
ΣX^2 = the sum of the squared raw scores
$(\Sigma X)^2$ = the square of the sum of the raw scores
n = the number of the scores in the distribution

Example:

X	X^2
6	36
10	100
8	64
4	16
$\Sigma X = 28$	$\Sigma X^2 = 216$

$$(\Sigma X)^2 = 28 \times 28 = 784$$

$$\sigma_x^2 = \frac{216 - \frac{784}{4}}{4}$$

$$= \frac{216 - 196}{4}$$

$$= \frac{20}{4}$$

$$= 5 \text{ square units}$$

It should be noted that the variance is a square measure rather than linear. To transform a square measure to linear it is necessary to calculate the positive square root.

The *standard deviation* of a distribution of scores is the square root of the variance. Hence, the standard deviation is the linear counterpart of the variance. It is obtained by the following formula.

Formula 3-4

$$\sigma_x = \sqrt{\sigma_x^2}$$

Where:

σ_x = standard deviation
σ_x^2 = variance

Example: The variance of the infant weights of 6 lb., 10 lb., 8 lb., and 4 lb. is 5 square units.

$\sigma_x = \sqrt{5 \text{ square units}}$
$\sigma_x = 2.24$

The standard deviation is a useful statistic for comparing differences in variability among two or more distributions. For example, if distribution A has a standard deviation of 3, while distribution B has a standard deviation of 5, then one would know that the variability in distribution B is greater than that for A.

The standard deviation also may be thought of as a unit of measurement along the baseline of a frequency distribution. For example, in a normal distribution there are about 3 standard deviations above the mean and 3 below. Therefore, the range of the distribution is made up of approximately 6 standard deviations and all deviations above the mean are positive, and those below the mean are negative. If a distribution has a mean of 20 and a standard deviation of 5, one could divide the baseline into standard units. To do this one would start at the mean and add one standard deviation (5) to the value of the mean (20) to obtain +1 standard deviation or 25. The raw score 25, then, is exactly one standard deviation above the mean. Likewise, scores that are 2 and 3 standard deviations above the mean are 30 and 35, respectively. To determine the value of –1 standard deviation one would subtract one standard deviation (5) from the mean (20) with the result 15, which is one standard deviation below the mean. The score values for –2 and –3 standard deviations would be 10 and 5, respectively. This is illustrated in Figure 3-8.

The standard deviation also is useful because in normal distributions it is known what percent of scores lie within specified standard deviations from the mean.

MEASURES OF CORRELATION

A number of procedures have been developed for assessing the quality of norm-referenced tests and test items that involve the use of the Pearson Product-Moment Correlation Coefficient or other measures of linear association. For this reason, Pearson Product-Moment correlation is discussed to present information necessary for understanding reliability and validity

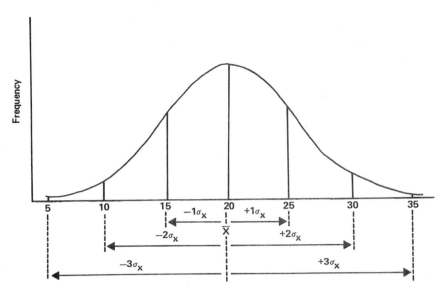

FIGURE 3-8. Illustration of standard deviation as units along the baseline of normal distribution with a mean of 20 and standard deviation of 5.

theory and the proper application and interpretation of correlation in measurement contexts.

The linear relationship of two sets of scores can be represented by a scatterplot or scattergram. Suppose two alternate forms of a 12-item professionalism scale were administered to a group of 8 nurses and resulted in scores on the two forms as shown in Table 3-2.

A two-dimensional representation of these scores is presented in the scatterplot shown in Figure 3-9. Although a scatterplot provides a good visual illustration of the relationship between two sets of scores, it often is desirable to summarize the extent of this relationship using a numerical index. The statistic most frequently employed to quantitatively summarize scatterplot information is the Pearson Product-Moment Correlation Coefficient (r_{xy}). Hence, r_{xy} is a quantitative measure of the linear relationship

TABLE 3-2 Hypothetical scores for 8 nurses on alternate forms of a 12-item professionalism scale

Nurse	Score	
	Form A	Form B
A	9	11
B	6	7
C	4	2
D	3	5
E	10	8
F	2	3
G	8	6
H	2	1

57

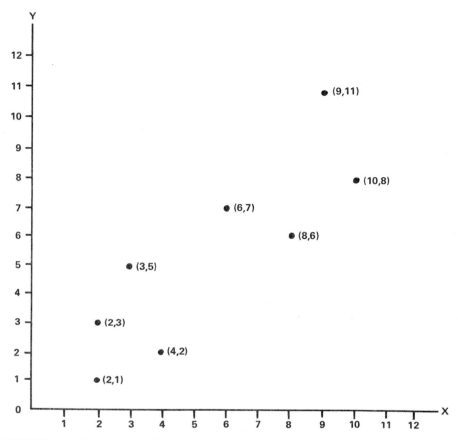

FIGURE 3-9. Scatterplot of scores presented in Table 3-2.

between two sets of scores. In other words, it measures the extent to which two sets of scores in two-dimensional space follow a straight line trend.

The value of r_{xy} lies between the interval −1.00 to +1.00. If r_{xy} of +1.00 was obtained, it would represent a perfect positive relationship between the two sets of scores and is illustrated by a scatterplot with a line that slopes downward from right to left as shown by scatterplot A in Figure 3-10. If the line slopes downward from left to right, as in scatterplot B in Figure 3-10, an r_{xy} of −1.00 would result. This represents a perfect negative relationship between the two sets of scores.

If the scores obtained from the same group of subjects on a measure are not perfectly correlated with the scores obtained on a second measure, patterns similar to those shown in scatterplots C and D in Figure 3-10 may occur. Scatterplot C in Figure 3-10 implies that increases in the value of one score (Y) tend to be associated with increases in the value of the other score (X). In scatterplot D, increases in the value of one score (Y) tend to be associated with decreases in the value of the other score (X). In other words, a positive linear relationship indicates that a person who scores high on one

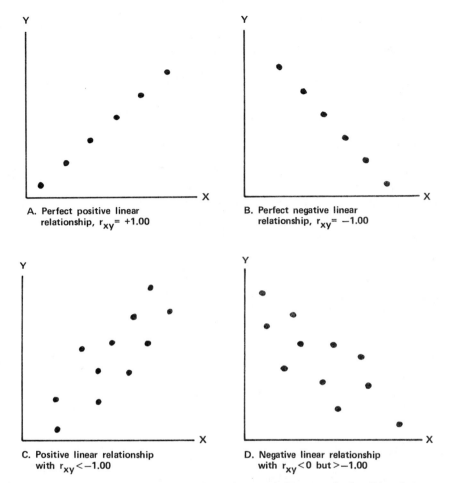

A. Perfect positive linear
relationship, $r_{xy}= +1.00$

B. Perfect negative linear
relationship, $r_{xy}= -1.00$

C. Positive linear relationship
with $r_{xy}<-1.00$

D. Negative linear relationship
with $r_{xy}<0$ but >-1.00

FIGURE 3-10. Examples of scatterplots of various linear relationships between two variables.

measure or test also is likely to score high on the other, and that a person who scores low on one test also is likely to score low on the other. A negative relationship suggests that a person who scores high on one test is likely to score low on the other. When a perfect correlation does not exist it results in a scattering of points away from the straight line which best summarizes the trend. In general, the more widely scattered the points, the closer r_{xy} is to zero.

Two types of scatterplot patterns will lead to an r_{xy} of zero (or a value very close to zero): (1) when there is no recognizable pattern in the scatterplots, or (2) when the pattern of the scatterplot is curvilinear, that is, seems to follow a well-defined curve.

An example of the former case is presented in scatterplot A in Figure 3-11, and an example of the latter case is illustrated by scatterplot B in Figure 3-11.

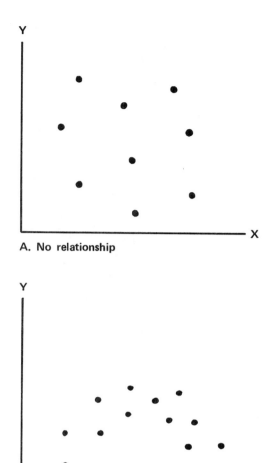

A. No relationship

B. Curvilinear relationship

FIGURE 3-11. Examples of scatterplots for which r_{xy} may be zero.

When the configuration is an amorphous glob, as in scatterplot A of Figure 3-11, an r_{xy} value of 0 is accurately reflected because there is no useful relationship between the two sets of scores. However, where a curvilinear relationship exists, as illustrated in scatterplot B of Figure 3-11, an r_{xy} value of 0 is quite misleading because a useful relationship may exist. Statistical indices are available that are appropriate for measuring the degree of curvilinear association between sets of scores, for example, eta (Guilford, 1965).

At this point, attention is given to interpretation of r_{xy}. It is useful to convert r_{xy} to a percentage in order to provide for further interpretation. This is done by squaring the r_{xy} value and by changing the result to a percentage. The value that results is the *percentage of explained variance* between two sets of scores. This means that scores obtained from one measure could be used to explain the variance in another measure and vice versa. For example, if the value of r_{xy} is $+.70$ then the percentage of explained variance is $r_{xy}^2 = (+.70)^2 = .49$ or 49%. This means that 49 percent of the variance in the scores from one measure or test would be explained on the basis of the scores from the other measure or test and vice versa.

Potential problems may influence the interpretation of r_{xy}. First, reducing the variability in the distribution of either or both sets of scores (X and/ or Y) tends to decrease the value of r_{xy}. This can occur when (1) there is loss of measurement information (e.g., when a nominal level measurement scale is employed rather than a higher level measurement scale) and (2) there is a restriction of range in the data, that is, when a homogeneous subset of data points in the scatterplot is used to calculate r_{xy} (Martuza, 1977, p. 76).

The effects of restriction of range can be illustrated by the scatterplot in Figure 3-12. Suppose the true association between X and Y in a population was as illustrated in Figure 3-12, but r_{xy} was calculated using individuals

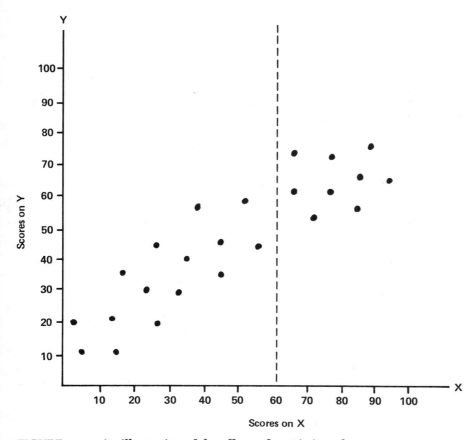

FIGURE 3-12. An illustration of the effects of restriction of range.

with scores of 60 or higher on variable X. The value of r_{xy} would be close to zero and, therefore, would misrepresent r_{xy}. This would happen because data points in the included portion of the scatterplot do not exhibit a strong linear trend. In most instances restriction of range will decrease the value of r_{xy}; however, in some instances it may be increased.

The second problem that may be encountered in the interpretation of r_{xy} is that measurement error can affect the value of r_{xy}. Random errors of measurement, that is, factors that can inadvertently increase or decrease the score values obtained from measurement, will distort the value of r_{xy}. When either or both sets of scores have been influenced to a large degree by random error, the true nature of their relationship will be distorted, and so will r_{xy}. The value of r_{xy} may be increased or decreased by random error of measurement. In most cases, however, a decrease in the value of r_{xy} will result. Random error of measurement is discussed more fully in subsequent sections of this chapter.

The Pearson Product-Moment Correlation Coefficient (r_{xy}) can be computed from raw scores in the following manner.

Formula 3-5

$$ r_{xy} = \frac{n\Sigma XY - (\Sigma X)(\Sigma Y)}{\sqrt{[n\Sigma X^2 - (\Sigma X)^2][n Y^2 - (\Sigma Y)^2]}} $$

Where:

ΣXY = the sum of the products of each person's X and Y scores
(ΣXY) = the sum of all X scores
(ΣY) = the sum of all Y scores
n = the number of subjects
ΣX^2 = the sum of all squared X scores
$(\Sigma X)^2$ = the square of the sum of all X scores
ΣY^2 = the sum of all squared Y scores
$(\Sigma Y)^2$ = the square of the sum of all Y scores

To illustrate the computation of r_{xy}, the scores presented in Table 3-2 will be used. Scores on Form A are designated as X and scores on Form B are designated as Y.

Subject	X	Y	XY	X^2	Y^2
A	9	11	99	81	121
B	6	7	42	36	49
C	4	2	8	16	4
D	3	5	15	9	25
E	10	8	80	100	64
F	2	3	6	4	9
G	8	6	48	64	36
H	2	1	2	4	1
	$\Sigma X = 44$	$\Sigma X = 43$	$\Sigma XY = 300$	$\Sigma X^2 = 314$	$\Sigma Y^2 = 309$

$(\Sigma X^2) = 1936$ $(\Sigma Y)^2 = 1849$

$$r_{xy} = \frac{n \Sigma XY - (\Sigma X)(\Sigma Y)}{\sqrt{[n \Sigma X^2 - (\Sigma X)^2][n \Sigma Y^2 - (\Sigma Y)^2]}}$$

$$= \frac{8(300) - (44)(43)}{\sqrt{[8(314) - (1936)][8(309) - (1849)]}}$$

$$= \frac{2400 - 1892}{\sqrt{(2512 - 1936)(2472 - 1849)}}$$

$$= \frac{508}{\sqrt{(576)(623)}}$$

$$= \frac{508}{\sqrt{358848}}$$

$$= \frac{508}{599}$$

$$= 0.85$$

If the value 0.85 for r_{xy} is squared, it can then be interpreted to mean that 72 percent of the variance in X may be explained or predicted on the basis of Y and vice versa. Several variations of r_{xy} can be employed. These coefficients are summarized in Table 3-3. Further information regarding these statistics and their formulas can be found in Agresti and Agresti (1979), Glass and Stanley (1970), Kirk (1968), or Nunnally (1978).

Waltz and Bausell (1981, p. 264) point out that some of the coefficients in Table 3-3, that is, phi, r_s, and r_{pb} are equal to r_{xy}: "That is, they are simply the Product Moment Correlation Coefficient formula applied to nominal and ordinal data." The remaining coefficients, r_{tet} and r_{bis}, are approximations of r_{xy}.

Now that an introduction to measurement and the basic statistical principles and procedures which undergird measurement has been provided, attention will be given to measurement theory.

MEASUREMENT ERROR AND RELIABILITY AND VALIDITY OF MEASURES

The goal of all measurement is to achieve accurate results. However, this is not completely possible because measurement error, to some extent, is introduced into all measuring procedures. There are two basic types of errors that affect the precision of empirical indicators: random error and systematic error. Random error, also termed variable or chance error, is caused by chance factors that confound the measurement of any phenomenon. An important characteristic of random error is that it occurs in an unsystematic

TABLE 3-3 Coefficients for use with various types of data*

		Variable X		
		Nominal	Ordinal	Interval or Ratio
Variable Y	Nominal	PHI (ϕ) CONTINGENCY (C) TETRACHORIC (r_{tet})	CURETON'S RANK BISERIAL (r_{rb})	BISERIAL (r_b, r_{bis}) POINT BISERIAL (r_{pb})
	Ordinal	CURETON'S RANK BISERIAL (r_{rb})	SPEARMAN RHO (P, r_s) KENDALL'S TAU (τ)	TAU (τ)
	Interval or Ratio	BISERIAL (r_b, r_{bis}) POINT BISERIAL (r_{pb})	TAU (τ)	PEARSON PRODUCT MOMENT (r_{xy})

*from Waltz and Bausell, 1981

manner in all measurement. A measuring device affected by random error will yield empirical indicators that will sometimes be higher and sometimes lower than the actual magnitude of the attribute measured. Assume that a nurse takes a patient's oral temperature six times during the course of a day. Also assume that on two measurement occasions the temperature is taken with the patient breathing through the mouth and on another measurement occasion the temperature is taken immediately after the patient has taken several sips of hot coffee. This is an example of random error because the temperature readings would sometimes be lower and sometimes higher than the patient's actual body temperature as a result of the introduction of various errors of measurement. Even if there were no fluctuations in the patient's true body temperature, the temperature readings obtained from measurement to measurement would not be consistent. Therefore, random error primarily affects the reliability, that is, the consistency of measurements, and consequently validity as well, because reliability is a necessary prerequisite for validity. However, one should recognize that this does not mean that the validity of measures is not affected at all by random error. The introduction of error always affects the validity of specific measures to some degree.

Systematic error, the second type of error that affects empirical measurements, has a systematic biasing influence on measuring procedures. Suppose a patient's thermometer always registers 0.4°F higher than the actual temperature. This is an example of systematic error because repeated temperature readings taken with this thermometer would always be 0.4°F higher than it really should be. A systematic increase of 0.4°F would always be introduced into the results. Hence, the extent to which the thermometer measures what it purports to measure, that is, temperature, is compromised.

Given the above information about the occurrence of random and systematic error, a central question arises as to how nurses can determine the extent to which a given tool or device measures the nursing concept under consideration. Stated in different terms, how well do the results of a measuring procedure represent a given nursing concept? For instance, how can one evaluate the extent to which an instrument designed to measure nursing professionalism accurately represents that concept? Reliability and validity of empirical measurements are two basic aspects of measurement that can be used to examine these questions. The occurrence of random error in measuring procedures is the central threat to the reliability of the measurement. In a similar manner, the validity of a measurement is more threatened by the occurrence of systematic error.

RELIABILITY AND RANDOM ERROR

The reliability of a measuring device is directly influenced by random error. There is an inverse relationship between the amount of random error introduced into measurement and the reliability of the measurement. The higher the reliability of the measurement, the less random error is introduced into the measuring procedure. A large amount of random error decreases the reliability of the measurement.

A measurement tool is reliable for a particular subject population to the extent to which it yields consistent results on repeated measurements of the same attribute. Because reliability refers to the consistency or stability of empirical indicators from measurement to measurement, it naturally follows that empirical indicators obtained from any measuring procedure are reliable to the extent that they are free of random errors. Because sets of measurements of the same attributes for the same objects or events will never exactly duplicate each other, unreliability in measurement is always present to some extent. Thus, the reliability of a measure is a matter of degree. While the amount of random error may be large or small, it is always present. If the random error is large, then the consistency of empirical indicators that result from repeated measurements will be poor and reliability will be compromised. If, however, there is only a small amount of random error, the stability of empirical indicators on repeated measurements will be high and reliability will be high. Stated in different terms, the more consistent and stable the results obtained from repeated measurements, the higher the reliability of the measuring procedure; but the less consistent and more variable the results, the lower the reliability.

The occurrence of random error is a common problem that affects the reliability of any measurement procedure. The following illustrations should clarify how random error is introduced into measurement procedures. First, suppose three nurses are given the task of independently measuring the height of two adult patients to the nearest one-eighth inch on the same day using the same device. It is probable that there will be noticeably different measurements of height obtained by these nurses as long as they are unaware of each others' results. Since height is not likely to change in the same day, obviously discrepancies between findings must be due to measurement errors. You can probably think of a number of chance factors that could influence the results, for example: (1) factors resulting from individual differences in patients, such as height of hair, (b) factors resulting from differences in the nurses' instructions to patients during the procedure, such as instructing patients to stand tall without slumping the back, or (c) differences in the nurses' procedure, such as location or placement of the device on the patients' heads.

Similarly, suppose a nurse takes the same patient's blood pressure twice with the patient lying in a recumbent position in a relaxed manner at a one-minute interval. It is likely that the two blood pressure readings will vary somewhat without any actual change in the patient's blood pressure. Differences in noise level in the room could affect auditory acuity during the repeated readings. Other factors that could affect the final results are variations in the nurse's eye level in relation to the column of mercury in the sphygmomanometer during readings and differences in the speed at which the blood pressure cuff is deflated on successive measurements.

In both of these examples, certain factors influenced the measuring procedure, which affected the results obtained. In each illustration, if random error had not occurred one could expect error-free results and results would have been the same across measurements. This is not the case in reality. A very important point should be made. Fluctuations in measurement results that occur due to random error do cancel each other out if many independent measurements are made. "They do not directly influence the meaning of the measurement but do directly affect the precision with which the characteristic of interest is being measured" (Martuza, 1977, p. 9). For example, if the heights of 20 adults were measured repeatedly for 3 days in succession, one would not expect each person's height to be precisely duplicated on repeated measurements. However, one would expect that the person who was the tallest on the first day would be among those measured the tallest on the second and third days. Although each person's height would not be exactly the same from measurement to measurement, it would tend to be consistent in relation to the heights of others in the group.

There are numerous sources of random error. Some examples are (a) the manner in which a measure is scored or coded, (b) characteristics or state of the subject or respondent (such as attention span, anxiety, or illness), (c) chance factors affecting the administration or appraisal of measurements obtained (such as fatigue of observers, different emphasis placed on different words by an interviewer, the amount of heat or lighting in the room, or luck in the selection of answers by guessing), and (d) characteristics of the measuring device, such as type of items employed in constructing the tool.

VALIDITY AND SYSTEMATIC ERROR

In addition to being reliable, it is desirable for a measuring procedure to be valid. Any measuring tool is valid to the degree that it measures what it purports to measure. Hence, an empirical indicator of a particular nursing concept is valid to the extent that it successfully measures the intended concept. For example, a rating scale designed to measure maternal behavior would be valid to the extent that it actually measures maternal behavior rather than reflecting some other phenomenon.

As noted above, the validity of a specific measuring device is influenced by the degree to which systematic error is introduced into the measuring procedure. There is an inverse relationship between the degree to which systematic error is present during a measuring procedure and the extent to which the empirical indicator is valid. The more systematic error is included in the measure, the less valid the measure will be, and vice versa. Therefore, validity is a matter of degree just as reliability is a matter of degree. The goal of obtaining a perfectly valid empirical indicator that represents only the intended concept is not completely achievable. As previously noted, systematic error causes independent measurements obtained by the same measuring device to be either consistently higher or lower than they ought to be. This clearly presents a problem with validity because there is a common systematic bias in all results obtained by the measuring device which influences the extent to which the attribute of interest is actually measured.

To illustrate the impact of systematic error on the validity of a measurement, suppose that an oxygen analyzer has an error in calibration such that it consistently registers the percentage of oxygen two points below the actual percentage of oxygen. Even though variations in the concentration of oxygen in a premature infant's isolette would be reflected in repeated measurements, each measurement would be two percentage points below the actual level due to systematic error in the measuring device, the oxygen analyzer. The effect is that a constant—two percentage points—would be subtracted from the value that would be obtained if the oxygen analyzer were properly calibrated. An inference about the absolute concentration of oxygen in the isolette would be invalid.

Similarly, if a measuring procedure that was designed to measure only nausea also measures anxiety, then this would present a problem of validity. The measuring procedure would not be a totally valid measure of nausea because it simultaneously measures anxiety. Thus, systematic bias has been introduced into the results, which do not accurately measure the concept of interest. However, this bias would be included in all measurements obtained with the tool.

There are a number of biasing factors that can contribute to systematic error in measurement. Usually the sources of systematic error are associated with lasting characteristics of the respondent or subject, the measuring tool, and/or the measuring process. The sources of systematic error do not fluctuate from one measurement situation to the next as is the case with random error. Examples of systematic sources of error associated with the respondent or subject are chronic illness, testwiseness, a negative attitude toward completing questionnaires or taking tests, and a poor comprehension of language used in the questionnaire or test items. Characteristics of measuring tools that may systematically bias measurements are the inclusion of items that measure knowledge, skills, or abilities that are irrelevant to the concept being measured and poor calibration of a measuring device. Another source of systematic error may be due to the measurement process itself; for example, observer or scorer bias (such as an observer's tendency to rate slim individuals higher than heavy individuals on items related to physical activity).

By now it should be clear that measurement error is central to questions related to reliability and validity. Any measuring tool is relatively reliable if it is affected to a minimal extent by random measurement error. Even though high reliability of a measuring instrument is a laudible goal, measures that are reliable are only a portion of the answer to measurement concerns. It also is important that a measuring tool be valid for the purposes for which it is used. Systematic error biases the degree to which an indicator measures what it is supposed to measure by reflecting some other phenomenon. Hence, validity is enhanced by the degree to which systematic error is kept to a minimum. While reliability focuses on the consistency of performance of the measuring device, validity is more of a theoretically oriented issue because it focuses on the crucial relationship between the concept and its empirical indicator (Carmines and Zellar, 1979).

Two important points should be made about the relationship of reliability and validity. First, a measuring procedure can be highly reliable but have low validity. Consistency of results does not necessarily mean that a tool effectively measures the concept that it is used to measure. Second, a measuring procedure that has low reliability when the measurement situation remains constant cannot have an acceptable degree of validity. The presence of large random error compromises the extent to which an empirical indicator represents the concept it is supposed to measure. Therefore, *reliability is a necessary but not sufficient condition for validity.*

CLASSICAL MEASUREMENT THEORY

The preceding section examined measurement error and related it to the concepts of reliability and validity. This section presents a discussion of classical measurement theory, which is a model for assessing random measurement error. As noted previously, random error is present in the measurement of any phenomenon. The basic tenet of classical measurement theory evolved from the assumption that random error is an element that must be considered in all measurement. The underlying principle of this theory is that every observed score is composed of a true score and an error score. The true score is the true or precise amount of the attribute possessed by the object or event being measured. The error score reflects the influence that random error has on the observed score. The basic formulation of classical measurement theory is as follows:

Formula 3-6 $O = T + E$

> Where:
> O = observed score
> T = true score
> E = error score

This equation simply indicates that every observed score that results from any measuring procedure is composed of two independent quantities: a true score, which represents the precise score that would be obtained if there were no errors of measurement; and an error score, which represents the contribution of random measurement error that happens to be present at the time the measurement is taken.

Consider the following examples as illustrations of true and error score components of the observed score. Suppose a nurse attempts to take the pulse of a patient for one minute and misreads the second hand on her watch. She counts the patient's pulse rate for 64 seconds rather than the intended 60 seconds, thereby increasing the patient's actual pulse rate of 82 (the true score) to 88 (the observed score). According to Formula 3-6, the error score in this instance is +6 beats, since this is the discrepancy between the patient's true pulse and observed pulse.

$$O = T + E$$
$$88 = 82 + (+6)$$

Suppose that the random error had been in the other direction and the nurse counted the patient's pulse rate for only 58 seconds rather than the intended 60 seconds. Although the patient's actual pulse rate was 82 (the true score), the observed pulse rate was 78 (the observed score). Therefore, the error score in this case is −4.

$$O = T + E$$
$$78 = 82 + (-4)$$

It should be noted that in reality one does not know the true score and the error score values. Only the observed score is known. The above examples are for the purpose of illustration only. Formula 3-6 assumes that the object or event being measured possesses a specific amount of the attribute of interest when the measurement is taken. The precise amount of the attribute is obscured because of random error, which either increases or decreases the results. The influence of the random error on the observed measurement is called the *error of measurement*. Classical measurement theory assumes that the observed score which is obtained when a measurement is taken is a combination of the true score and the error of measurement.*

True scores are conceived to be unobservable quantities that cannot be directly measured. When an attribute is measured, the true score is assumed to be fixed. If it were possible for the true score to remain constant while the attribute of interest was measured an infinite number of times variability in observed scores would result from the impact of random error of measurement that would occur by chance when each measurement was taken. Random disturbances in the observed score due to random error mean that some observed scores would be higher than the true score, while other observed scores would be lower than the true score. Classical measurement theory assumes that the mean of error scores is zero and that the correlation between the true score and error score is zero. Therefore, distributions of random error can be expected to be normally distributed; hence, the distribution of observed scores would be normally distributed. The effects of random error can be expected to cancel each other out if many independent measures of the same attribute of an object or event are made and averaged. An average or arithmetic mean of observed scores would be the true score. Such a hypothetical dispersion of observed scores about the true score is illustrated in Figure 3-13.

The more widely dispersed observed scores are about the true score, the larger is the error of measurement. If the true score were known and could

---

*The implication of this assumption is that systematic errors become part of the true score and affect validity but not reliability.

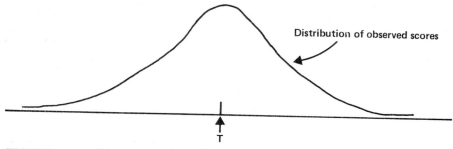

FIGURE 3-13. The true score and hypothetical distribution of observed scores for a person at a specific point in time.

be subtracted from each observed score, the results would be a set of deviation scores, which would be the errors of measurement. Since the true score is considered fixed and the dispersion of observed scores is due to errors of measurement, subtraction of true scores from observed scores would result in a normal distribution of error scores (errors of measurement) (Fig. 3-14).

The standard deviation of this distribution of error scores would be an index of the amount of measurement error. This standard deviation of error scores is termed the *standard error of measurement*.

If it were possible to have a measuring procedure that was perfectly reliable, the observed score and the true score would be the same. There would be no error of measurement and, therefore, no error score. In such a case the standard error of measurement would equal zero. The more reliable a measuring procedure is, the smaller will be the standard error of measurement. The less reliable the measuring procedure, the larger the standard error of measurement. The size of the standard error of measurement is an indicator of the amount of error involved in using a particular measuring procedure.

OBSERVED SCORE VARIANCE

If a large number of persons were measured with respect to the same attribute, the observed scores would not be the same. This is true because there would be real differences in the amount of the attribute possessed by different individuals, and because there would be differences in the effects of

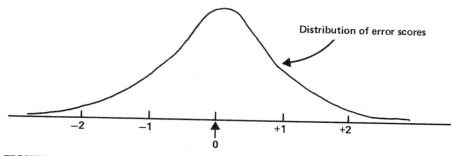

FIGURE 3-14. Hypothetical distribution of errors of measurement.

random error on each observed score. Since each persons's observed score is composed of true score and error score components, three different score distributions would result: (1) a distribution of the observed scores; (2) a distribution of true scores; and (3) a distribution of error scores. Figure 3-15 illustrates these distributions of scores. Each person's observed, true, and error scores (e.g., for individuals J and L) are represented in each of the three distributions.

Remember that true scores and error scores are not observable. Only the values of the observed scores are known. Classical measurement theory assumes that the correlation between the true score and error score is zero. If this is the case, the following formula holds.

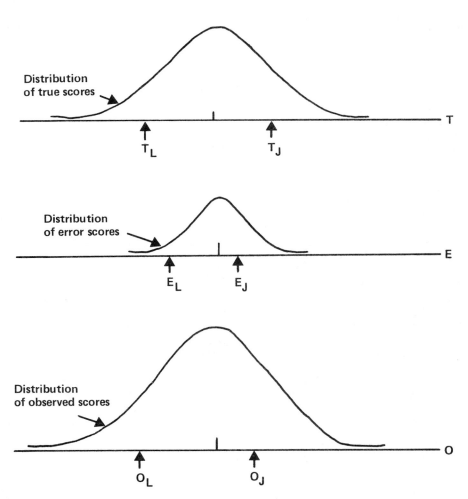

FIGURE 3-15. Distributions of true scores (T), errors sources (E), and observed scores (O) for a population of persons measured for the same attribute.

Formula 3-7 $\text{Var (O)} = \text{Var (T)} + \text{Var (E)}$

Where: Var (O) = variance of the observed score distribution also noted
as σ_O^2

Var (T) = variance of the true score distribution also noted as σ_T^2

Var (E) = variance of the error score distribution also noted
as σ_E^2

The basic variance formula, Formula 3-7, holds only when true scores
and error scores are not correlated; that is, when the true score cannot be
used to predict the error score and vice versa.

THE STATISTICAL DEFINITION OF RELIABILITY

Formula 3-7 can be converted to illustrate the statistical definition of reliability. In order to do this, each term in Formula 3-7 is divided by Var (O).
The result is as follows:

$$\text{Var (O)} = \text{Var (T)} + \text{Var (E)}$$

$$\frac{\text{Var (O)}}{\text{Var (O)}} = \frac{\text{Var (T)}}{\text{Var (O)}} + \frac{\text{Var (E)}}{\text{Var (O)}}$$

Formula 3-8 $$1.00 = \frac{\text{Var (T)}}{\text{Var (O)}} + \frac{\text{Var (E)}}{\text{Var (O)}}$$

Note that Var (O)/Var (O) is equal to one. The expression Var (T)/Var (O)
is the statistical definition of reliability. It is representative of the proportion of variation in the observed score distribution that results because of
true score differences among respondents or subjects. The second ratio in
Formula 3-8, Var (E)/Var (O), is the statistical definition of unreliability. It
is a representation of the proportion of variation in the observed score distribution that is due to random errors of measurement. A variance ratio is
equivalent to a squared Pearson r (coefficient of correlation). Therefore, Var
(T)/Var (O) may also be written as $r_{(T,O)}^2$, which is the squared correlation of
true scores with observed scores. The second ratio Var (E)/Var (O) may be
written as $r_{(E,O)}^2$, which is the squared correlation of error scores with observed scores. Thus, $r_{(T,O)}^2$ is also a statistical representation of reliability
and is termed the reliability coefficient. Similarly, $r_{(E,O)}^2$ is a statistical representation of unreliability.

The square root of the reliability coefficient is the correlation between
observed scores and true scores for a test or measure. This is usually called
the test's *reliability index*. Since a reliability coefficient is conceptually a
squared value, the statistic used to estimate it empirically is never squared
in practice. Reliability also can be expressed in terms of error variance.
Referring to Formula 3-8:

$$1.00 = \frac{\text{Var (T)}}{\text{Var (O)}} + \frac{\text{Var (E)}}{\text{Var (O)}}$$

If Var (T)/Var (O) were transposed to the left side of the equation and 1.00 to the right side, it can be seen that:

Formula 3-9
$$\frac{\text{Var (T)}}{\text{Var (O)}} = 1.00 - \frac{\text{Var (E)}}{\text{Var (O)}}$$

Hence, the reliability of the observed score (O) as a measure of the true score (T) is equal to 1.00 minus the error variance. It is obvious then that the reliability of a measure varies between 0 and 1. If the observed score is highly contaminated with random error, then the reliability is decreased and becomes closer to zero. Conversely, if only a small amount of random error occurs in the measurement of a phenomenon, the reliability increases and is closer to 1.00. Reliability coefficients provide an indication of the significance of interindividual differentiation in observed scores. If a reliability coefficient is high, then more credence can be given to interindividual differences in observed scores. A low reliability coefficient reduces the credibility. The variance of error of measurement indicates intraindividual variability in the person's observed score due to the introduction of random error when the measurement was taken (Stanley, 1971, p. 373). When the variance of error of measurement is large, this means that a large amount of random error was introduced into individual scores.

If a nursing instructor used an achievement test with an estimated reliability of 0.85 to test her students' knowledge of surgical nursing, this would indicate two things. First, 85 percent of the variance in the distribution of observed scores is due to actual differences in knowledge among the nursing students tested. Second, the remaining 15 percent of variance in the observed score distribution resulted from random errors of measurement, for example, misinterpretation of items or guessing.

The derivation of the statistical definition of reliability for a distribution of scores on a single measurement of a group of persons has been shown. However, it is optimal to compute the reliability coefficient directly with at least two observed scores per subject. When the observed score is a composite of more than one part of a measure, then the consistency among several parts can be examined and a reliability estimate obtained. For example, if a test contained two or more items, one could study how scores on items of the test co-vary with each other and determine the consistency of the test.

Two conceptual models which have evolved from classical measurement theory are commonly used for the discussion of measurement error: (1) the model of parallel measures, and (2) the domain-sampling model. Both are basic models for the computation of reliability coefficients.

THE MODEL OF PARALLEL MEASURES

This model purports to determine a measure's reliability by correlating parallel measurements. It is assumed that two measures of the same thing are parallel if: (a) they have the same correlation with a set of true scores; (b) variance in each measure that is not due to true scores is strictly the result of random error of measurement; and (c) they have the same standard deviation. For example, if two devices designed to measure depression are parallel, they would yield the same true scores when used in the same measurement situation. The differences in the observed scores on the measures would be due only to random error. Since random errors tend to cancel each other out, the standard deviation of both tests would be the same because the standard deviations reflect true score variance.

The model of parallel tests assumes that the correlation between any two tests of a domain is a complete and precise determination of the reliability coefficient rather than only an estimate. A major limitation of this model is that it disregards the fact that reliability cannot be precisely determined by a sampling of items in a content domain.

Nunnally (1978, p. 203) points out that the model has limitations because it offers a conceptual dead end for the development of theories of measurement error since true scores are defined by only two tests. He contends that if there are three supposedly parallel tests rather than two and the three correlations among them are different, what then is the reliability? Since the model explicitly assumes that all parallel tests have the same reliability, one is placed in a dilemma. However, this is no problem for the domain-sampling model with which this possibility is admitted and an estimate of the reliability of any one measure is the average of its correlations with other measures.

THE DOMAIN-SAMPLING MODEL

The domain-sampling model considers any measure to be composed of a random sample of items from a hypothetical content domain which it purports to measure. According to this model, if a 50-item nursing test was designed to measure knowledge of pulmonary physiology, it could be considered to consist of a random sample of 50 items from a domain of all possible items which could test knowledge in this content area. A number of other tests could also be devised by randomly sampling the same domain. Each of the tests that would result from sampling the same domain would have somewhat different means, standard deviations, and correlations because of random error in the sampling of items. Tests or measures composed of items randomly taken from the same content domain are considered randomly parallel tests.

The domain-sampling model indicates that the goal of any measure is to estimate the score a person would obtain if examined on all possible items within the content domain. The score that an individual would obtain if it were possible to be measured with a test composed of all possible items from a domain would be the *true score*. This is sometimes referred to as the domain score. In reality, it is not possible to obtain a domain score. In most instances there are an infinite number of items in a content domain. It also is difficult to randomly sample a domain. Most test items are constructed for each specific measure. However, actual applications of the domain-sampling model do result in accurate predictions.

According to the domain-sampling model, *the extent to which any sample of items from the domain is correlated with the true score is an indication of its reliability.* If a sample of items has a low correlation with the true score or domain score, then the reliability also would be low. Conversely, a high correlation between a sample of items from the domain and the true score means that the reliability of the sample is high. The domain-sampling model is applicable regardless of the number of items in the sample. Reliability estimates can be obtained if there is only one item in the item sample, or if there are many items.

The only assumption of this model is that the average correlation of each item with all the others in the domain is the same for all items. The degree to which items in the domain measure the same attribute would be indicated by the average correlation of items in the domain. The wider the dispersion of correlations of items about this average, the less likely would the items in the domain measure a common attribute. When the average correlation of items in the domain is zero or close to zero, the items do not have a common element and do not measure one attribute. It is, therefore, desirable for item correlations in the domain to be relatively homogeneous, positive, and greater than zero. When item correlations in the domain are more homogeneous, the more precise are reliability estimates. The degree of variance in the correlations among items in the domain is a reflection of random error connected with the average correlation for a particular sampling of items. Errors that would cause variation from item to item, such as guessing, would reduce item correlations and thereby reduce reliability.

Thus far, the discussion of the domain-sampling model has primarily focused on the correlations of single items in the domain. However, these concepts can be extended to whole tests as well. It was noted earlier that this model views tests as consisting of a random sample of items from a content domain. A number of tests generated from the same domain using random selection of items would be considered randomly parallel tests. Each would have means, standard deviations, and correlations with true scores that would differ by chance only. If it were possible to randomly select test items from the domain, the average correlation of a single test with a number of other randomly parallel tests would be an estimate of the average correlation of the test with all other tests in the domain. Conceptually, this would result in the reliability for the tests.

Since a whole test is a summation of its items, the average correlation among whole tests will be larger than the average correlation among items. This will result in higher correlations with true scores for the whole test. The domain-sampling model assumes that the reliability of scores obtained on a sample of items from the domain increases as the number of items sampled from the domain increases. Therefore, longer tests have higher reliability coefficients than shorter tests. However, Nunnally (1978, p. 208) noted that tests that have as few as 10 items may have rather precise reliability.

On initial examination the model of parallel measures and the domain-sampling model appear quite different. However, Nunnally (1978) notes that the model of parallel measures is a special case of the domain-sampling model. Whereas the basic assumptions of the parallel measures model result in a specification of a characteristic of measurement error, the domain-sampling model estimates the same characteristic. Any formula obtained from the parallel measures model can be matched by a formula from the domain-sampling model which is based on estimation. However, the reverse does not hold true. There are many principles and formulas emanating from the domain-sampling model that cannot be provided for by the model of parallel tests.

The model of parallel measures and the domain-sampling model are the most well-known conceptual approaches to measurement. Both have evolved from classical measurement theory and have proven to be useful and understandable approaches to the discussion of measurement error. Although classical measurement theory is widely used, the binomial model is a competing perspective that has gained popularity, particularly in terms of its potential usefulness in the criterion-referenced measurement framework.

THE BINOMIAL MODEL: AN ALTERNATIVE APPROACH TO MEASUREMENT

Whereas classical measurement theory assumes that errors are normally distributed about the true score, the binomial model purports that errors have a binomial distribution. Hence, errors may be positively or negatively skewed about the true score. The direction of skewness of the binomial distribution would depend upon whether the person had a low, average, or high probability of correctly responding to items drawn from the content domain.

The basic assumption of the binomial model is that a binomial distribution of scores, that is, a skewed distribution, would result for each person on repeated measurements. An individual who had a very high true score for the domain would have a high probability of correctly answering items drawn randomly from the domain. Conversely, the person with a low true score would have a low probability of correctly answering items drawn at random from the domain. Individuals with high and low true scores would be more likely to have observed scores that regress toward the average score for the domain. A person with a high true score would have a distribution of observed scores skewed toward the left, while a person with a low true score would have a distribution of observed scores skewed toward the right. An individual with an average true score would be expected to have a symmetrical distribution of observed scores approximating the normal distribution. Distributions for individuals with low, average, and high true scores are illustrated in Figure 3-16.

The individual with an average true score would be expected to have a standard deviation for observed scores that would be larger than for those with high or low true scores. There would be less variation in the observed scores of persons with extremely high and extremely low true scores, since variation in scores increases as the true score approaches the average score.

This model is more true to life, since it depicts the standard error of measurement in relation to the point on the continuum at which true scores are located. In reality the standard error of measurement is not the same at all points on the continuum of true scores nor are errors normally distributed for true scores above or below the average. The amount of skewness for persons at either end of the true score continuum would be inversely related to the number of test items. However, when measures have less than 20 items, the skewness might be unnoticeable. Nunnally (1978) notes that

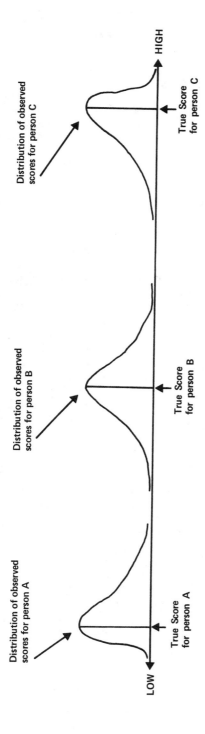

FIGURE 3-16. True scores and binomial distributions of observed scores for low (Person A), average (Person B), and high (Person C) scores.

application of the binomial model would in most instances result in negligible modifications of statistics deduced from classical measurement theory.

SOURCES OF VARIANCE IN SCORES

There are many sources of variation in scores obtained from measurement. In previous sections of this chapter, a discussion of random and systematic sources of error emphasized how error variance can affect the reliability and validity of measures. The goal of measurement is to obtain measurements in a manner such that variance that results from error is kept at a minimum. It is desirable that variance reflected in scores be due to actual differences in score values.

TRUE SCORE VARIANCE

For the most part, variance within a set of scores for a group of individuals occurs because different persons manifest different amounts of the attribute of interest. It should be kept in mind that the importance of the reliability coefficient for a measure is that it reflects the proportion of the variance in scores that is due to true differences within the particular population of individuals on the variable being evaluated. Therefore, it is desirable that measures be constructed and used so that they will be sensitive to real variations in true scores of individuals. The size of variation in true scores between persons is primarily determined by two factors: (1) the frequency of correct or appropriate responses to items, and (2) the correlations between the individual items. A measure will be most sensitive to real differences between persons when variance of the individual items is greatest—that is, when the probability of a correct response is 0.5 for any item chosen at random from the domain. When test items are either too easy or very difficult, score variance between individuals will be small, because such items do not distinguish variations in the attribute of interest well. This also is true for measures such as opinionaires and attitude scales that have no correct answers. Each individual can be perceived as having a set probability of either agreeing or disagreeing with each statement. If statements are constructed in a manner such that true differences in opinions or attitudes are not elicited, then variations in scores will be small. True score variance also will be increased when the correlations between items in the domain are large and when the number of items in a measure is large.

It is desirable for measurements to have true score variance, particularly in the norm-referenced case. The magnitude of reliability coefficients depends upon the dispersion of true scores between individuals. Restriction of the range of variability is likely to lower the reliability of a measure in the manner noted earlier in the discussion of measures of correlation.

ERROR VARIANCE WITHIN A SET OF SCORES

Error variance within a set of scores obtained on a specific occasion occurs for many reasons. For any measure, error variance due to such factors as general ability to comprehend instructions, testwiseness, and shrewdness in guessing is likely to affect scores. This type of systematic error results from lasting characteristics of each individual and results in stable individual differences in scores. Other such sources of systematic error include familiarity of the subject with test format, the nature of items, and level of comprehension of words, formulas, and generalizations that must be applied to correctly respond to certain items. Temporary characteristics of the individual can result in random error. Fatigue, emotional strain, and condition of the testing environment could result in an inability to concentrate, inadvertent skipping of items, misreading of items, and fluctuations in memory. Differences in standards and approaches to scoring would reduce correlations between items and thereby reduce reliability estimates. Errors in scoring could be assessed within a test if scoring errors tended to reduce correlations among items.

VARIATION IN SCORES BETWEEN MEASUREMENTS

In some instances two randomly parallel tests are administered either simultaneously at the same testing period or at separate short time intervals, for example, two-week intervals. If the attribute of interest is such that there should not be noticeable variations for individuals tested, then the correlation between the two sets of scores should be nearly perfect. This may not be the case, however. Sets of scores on randomly parallel tests, also termed alternative forms, may not be highly correlated for four major reasons. First, randomly parallel tests may not be truly parallel. There may be actual differences in the content of the two tests. The domain-sampling model envisions that randomly parallel tests are composed of items randomly selected from the same content domain. Since this is not possible in reality, some tests which are developed as parallel measures of an attribute may not be really parallel. Some aspects of the content domain may receive more emphasis in one test than the other, or one test may be constructed in a manner such that the use of certain words or terminology is emphasized more than in the other measure. The correlation between scores on the two tests might be less because of these differences.

A second reason that variation may occur between measurements is because the conditions under which the tests were administered are markedly different and thereby influence the scores. Different environmental conditions such as a very hot room or noisy distractions may be present at one testing situation and not at the other. Temporary factors that can affect performance have already been discussed. If an entire group of persons were tested together on both occasions under markedly different conditions, then the effect could be that a number of persons in the group would have quite different observed scores on the two testing occasions. This would decrease the correlation between scores.

Differences in scoring from one occasion to another is a third factor that might lessen correlations of scores between measurements. The use of different criteria for scoring either by the same scorer or two or more different scorers might give somewhat different scores for the same person. This is particularly likely to happen when one scorer or rater is used on one occasion and a different scorer or rater is used on a subsequent occasion.

Finally, another factor that can cause variation in scores from one occasion to another is that the object or event actually changes with regard to the attribute being measured. For example, a group of diabetic patients who are tested at two-week intervals regarding their knowledge of self-care might actually have a change in knowledge which increased their scores on the subsequent testing. Another example is that an attitude scale used to determine the attitudes of student nurses toward the elderly might be given at three-week intervals. There could be a general increase or decrease in the scores on the measure if the group of students had experiences with elderly persons that changed their attitudes. In such cases, correlations between the two sets of scores would be lower than if no change in the attribute of interest had occurred.

THE RELIABILITY OF CHANGE SCORES

In some cases, it is desirable to determine the reliability of change scores, such as when one is considering a pretest and a post-test to determine whether there has been a change in the amount of a specific attribute of interest. In such an instance, the change score would be the post-test score of a subject minus his pretest score. To illustrate: a nurse wants to determine if the level of preoperative patient anxiety for a group of patients will decrease after a planned patient teaching program is given. Two parallel forms are used: one to measure patient anxiety prior to the teaching program, and one to measure patient anxiety after the patient teaching program is completed. The *raw change score* of each patient would be the difference score between his post-test and pretest scores. How will the nurse know if any changes that are exhibited are reliable?

One should keep in mind that errors of measurement previously discussed that could increase or decrease both sets of observed scores could have a significant impact on change scores, resulting in an interpretative problem. The obtained difference score equals true score difference plus error of measurement difference. Although the post-test score minus pretest score seems to be the best way to measure change, it is not the best estimator of true change. Errors of measurement that are present in the pretest and post-test measurement procedures can seriously affect the difference score. Two commonly discussed problems associated with the measurement of change are the reliability of the difference score and the systematic relationship between measures of change and initial status.

The reliability of difference scores depends upon the variance and reliability of the pretest, corresponding values for the post-test, and the correlation between the pretest and post-test. When the correlation between the pretest and post-test is high, the difference score reliability tends to be low. For example, for a pretest and post-test with a common variance and a common reliability of 0.8, the reliability of the difference score would be 0.60, 0.50, 0.33, and 0.00 when the pretest-post-test correlation was 0.5, 0.6, 0.7, and 0.8, respectively (Linn, 1979, p. 4). Hence, for the measurement of change, the lower the correlation between pretest and post-test scores, the higher the reliability of the measure of change. However, this fact causes a dilemma because the low correlation provides less confidence that one is measuring the same thing on each occasion.

The second problem that is frequently encountered with difference scores is that they generally are correlated with pretest scores. This is a disadvantage because a goal in the use of difference scores often is to compare the gains of individuals or groups that started with unequal pretest scores by removing initial differences. The problem arises from the fact that the sign of the correlation between the difference and pretest scores depends upon the variances of the pretest and post-test. Where the variances for the pretest and post-test are equal, a negative correlation is to be expected. In this case, persons or groups with low pretest scores will tend to have larger gains than those with high pretest scores, and the initially lower scoring group has a built-in advantage. On the other hand, if the post-test variance is enough larger than the variance for the pretest, the correlation between the difference score and the pretest will be positive rather than negative. Where the correlation is positive, there is a built-in advantage to the group scoring higher on the pretest when comparisons are made in terms of simple difference scores (Linn, 1979, p. 5). Given the problems associated with using difference scores for the measurement of change, several alternatives have been offered: (a) residualized change scores; (b) estimated true change scores; and (c) standardized change scores.

Residualized change scores have come into use because of the desire to obtain gain scores that are uncorrelated with initial status or pretest scores. However, they are not true measures of change (Cronback and Furby, 1970). They are measures of whether a person's post-test score is larger or smaller than the predicted value for that person. *Residualized change scores* are based on the assumptions of classical test theory regarding true score and error score components of observed scores and involve using the linear regression of the post-test on the pretest in order to determine predicted values. Major limitations to using residualized change scores are that they can be used only with measures taken at two points in time, and they are not really growth measures or change scores.

Estimated true change scores are corrected measures of change. Cronbach and Furby (1970) as well as several other authors have described procedures for estimating true change. They require estimates of reliability for the pretest and post-test for the sample involved. This is viewed as a major drawback of this approach, because good reliability estimates for the sample often are not available (Linn, 1979).

The use of standardized change scores has been suggested as an alternative to raw difference scores by Kenny (1975). *Standardized change scores* simply are difference scores that have been standardized. This means that difference scores have been converted such that score distributions have means of zero and unit variances. Hence, standardized change scores will have a negative correlation with initial status or pretest scores, because they are based on pretest and post-test scores with variances that have been set equal.

Further information regarding the alternatives to using raw change scores can be found in Cronbach and Furby (1970) and Kenny (1975). Specific alternatives to the measurement of change have advantages and disadvantages. Selection of an alternative approach should depend upon the nature of the study and the purposes for which change is to be measured.

Since change scores are fraught with many problems, we discourage their use and encourage the selection of alternative approaches to measurement whenever possible.

SUMMARY

This chapter presented the basic principles of statistics and measurement theory. Measurement is a process that involves employing rules to assign numbers to phenomena. The rules for assigning numbers to phenomena have been categorized hierarchically as either nominal, ordinal, interval, or ratio. The numbers that result from measurement are referred to as scores. The use of statistical procedures facilitates a better understanding of groups of numbers by providing numerical summaries of scores or data.

A distribution of scores may be described by its shape, measures of central tendency, and dispersion. A distribution's shape may be symmetrical or asymmetrical. The extent to which a distribution departs from symmetry is referred to as its degree of skewness. The peakedness of a distribution is referred to as kurtosis. The mode, median, and mean are three statistical indices of the central tendency of a distribution of scores. The dispersion or amount of spread of a distribution is indicated by its range, variance, and standard deviation. The range is the distance from the lowest to the highest score in a distribution. The variance and standard deviation represent the amount of scatter among the scores within a distribution. The Pearson Product-Moment Correlation Coefficient (r_{xy}) is a statistic often used to summarize the relationship between scores within two separate distributions.

Whenever a measurement is obtained, error is introduced into the results to some degree. The two types of error of measurements are random error and systematic error. Random error results from chance factors that affect measurements and systematic error arises from factors within the measuring tool, measurement process, or subject. Random error primarily affects the reliability of measurements, while systematic error primarily influences the validity of measurements.

Classical measurement theory is a model for assessing random measurement error. It purports that every observed score consists of a true score, which is the precise amount of an attribute possessed by an object, and an error score, which reflects the influence of random error. The model of parallel measures and the domain-sampling model are two approaches to reliability based on classical measurement theory. The model of parallel measures purports to determine reliability by correlating parallel measurements. The domain-sampling model provides for an estimate of reliability via an average of item correlations between measures.

The binomial model is an alternative approach to measurement which assumes that the error component of an observed score is binominally distributed about the true score. This model purports that a skewed distribution would result for persons on repeated measurements. The degree of skewness of the distribution would depend on the persons's probability of correctly answering items in a content domain.

Variation in scores between measurements is due to actual changes in the true score or to variation in the amount of error introduced into measurements. It is problematic to use post-test minus pretest difference scores to assess change in true scores, because there is a systematic relationship between measures of change and the initial status, and the reliability of difference scores may be compromised by psychometric properties of the pretest and post-test. Alternative approaches to the measurement of change include residualized change scores, estimated true change scores, and standardized change scores.

REFERENCES

AGRESTI, A AND AGRESTI, BF: Statistical Methods for the Social Sciences. Dellen Publishing Company, San Francisco, 1979.

CARMINES, EG AND ZELLER, RA: Reliability and Validity Assessment. Sage Publications, Beverly Hills, CA, 1979.

CAMPBELL, NR, et al: "Final report." Advancement of Science 2:331–349, 1940.

CRONBACH, LJ AND FURBY, L: "How we should measure "change"—Or should we?" Psychological Bulletin 74:68–80, 1970.

GLASS, GV AND STANLEY, JC: Statistical Methods in Education and Psychology. Prentice Hall, Englewood Cliffs, NJ, 1970.

GUILFORD, JP: Fundamental Statistics in Psychology and Education, ed. 4. McGraw-Hill, NY, 1965.

KENNY, DA: "A quasi-experimental approach to assessing treatment effects in the nonequivalent control design." Psychological Bulletin 82:345–362, 1975.

KIRK, RE: Experimental Design: Procedures for the Behavioral Sciences. Brooks Cole, Monterey, CA, 1968.

LINN, RL: "Measurement of change." In Educational Evaluation Methodology: The State of the Art. Second Annual Johns Hopkins University National Symposium on Educational Research, Baltimore, 1979.

MARTUZA, VR: Applying Norm-Referenced and Criterion-Referenced Measurement in Education. Allyn and Bacon, Boston, 1977.

NUNNALLY, JC: Psychometric Theory, ed. 2. McGraw-Hill, New York, 1978.

STANLEY, JC: "Reliability." In THORNDIKE, RL (ed.): Educational Measurement, ed. 2. American Council on Education, Washington, DC, 1971.

STEVENS, SS: "On the theory of scales of measurement." Science 103:677–680, 1946.

WALTZ, CF AND BAUSELL, RB: Nursing Research: Design, Statistics, and Computer Analysis. F.A. Davis Company, Philadelphia, 1981.

4

NORM-REFERENCED MEASUREMENT

In Chapter 1, it was noted that norm-referenced measures are employed when the interest is in evaluating a subject's performance relative to the performance of other subjects in some well-defined comparison group. This chapter focuses on the design and interpretation of norm-referenced measures in nursing.

DESIGNING NORM-REFERENCED MEASURES

Essential steps in the design of a norm-referenced measure are: (1) selection of a conceptual model for delineating the nursing aspects of the measurement process; (2) explication of objectives for the measure; (3) development of a blueprint; and (4) construction of the measure, including administration procedures, an item set, and scoring rules and procedures. Since selection of a nursing conceptual model is addressed in Chapters 1 and 2 and the Appendix, the focus here will be on steps 2 through 4.

EXPLICATING OBJECTIVES

The first step in the design of any measure is to clarify the purposes for the measurement. When a conceptual model serves as the basis for the tool's development, this step is more easily undertaken than when one is not. For example, suppose one is interested in measuring job satisfaction of nurse educators and one conceptualizes job satisfaction as the subjective response of individuals to their job—that is, to a position of employment for which remuneration is received. Furthermore, assume that: (1) job satisfaction generally encompasses a continuum of affective response, which ranges from feelings of extreme contentment and gratification to feelings of extreme discontent; thus, the concept does not necessarily designate a positive state, but a continuum of feeling states; and (2) given the complexity and multi-dimensionality of the work situation, the individual's level of satisfaction with certain aspects or characteristics of the job (e.g., the level of responsibility or the nature of the tasks performed) may differ from the individual's level of satisfaction with other characteristics (e.g., working conditions, salary).

On the basis of this conceptual definition of job satisfaction the investigator is directed to operationalize job satisfaction in the following manner:

(1) use an affective-subjective type of measure, most appropriately self-report;

(2) include in the measure multiple items reflecting salient job characteristics or conditions; and

(3) provide for respondents to indicate various levels of satisfaction/dissatisfaction with each of the items or job conditions on the measure.

Hence, the objective for the measure becomes: Given a set of job conditions characteristic of academia in nursing, subjects will rate their level of satisfaction/dissatisfaction with each condition.

It should be apparent that this objective derives from and is consistent with the conceptual definition of job satisfaction; defines the relevant domain of content to be assessed by the measure as specific and varied job conditions characteristic of academic settings in nursing; and specifies the type of behavior the subject will exhibit to demonstrate that the purpose for the measure has been met—that is, will indicate (rate) the level of satisfaction with each job condition. To meet this objective, the investigator looks to the conceptual framework as well as empirical findings from studies defining job satisfaction in a similar manner to identify and list a number of job conditions salient to the measurement of job satisfaction in nursing education. This preliminary list is then subjected to scrutiny by experts in nursing education who may add and/or delete conditions. Each of these conditions then becomes an item on the measure. Hence, each item included on the measure should be specific and relevant to the objective for the measure and should be linked to the conceptual definition, that is, items that do not relate directly to the objective for the measure are superfluous and if included will tend to decrease validity.

To assess the level of job satisfaction, the investigator employs a 4-point rating scale, ranging from very dissatisfied (1) to very satisfied (4). A portion of the resulting measure of job satisfaction is illustrated in Figure 4-1. It should be apparent from this example that objectives provide the link between theories and concepts and their measurement. Unless objectives for the measure are explicated prior to its construction, there is a high probability that the resulting tool or method will be irrelevant and invalid for the purpose intended. Not only is it important to explicate objectives, but it is also paramount that they be stated correctly. A poorly stated objective can be more troublesome than having no objective stated at all. For this reason, attention now turns to approaches for writing objectives that have gained favor with use.

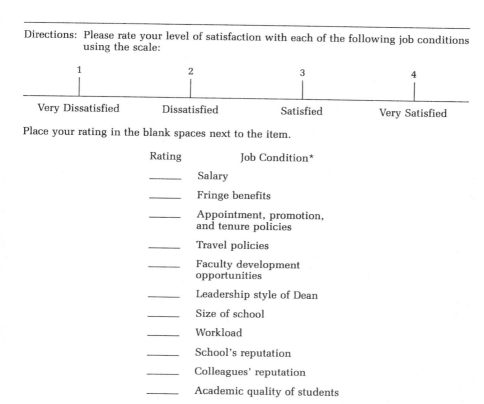

Directions: Please rate your level of satisfaction with each of the following job conditions using the scale:

1	2	3	4
Very Dissatisfied	Dissatisfied	Satisfied	Very Satisfied

Place your rating in the blank spaces next to the item.

Rating   Job Condition*

_____   Salary

_____   Fringe benefits

_____   Appointment, promotion, and tenure policies

_____   Travel policies

_____   Faculty development opportunities

_____   Leadership style of Dean

_____   Size of school

_____   Workload

_____   School's reputation

_____   Colleagues' reputation

_____   Academic quality of students

*Conditions included here are limited and intended only to exemplify a few of the many conditions relevant to job satisfaction in nursing education.

FIGURE 4-1. A sample measure of job satisfaction.

Behavioral objectives are usually stated by using one of two approaches. The first approach is best characterized by the work of Mager (1962). In this view an objective has essentially four components: (1) a description of the respondent; (2) a description of the behavior the respondent will exhibit to demonstrate accomplishment of the objective; (3) a description of the conditions under which the respondent will demonstrate accomplishment; and (4) a statement of the standard of performance expected to indicate accomplishment. This format for writing objectives is particularly useful when constructing measures of cognition, especially in a criterion-referenced framework, because it forces one to explicate clearly the standard of performance expected prior to the construction of items. Figure 4-2 illustrates Mager's approach to the formulation of an objective for measuring cognition in a nursing research course.

The second approach reflects the views of scholars like Tyler (1950) and Kibler (1970). Although similar to Mager's approach, in this case a behavioral objective is composed of only three components: (1) a description of the respondent; (2) delineation of the kind of behavior the respondent will

Objective: Given a novel research report, the nursing student will provide a critique of the contents of the report in terms of the 7 criteria outlined in class.

Component	Example
1. Description of respondent	Nursing student enrolled in the research course
2. Description of behavior to be exhibited if objective is accomplished	Provide a critique of the contents of the report
3. Description of conditions under which respondent will demonstrate accomplishment	Given a novel (i.e., one not familiar to the student) research report
4. Statement of standard of performance expected to indicate accomplishment	Provide critique in terms of the 7 criteria outlined in class

FIGURE 4-2. Formulation of an objective to measure cognition in a nursing research course using Mager's approach.

exhibit to demonstrate accomplishment of the objective; and (3) a statement of the kind of content to which behavior relates. This approach to objective explication is quite useful within a norm-referenced measurement context, because it results in an outline of content and list of behaviors that can then be readily used in blueprinting, which is discussed in the next section of this chapter. Figure 4-3 illustrates the same objective written according to the Tyler-Kibler scheme.

In Figure 4-3 reference is made to Bloom's taxonomy (1956). A taxonomy is a useful mechanism for defining the critical behavior to be assessed by an objective in such a manner that all who use the same taxonomy or classifying scheme will assess the same behavior in the same way, thus increasing the reliability and validity of measurement. Numerous taxonomies have been proposed for the cognitive, affective, and psychomotor domains. Attention here will focus briefly on those that have gained favor through empirical use: (1) Bloom's taxonomy of the cognitive domain; (2) Kratwohl's taxonomy (1964) for the affective domain; and (3) Fitts's scheme (1962, 1964) for the psychomotor domain.

Table 4-1 presents a simplified version of the taxonomy of the cognitive domain. In Bloom's framework, the mental operations are grouped into a small number of simple to complex hierarchically ordered categories: knowledge, comprehension, application, analysis, synthesis, and evaluation. Hence, each subsequent level of mental activity involves the mental operations required at the preceding levels. For example, to be able to analyze, the respondent must first be able to know, comprehend, and apply.

A simplified version of the taxonomy for the affective domain appears in Table 4-2. As with the cognitive taxonomy, levels are hierarchical in nature, and performance at higher levels allows one to assume that the respondent can perform at lower levels as well.

Taxonomies for assessing the psychomotor domain are far less developed than for the other two; however, the approach by Fitts, which is summarized in Table 4-3, shows some promise in this area and is included for

Objective: The nursing student provides a critique of the contents of research reports	
Component	**Example**
1. Description of respondent	Nursing student enrolled in the research course
2. Description of behavior to be exhibited if objective is accomplished	Provides a critique of the contents of the report (evaluation level of Bloom's Taxonomy)
3. Statement of the kind of content to which behavior relates	A content outline of guidelines for critiques that was presented in class with 7 criteria for doing critiques of research reports included

FIGURE 4-3. Formulation of an objective to measure cognition in a nursing research course using the Tyler-Kibler scheme.

this reason. Fitts (1962, 1964) identifies three phases of skill development: cognitive, fixation, and autonomous. Phases overlap to some extent—that is, they are not distinct units—and movement from one phase to another is a continuous process. As a subject proceeds from early to later phases, the performance of the skill becomes progressively more automatic and more accurate and demands less concerted effort on the part of the subject, allowing attention to be given to other activities concurrently.

From the tables it should be apparent that the use of taxonomies in explicating and measuring objectives provides several advantages. A critical aspect of any behavioral objective is the word selected to indicate expected behavior. A behavioral term by definition is one that is observable and measurable (i.e., behavior refers to any action on the part of an individual that can be seen, felt, or heard by another person). Cognitive and affective objectives, although they are concerned with thinking and feeling, which themselves are not directly observable, are inferred from psychomotor or behavioral acts. In reality, the same behavioral term can be seen, felt, or heard differently by different people. Similarly, since it is impossible to measure every action inherent in a given behavior, different people frequently define the critical behavior to be observed, using a given objective, quite differently. When taxonomies are employed, action verbs and critical behaviors to be observed are specified, hence, decreasing this possibility and increasing the probability that the resulting measure will be reliable and valid.

A measurement must match the level of respondent performance stated in the behavioral objective; that is, a performance verb at the application level of the cognitive taxonomy must be assessed by a cognitive item requiring the same level of performance. Any discrepancy between the stated objective and the performance required by the instrument or measurement device will result in decreased reliability and validity of the measurement process. For example, if the objective for the measurement is to ascertain the ability of practicing nurses to apply gerontological content in their work with aging clients (application level of Bloom's) and if the measure constructed to assess the objective simply requires them to state in their own words some principles important to the care of the gerontological pa-

TABLE 4-1 A Simplified version of the taxonomy of the cognitive domain*

Mental Operation		Examples		Comments
Level	**Action Verbs**	**Objective**	**Measurement**	
Knowledge: Measures the subject's ability to recall or recognize information in essentially the same form as it was presented. The essential learner behavior is remembering.	Action verbs at the knowledge level usually include: Cite Read Classify Recall Complete Recite Correct Recognize Identify Show Label State List Tell Mark Write Name	The subjects will list the steps necessary for inserting a Foley catheter.	PLC†: The inservice instructor has outlined the procedure for inserting a Foley catheter. Question: List the steps necessary for inserting a Foley catheter.	This is the lowest level of mental activity. The PLC reflects the information to be acquired by the subjects that is part of the objective stated during the program's development.
Comprehension: Measures understanding at the most rudimentary level, i.e., the subject's ability to use previously acquired information to solve a problem. 1. Translation: Ability to paraphrase, present in a different language, or recognize paraphrases or symbolic changes.	Action verbs at the comprehension level usually include: Conclude Convey meaning of Decode Describe in own words Explain Extrapolate Give reasons Illustrate Interpret Reformulate Restate Rewrite Summarize Tell why Translate	The subjects will explain in their own words how a health history is elicited from a patient.	PLC: The instructor has explained how a health history is elicited from a patient. Question: The instructor assigns subjects to play roles of nurse and patient. In a sociodrama the subjects are to act out these roles as explained to them by the instructor.	At this level, the subject must remember the information and use it to solve a novel problem. A key feature at this level is that the item or the context in which it is asked is structured in such a way that the respondent is made aware of the information required to solve the problem. Items are designed to determine whether the learner can solve a novel problem if the information to be used is specified.

2. Interpretation: Measures the subject's ability to make an inference based on the information in a communication to explain what is meant by the communication or to summarize the information in the communication.	Given a case history and a series of x-ray pictures on a patient, the learners will make conclusions about the disease process on the basis of the data.	PLC: The learners have been taught to read x-ray pictures. The instructor then presents the learner with a case history and a series of x-ray pictures on the patient. Question: (True or False) After the first 4 weeks of chemotherapy, the patient's disease process was beginning to clear.	In Bloom's taxonomy there is a third type of comprehension, which is not dealt with in this simplified version because it is so similar to translation and interpretation. In this simplified version, extrapolation is subsumed under interpretation.
Application: Requires the subjects to use previously acquired information in solving a novel problem. Neither the question nor the context in which it is asked helps the respondents decide what previously acquired information must be used to solve the problem. Questions aim at determining whether subjects are able to select the appropriate knowledge as well as use it correctly in solving a new problem.	Action verbs at the application level include: Administer Adopt a plan Apply Carry out Compute Demonstrate Employ Make use of Perform Plot Put in action Put to use Using the *Physicians' Desk Reference* (PDR), the subjects will find the page on which each of the following is described: insulin, penicillin, sulfa	PLC: In pharmacology class the instructor has taught the learners how to use the index of the PDR. Later, on the ward, the instructor asks: Can you find information about the side effects of insulin?	Note that if this question were a comprehension item, the instructor would have told the learners to use the index of the PDR. Application items like comprehension items require the learners to use previously acquired information to solve a novel problem. Unlike the comprehension item, an application item does not identify for the learners the previously acquired information to be used in solving the problem. Thus, questions at the application level are aimed at determining if the respondents are able to select as well as use knowledge correctly in solving a new problem.

TABLE 4-1 Continued

Mental Operation		Examples		Comments
Level	Action Verbs	Objective	Measurement	
Analysis: May require the subjects to (1) identify a logical error in a communication (e.g., a contradiction, an error in deduction, an erroneous causal inference) or (2) identify, classify, and/or recognize the relationships among the elements (i.e., facts, assumptions, hypotheses, conclusions, ideas, etc.) in a communication. Items at this level usually assume specific training in a logical process to be used.	Action verbs at the analysis level include: Analyze Arrange in order Combine Compare Contrast Criticize Deduce Designate Detect Determine Distinguish Formulate	After watching a film on the effects of pollution on our environment, the respondents will list at least 15 statements made by people in the film about the effects of pollution on the environment. The respondents will underline each statement that is based on fact; they will not mark statements that are opinions.	PLC: The subjects are instructed to watch a 15-minute film on the effects of pollution on our environment. Question: List all of the statements made by people in the film about the effects of pollution on the environment. Underline each statement that is based on fact. Do not mark statements that are opinions.	
Synthesis: Requires the respondent to produce or create: (1) a unique verbal or written communication, or (2) a plan or procedure for accomplishing a particular task.	Action verbs at the synthesis level include: Construct Propose Develop Reorganize Form Restructure Compose Devise Formulate hypotheses Design Fabricate Integrate	The learner will design an experiment using a valid experimental design that will demonstrate the effect of oral intake on the accuracy of oral temperature readings.	PLC: The learners have read that oral intake prior to an oral temperature reading affects the accuracy of the measurement. Question: How can we experimentally demonstrate the effect of oral intake on the accuracy of oral temperature readings?	

Evaluation: Requires the subjects to judge the value of ideas, people, products, methods, etc., for a specific purpose and state valid reasons for their judgment (i.e., the learners must state the criteria upon which the judgment is based).	Action verbs at the evaluation level include: Appraise, Ascertain value, Assay, Assess, Diagnose, Evaluate, Fix value of, Judge, List in order of importance, Rank in order of importance	After observing a demonstration of two contrasting ways of handwashing, the learners will select the most acceptable one for dermatology clinic patients and state reasons for the selection.	PLC: The instructor demonstrates two contrasting ways of handwashing. Question: Which do you think is the most acceptable for handwashing among dermatology patients? Tell why you chose the one you did.

*Portions of the material in this table are adapted from Staropoli and Waltz, *Developing and Evaluating Educational Programs for Health Care Providers.* F.A. Davis, Philadelphia, 1978, with permission.
†PLC refers to the prior learning condition.

TABLE 4-2 A simplified version of the taxonomy of the affective domain

Affective Levels		Examples		Comments
Level	Action Verbs	Objective	Measurement	
Receiving (Attending): Measures the respondent's awareness and/or willingness to receive specified stimuli. Indicates the respondent is capable of directing attention toward specified materials or behavior.	Action verbs at the receiving level include: Accept Limit Attempt Listen Comply List Define Observe Identify Recognize Refrain Reject	The respondent will listen carefully and respectfully to all opinions rendered by patients concerning abortion.	Over time the respondent consistently demonstrates behavior indicating he is listening (eye contact, nondirective responses, etc.) respectfully to patient opinions re: abortion.	
Responding: Measures the respondent's tendency to respond in a favorable manner to specified stimuli. Response behavior indicates that the respondent has become adequately involved or committed to a specified stimulus. If the respondent consents, seeks, and/or enjoys working with a specified activity, he/she is responding favorably.	Action verbs at the responding level include: Ask Inquire Challenge Offer Choose Query Cite Question Consult Read Delay Repeat Doubt Select Hesitate Try	The respondent will willingly comply with agency suggestions concerning courtesy toward the client's family.	The respondent seeks out agency suggestions concerning courtesy toward clients' families and performs consistently within agency expectations.	

Description	Action Verbs	Objective	Behavioral Example
Valuing: Measures reflect that the respondent displays behaviors with acceptable consistency under appropriate circumstances to indicate the adoption of a certain value or ideal. In demonstrating the value behavior, the respondent can select from among differing values on specified topics and may demonstrate a high degree of commitment, conviction, or loyalty to the accepted value.	Action verbs at the valuing level include: Consider Display Examine Express Insist Join Participate Persist Practice Pursue Qualify Seek Specify Support Test Undertake Volunteer Weigh	The learner will volunteer for a classroom debate and enthusiastically support a pro or con position concerning euthanasia.	The learner volunteers for a classroom debate and enthusiastically supports the position he or she has chosen to debate.
Organization: Measures reflect the learner is able to classify a value concept by (1) determining, analyzing, comparing its characteristics and (2) placing all previously classified values into a harmonious and ordered relationship, thus building a personal value system.	Action verbs at the organization level include: Adapt Analyze Compare Contrast Criticize Deduce Demonstrate Order Propose Designate Design Determine Diagnose Gather Identify Investigate Organize	The respondent will design a plan of physical exercise to be incorporated into his weekly schedule of activities.	The respondent designs and incorporates the physical exercise plan into his weekly schedule.
Characterization by a Value or Value Complex: Measures indicate the respondent is able to respond to the complex world and environment about him in a consistent, predictable, and comprehensible manner.	Action verbs at the characterization level include: Construct Design Develop Evaluate Formulate Plan Revise Synthesize	The respondent will solve problems in terms of patient consequences rather than in terms of rigid principles or emotional feelings.	The respondent consistently solves problems in terms of patient consequences rather than rigid principles or emotional feelings.

TABLE 4-3 Fitts's phases of complex skill development

Phase of Development	Examples		Comments
	Objective	Measurement	
1. Cognitive: Measures indicate that the subject tends to intellectualize the skill and makes frequent errors in performing it.	The subject does a physical assessment of a newly diagnosed diabetic patient.	Observation of subject's performance reflects a preoccupation with the examination, and attention to proceeding according to the outline in the procedure manual even when deviation in the sequence of events appears appropriate. Interpersonal interaction with the patient is limited and the subject makes frequent errors and eye contact with the observer each time an action is taken.	At this phase subjects dwell on the procedure and plans that guide the execution of the skill.
2. Fixation: Measures indicate a tendency to practice correct behavior patterns; errors are fewer than during phase 1 and decrease with practice.	The subject does a physical assessment of a newly diagnosed diabetic patient.	Observation of subject's performance reflects less preoccupation with the skills and the observer, fewer errors are noted, and a pattern for proceeding with the examination has emerged.	At this phase practice of the skill is important, and errors decrease with practice.
3. Autonomous: Measures indicate increasing speed of performance, errors occur infrequently, individual is able to resist stress and interference from outside activities and is able to perform other activities concurrently.	The subject does a physical assessment of a newly diagnosed diabetic patient.	Observation of subject's performance reflects few errors, a pattern of performance that is less rigid than during the preceding stages, interpersonal communication between patient and provider is high and elements of the health history are considered and elicited in conjunction with the physical	At this phase, the skill becomes automatic and attention focuses on other aspects of the patient.

tient (comprehension level of the taxonomy), then the outcomes of the measurement are not valid, in that this tool does not measure what is intended. When taxonomies are employed, this type of discrepancy between the level of objective and level of performance measured is less apt to occur than when taxonomies are not employed.

BLUEPRINTING

Given a set of objectives reflecting the process or outcomes to be assessed by the measure and a content outline representative of the domain of interest, the next step is to develop a blueprint to establish the specific scope and emphasis of the measure. Table 4-4 illustrates a blueprint for an examination in nursing research. The five major content areas to be assessed appear as column headings across the top of the table; critical behaviors to be measured are listed on the left hand side of the table as row headings. Each intersection or cell thus represents a particular content-objective pairing,

TABLE 4-4 Blueprint for an examination in nursing research

Content \ Objectives	I Hypothesis Testing	II Univariate Statistics	III Bivariate Statistics	IV Reliability and Validity of Measures	V Overview Multivariate Statistics	Total
Generates testable hypotheses on the basis of nursing theory and practice	10	4	4	5	2	25
Produces a plan or procedure for testing a research hypothesis using univariate and bivariate statistics	5	20	20	5	—	50
Selects and uses appropriate statistical procedures for determining instrument reliability and validity	2	5	5	3	—	15
Comprehends multivariate statistics	—	—	—	—	10	10
Total	17	29	29	13	12	100

and values in each cell reflect the actual number of each type of item to be included on the measure. Hence, from the table it can be seen that four items will be constructed to assess the content-objective pairing—univariate statistics/generates testable hypothesis—on the basis of nursing theory and practice. The scope of the measure is defined by the cells, which are reflective of the domain of items to be measured, and the emphasis of the measure and/or relative importance of each content-behavior pairing is ascertained by examining the numbers in the cells. From the blueprint, one can readily tell about what topics questions will be asked, the types of critical behaviors subjects will be required to demonstrate, and what is relatively important and unimportant to the constructor. Tables 4-5 and 4-6 present additional examples of blueprints that vary slightly in format. In Table 4-5, the blueprint for an examination in nursing research is defined by topic area and objectives, but in this case, rather than listing the critical behaviors to be assessed, the performance expectations are specified using the levels of Bloom's taxonomy. In Table 4-6, objectives are defined in terms of the steps of the nursing process, content is defined by components of the nursing conceptual model used, and numerals in the cells represent percentages of each type of item to be included rather than actual number of items.

Given the blueprint, the number (or percentage) of items prescribed in each cell would be constructed. Content validity (discussed in more detail in Chapter 5) could then be assessed by presenting content experts with the blueprint and the test and having them judge the adequacy of the measure as reflected in the blueprint—that is, whether or not the domain is adequately represented—to ascertain that the most appropriate elements are

TABLE 4-5 Blueprint for an examination in nursing research

Objectives / Content	Knowledge	Comprehension	Application	Analysis	Synthesis	Total
I Hypothesis Testing	—	—	2	—	15	17
II Univariate Statistics	—	—	5	—	24	29
III Bivariate Statistics	—	—	5	—	24	29
IV Reliability and Validity of Measures	—	—	3	—	10	13
V Multivariate Statistics	—	10		—	2	12
Total	—	10	15	—	75	100

TABLE 4-6 Blueprint for a measure of clinical performance

Objectives (Nursing Practices) / Content (King's* Model)	I Assessment	II Planning	III Implementation	IV Evaluation	Total
(1) Nurse Variables a. perception b. goals c. values d. needs e. expectations	5%	5%	5%	5%	20%
(2) Patient Variables a. perception b. goals c. values d. needs e. expectations f. abilities	10%	10%	30%	20%	60%
(3) Situational Variables a. structure b. goals c. groups d. functions e. physical resources f. economic resources g. climate	10%	5%	2%	2%	20%
TOTAL					100%

*King, I. "A Conceptual Frame of Reference for Nursing." *Nursing Research,* 1968, 17, 27–31.

being assessed; the fairness of the measure, that is, it does not give unfair advantage to some subjects over others; and the fit of the method to the blueprint from which it was derived.

CONSTRUCTING THE MEASURE

The type of measure to be employed is a function of the conceptual model and subsequent operational definition of key variables to be measured. If, for example, one conceptualizes job satisfaction as a perceptual phenomenon, the measurement will require use of an affective or typical performance instrument. If, on the other hand, job satisfaction is conceptually defined as a cognitive phenomenon dependent upon one's understanding and comprehension of factors in the work setting, a maximum performance or cognitive measure is appropriate. The essential characteristics of the types of measures are presented in Chapter 1 and will not be given further attention here.

Regardless of type, every measure is composed of three components: (1) directions for administration; (2) a set of items; and (3) directions for obtaining and interpreting scores.

ADMINISTRATION. Clemans (1971) presents a comprehensive set of considerations to be made in preparing instructions for the administration of a measure. More specifically, he advocates the inclusion of the following information:

(1) A description of who should administer the measure
   — a statement of eligibility
   — a list of essential characteristics
   — a list of duties
(2) Directions for those who administer the measure
   — a statement of the purposes for the measure
   — amount of time needed for administration
   — a statement reflecting the importance of adhering to directions
   — specifications for the physical environment
   — a description of how material will be received and stored
   — specifications for maintaining security
   — provisions for supplementary materials needed
   — recommendations for how to respond to subjects' questions
   — instructions for handling defective materials
   — procedures to follow when distributing the measure
   — a schedule for administration
   — directions for how to collect completed measures
   — specifications for the preparation of special reports (e.g., irregularity reports)
   — instructions for the delivery and/or preparation of completed measures for scoring
   — directions for how to return or dispose of materials
(3) Directions for respondents
   — a statement regarding information to be given to subjects prior to the data collection session (e.g., materials to be brought along and procedures for how, when, and where data will be collected)
   — instructions regarding how to complete the measure, including a request for cooperation, directions to be followed in completing each item type, and directions for when and how to record answers
(4) Directions for users of results
   — suggestions for how to use results
   — instructions for how to disseminate results (p. 196).

The importance of providing this information as an essential component of any measure cannot be overemphasized. Errors in administration are an important source of measurement error, and their probability of occurrence is greatly increased when directions for administration are not communicated clearly and explicitly in writing. Those readers who desire further specifics on the topic of administration procedures will find Clemans's work extremely useful.

ITEMS. Within the context of a given type of measure, there are a variety of specific item formats available, each with its own unique advantages and disadvantages in light of the specific purposes for and characteristics of the setting in which measurement is to occur. Most importantly, an item should be selected because it elicits the intended outcome, that is, the behavior specified by the objective(s). For example, if the objective of a measurement is to assess clinical performance, the item format should elicit performance by respondents in the clinical area. A written multiple-choice test or attitude survey would not be likely to elicit clinical performance on the part of subjects and hence would not be an appropriate item format for this measurement objective. Similarly, if a cognitive measure derived from behavioral objectives at the synthesis level of Bloom's taxonomy was composed of a set of true-false items, the behavior specified by the objective and the outcome elicited would be incongruent; that is, at the synthesis level respondents are required to construct or create something new, while true-false items only require them to select from one of two options on the basis of recall or comprehension.

Conditions surrounding the measurement will also establish parameters for what is an appropriate and useful item format. For example, if a measure is to be administered to diabetics with impaired vision, item formats requiring the reading of lengthy passages would be impractical. Similarly, measures to be administered to patients in acute care settings should be for the most part short and easily administered and understood, to avoid fatigue on the part of respondents and/or to be economical of time so as not to conflict with ongoing care activities. The important point is that the personal characteristics of the respondents, such as ability to read, ability to perform physical skills, computational skills, and communications skills, must be considered, and an item format must be selected that enhances their ability to respond rather than one that hinders some or all of the subjects.

Other factors in the measurement setting are also important in selecting the format. If an instrument is to be administered by individuals without training or experience in measurement or if it is to be employed by a variety of different people, the format should be selected with an eye to easy administration. For example, an instrument employing only one item format would be likely to require less time and less complex directions with less probability of being misinterpreted than one employing a number of different item formats. If tables or other illustrations are to be used on the tool, resources should be available for preparing them correctly and to scale; that is, incorrectly or inadequately prepared illustrative materials will increase measurement error and reduce reliability and validity as well as serve to decrease the subjects' motivation to respond. If space is limited or reproduction of the tool is apt to be problematic, items requiring lengthy explanations or repetitions of rating scales or other content on each page of the tool are impractical. If scoring is to be undertaken by a few individuals without the advantage of computers, an item format that is automatic and requires little or no judgment on the part of the scorer is indicated, for example, multiple choice or short answers. When computer scoring is employed, attention should be paid to requirements imposed by available computer programs as well as by scan sheets and the like. For example, if the computer scoring sheet provides for only four response options, an item format requiring four or fewer options is required.

There are as many different sets of conditions to be considered as there are varied measurement settings, and for this reason, only a few of the more frequently overlooked have been included here. In all cases, it is essential that careful analysis of the measurement situation be made and an item format be selected that capitalizes on the factors inherent in a given situation.

All items can be thought of on a continuum ranging from objective to subjective. Objective items—those allowing little or no latitude in response and hence, requiring no judgment in scoring—are often referred to as *selection-type items*. Examples of selection-type item formats are true-false, matching, multiple choice, and scaled response. These items are so named because they require the subjects to choose their responses from a set of options presented to them. Table 4-7 illustrates some of the more common varieties of selection-type items. The multiple choice format is one of the most objective available and for this reason is employed widely, especially for cognitive tools. The multiple choice items presented in Table 4-7 exemplify the desirable characteristics of multiple choice items. Perhaps because such items are so extensively used, they also tend to be extensively abused, and it is for this reason that some of the most frequently encountered pitfalls in constructing multiple-choice items are highlighted in Table 4-8.

From Table 4-8 it becomes apparent that if pitfalls are to be avoided, certain considerations must be made when a multiple choice format is employed.

1. Items should be expressed as clearly as possible, and whenever possible, words with precise meanings chosen.

2. Complex or awkward word arrangements or nonfunctional words should be avoided. Nonfunctional words are those that do not contribute to the basis for choosing a given response.

3. All qualifiers needed to provide a reasonable basis for responding should be included, that is, to whom and for what purpose.

4. Unessential specificity in the item stem or response should be avoided.

5. The level of difficulty of the item needs to be adapted to the level of participants and should be in concert with the purpose of the measurement.

6. Irrelevant clues to the correct response should be avoided. Irrelevant clues include pat verbal associations, grammatical constructions, the correct response being consistently stated more precisely and at greater length than the distractors, and systematic formal differences between the answer and distractors (i.e., common elements in the stem and response, including interrelated items in the statement or response of one question that give a clue to another question).

7. The content of questions should be exposed to expert editorial scrutiny prior to administration of the measure, even for piloting purposes.

8. Specific determiners (all, none, certainly, never, always) and stereotyped phraseology should be avoided.

Subjective items allow more latitude on the part of respondents in constructing their answer and therefore require more judgment to be executed on the part of the scorers. *Supply-type items*—so named because they require the subject to respond by supplying words, statements, numbers, or symbols—best characterize subjective items. The more frequently encountered supply-type item formats are exemplified in Table 4-9.

When a norm-referenced measure is employed, one designs items that are likely to make fine distinctions between respondents with differing levels of the attribute being measured, so that the distribution of responses to the measure will resemble a normal curve with a few high and low scores and with most scores falling in the middle range. Hence, one wants to avoid items that are too easy or too difficult for most respondents.

The difficulty of an item is defined as the percentage of respondents answering that item correctly or appropriately. In other words, if a cognitive test item is answered correctly by 40 of 100 respondents, the item has a difficulty level of 40 percent or 0.40. Hence, difficulty may vary from 0, in the case where no one responds correctly, to 1.00, in the case where all respondents respond correctly. When affective or performance measures are employed, the term appropriately or as expected is more meaningful than the term correct; that is, if subjects' responses are to be compared with a well-defined referent group, for example, first level baccalaureate nursing students, one might define what is appropriate on a performance measure on the basis of the behavior one would expect to see in the comparison or referent group. Similarly, if one is measuring attitudes toward gerontology patients, one might define appropriate on the basis of having responses that reflect those behaviors deemed acceptable or desirable by program planners.

Item difficulties for norm-referenced measures as a whole usually range from 0.30 to 0.70 (Martuza, 1977, p. 179). Several factors come into play in determining the optimum difficulty level for a given item, for example, the nature of the trait being measured, the item's correlation with other items on the instrument, and the specific objectives for the measure. Tinkelman (1971) suggested the following guidelines for determining item difficulty level.

1. In a situation in which the measure is designed to differentiate subjects' competence in a field, there is no standard of passing or failing, scores are interpreted as percentile norms or other measures of relative standing in a group, and intercorrelations among items are low. A 0.50 level of average item difficulty and a narrow range of difficulty among items are desirable in order to increase the variance of scores and increase reliability.

2. In situations in which guessing may come into play, the optimum item difficulty level should be such that the proportion of right or appropriate answers by the average subject would be 0.50 after correction for chance, that is, the average item difficulty level before correction for chance would be halfway between the chance probability of success and 1.00 (Lord, 1952). For example, for a 4-option multiple-choice test, the chance probability of success is 0.25. The difficulty level midway between 0.25 and 1.00 would be 0.65.

3. In general, the measure's reliability and the variance of scores increase as the variance of the item difficulties decreases. Thus, it is generally desirable that the items on a measure have a fairly narrow range of difficulty around the average difficulty level.

4. In the case of homogeneous measures (in which high intercorrelations exist between items) or in cases in which heterogeneous groups of subjects respond, a wider spread of difficulty is indicated.

TABLE 4-7 Selection-type item format

Format	Example	Comments
Alternate-Choice		Consists of a statement to be responded to by selecting from one of two options. Format provides for presentation of a large number of items in relatively short periods of time, therefore allowing broader, more representative sampling from the domain. There is a tendency, however, to select materials out of context, resulting in ambiguity and/or measurement of trivia. More in-depth discussion of these items may be found in Wesman, 1971; Ebel, 1975; Martuza, 1977; King, 1979; Gronlund, 1976.
1. True-False	Moderate excesses of digitalis cause premature heartbeats and vomiting. T or F I usually feel in control of my life. T or F	Consists of a declarative statement that is True or False.
2. Right-Wrong	The median is determined using the formula: $$M = \frac{EX}{N}$$ R or W The turnover among nurses in this hospital is largely the result of their feeling undervalued by administration. R or W.	Consists of a statement, question, equation, or the like that is identified as Right or Wrong by the respondent.
3. Yes-No	Is it more appropriate to serve shredded wheat than Wheatena for breakfast to a patient on a 250 mg sodium diet? Y or N Is it more desirable for a faculty member in this institution to spend time conducting research than consulting in that person's specialty area? Y or N	Consists of a direct question to be answered by a Yes or No.

4. Cluster

Pulse pressure is:

1. the difference between venous and systolic pressure.   T or F
2. the difference between arterial and venous pressure.   T or F
3. the difference between diastolic and systolic pressure.   T or F
4. pressure and expansion of the artery as blood flows toward the capillaries.   T or F
5. all of the above.   T or F

Consists of an incomplete statement with suggested completions, each of which is to be judged True or False.

5. Correction

Lightening usually occurs approximately *4 weeks* before delivery. _____

I am *satisfied* with the policies in this School of Nursing. _____

Combines selection and supply by presenting a statement and directing the respondent to correct false statements by substituting appropriate word(s).

Matching

Consists of a list of words or statements, a list of responses, and directions for matching responses to words or statements. Imperfect and association type are preferred, because they allow assessment of higher level behaviors. Because homogeneity is paramount in writing such items, the desire for homogeneity when heterogeneity is more appropriate may result in a shift in emphasis away from that desired. Additional information regarding this type of item is available in Wesman, 1971; King, 1979; Gronlund, 1976.

1. Perfect matching

On the line before each poison, place the number of the symptoms that usually characterize it.

Poisons

___ a. acids
___ b. rat poisons
___ c. cocaine
___ d. carbon monoxide

Symptoms

1. diarrhea, garlic breath
2. restlessness, rapid pulse
3. drowsiness, flushed cheeks
4. dyspnea, cyanosis

Each response matches one and only one word or statement.

TABLE 4-7 Continued

Format	Example	Comments
2. Imperfect matching	Match each term with its definition: ___ mode ___ median ___ mean 1. score that separates upper 50% of scores in the distribution from the lower 50% of the scores 2. score obtained by the largest number of respondents 3. largest number of respondents selecting a given score 4. sum of scores in a distribution divided by the total number of scores 5. the average	Some responses do not match any of the words or statements.
3. Statement classification	Judge the effects of the nurse's intervention on the patient's physical comfort in each of the numbered situations, using the following: a. Nursing intervention would tend to reduce the patient's physical comfort. b. Nursing intervention would tend to increase the patient's physical comfort. c. Nursing intervention would tend to have little or no effect on the patient's physical comfort. ___ 1. A primigravida in the first stages of labor is encouraged by the nurse to walk around the corridors. ___ 2. As labor progresses, the nurse remains with the primigravida, directing her attention to the fact that labor is progressing as expected. ___ 3. As labor progresses, the nurse teaches the patient various breathing and relaxing techniques. ___ 4. The nurse assesses and records the frequency, duration, and intensity of the contractions at regular intervals. ___ 5. The nurse encourages the patient to void at regular intervals.	Requires respondent to use higher level mental operations such as analysis, evaluation.

Multiple Choice*

		Components of a multiple choice item are: (1) stem—which is an introductory statement or question; and (2) responses or suggested answers. Readers are referred to Ebel, 1975; Wesman, 1971; Martuza, 1979; King, 1979; Staropoli and Waltz, 1978; and Gronlund, 1976, for further reading.
1. Correct answer	The basic service unit in the administration of public health is: a. the federal government. b. the state health department. c. the local health department. d. the public health nurse.	Items that require or permit a correct answer are those that eliminate the need for the respondent to make a judgment regarding the correctness of his response, i.e., matters of fact provide a suitable basis for such items.
2. Best answer	The primary responsibility of the instructor in health services is: a. to provide an emotional and social environment that adds a wholesome and healthful tone to the child's school day. b. to provide emergency or first aid care when a child becomes ill or injured in school. c. to provide up-to-date material about health as part of the curriculum. d. to screen for abnormalities and sickness and record the findings.	For many of the important questions that need to be asked it is impossible to state an absolutely correct answer within the reasonable limits of a multiple choice item. Even if space limitations were not a factor, two experts would probably not agree on the precise wording of the best answer. The use of this type of item, which has one best answer, permits the item writer to ask more significant questions and frees the writer from the responsibility of stating a correct answer so precisely that all authorities would agree that the particular wording used was the best possible wording.
3. Based on opinion	Advocates of the specialized approach to school nursing point out that: a. the health of the child cannot be separated from that of the family and community as a whole. b. specialized nursing care for the child cannot be separated from that for the family and community as a whole. c. a specialized program offers greater diversity and challenge to a well-prepared community health nurse. d. specialized nursing in the school allows the nurse to function without the disadvantages of a dual channel of administrative responsibility.	The responses to this question represent generalizations on the basis of literature written by the advocates of the specialized approach to school nursing. No authoritative sanction for one particular generalization is likely to be available, yet respondents familiar with this literature would probably agree on a best answer to this item.

TABLE 4-7 Continued

Format	Example	Comments
4. Novel question	The problem of air pollution is most likely to be reduced in the future by which of the following: a. urban population will wear air purifying equipment. b. cities will be enclosed to facilitate air purification. c. development of processes that will not produce air pollutants. d. use of nonpollutant fuels.	Requiring the respondent to predict what would happen under certain circumstances is a good way of measuring understanding of the principle involved.
5. Selective recall	The U.S. Public Health Service was reorganized in 1966 to: a. include the UNICEF program. b. include the Agency of International Development. c. combine the Voluntary Agency Services with the official ones. d. provide leadership in control of disease and environmental hazards and in development of manpower.	Unless this item had been made the specific object of instruction, it will function to assess the learner's ability to recall a variety of information about the Public Health Service, to select that which is relevant, and to base a generalization upon it.
6. Descriptive response	The child's socialization may be defined as: a. a behavioral process in which behavior conforms to the social practices of family and extra family groups. b. a process of developing an effective set of performances characteristic of self-control. c. the genetically determined or hereditary mechanisms that determine the individual's physical traits. d. all of the above.	Inexperienced item writers tend to seek items having very short responses. This can seriously limit the significance and scope of the achievements measured. In an item measuring the ability to define an important term, it is usually better to place the term to be defined in the item stem and to use definitions or identifications as the responses. The same principle should be applied to other items, i.e., one word responses need not be avoided altogether, but they should seldom be prominent in any measure.
7. Combined response	A school community safety program should be concerned with: a. teaching children how to avoid accidents. b. teaching adults and children to eliminate physical hazards that endanger them.	A difficulty with four-option multiple choice items is that of securing four good alternatives. One solution to this problem is to combine questions with two alternatives each to give the necessary four alternatives.

	c. eliminating physical hazards that endanger children and teaching them to avoid accidents. d. teaching children and adults to avoid accidents and eliminating physical hazards that endanger them.	
8. Combined question and explanation	When was the World Health Organization created and why? a. 1954, to prevent the spread of disease from one continent to another. b. 1948, to achieve international cooperation for better health throughout the world. c. 1945, to structure health privileges of all nations. d. 1948, to provide for a liberated population and aid in the relief from suffering.	This is a variation of the item type in which essentially two or more alternatives each are combined to give four alternatives.
9. Introductory sentence	When a group is working as a health team, overlapping of activities may occur. What is essential if this is to be prevented? a. auxiliaries will work within a fairly circumscribed field. b. the public health nurse will assume responsibility for all phases of the nursing team's activities. c. the functions of all personnel will be defined. d. maximum skills of each team member will be used.	The use of a separate sentence frequently adds to the clarity of the item stem if it is necessary to present background information as well as to ask the question itself. Combining these two elements into a single question-sentence probably would make it too complex.
10. Necessary qualification	Generally speaking, the environmental health program personnel in urban centers are: a. persons with professional training in civil or sanitary engineering. b. sanitary inspectors, or nonengineering personnel with indoctrination and orientation by the health department. c. public health engineers whose training embraces the public health aspect of both sanitary engineering and sanitary inspection. d. all of the above.	If this question asked only about environmental health program personnel in general, without qualifying *urban* personnel, it would be difficult for the respondent to give a firm answer to the question, given the existing differences between the environmental health programs in other than urban areas, i.e., county, state, federal.

TABLE 4-7 Continued

Format	Example	Comments
11. None of above and/or all of above as options.	A necessary requirement for receiving funds under the Comprehensive Health Planning Act of 1966 is that: a. state boards of health must have at least 10% lay representation. b. the council responsible for developing a comprehensive health plan for the state must have 50% consumer participation. c. health and welfare councils, whether or not actively involved in health planning on the state level, must have at least 25% lay representation. d. none of the above.	Whenever each of the responses can be judged unequivocally as correct or incorrect in response to the question posed in the item stem, it is appropriate to use none of the above as a response. It would be appropriate to use all of the above in a similar situation in which more than one perfectly correct answer is possible.
12. True statements as distractors.	The general purpose of parent education programs is: a. to teach parents information they need to know throughout their children's changing developmental stages. b. to help parents reinforce their understanding and strengths in regard to themselves and their children. c. to develop attitudes of healthy family life in parents of young children. d. to cover a wider range of subject matter, format, and method than is possible on an individual basis.	It is not necessary for the incorrect options to a test item to be themselves incorrect statements. They simply need to be incorrect answers to the stem question. Judgments concerning the relevance of knowledge may be as important as judgments concerning its truth. This is particularly useful as a technique for testing achievement which is sometimes thought to be testable only by using essay measures.
13. Stereotypes in distractors.	The particular process of interaction between the organism and its environment that results in a specifiable change in both is referred to as: a. homeostasis. b. human behavior. c. operant behavior. d. developmental dynamism.	Phrases such as operant behavior and homeostasis, which a respondent may have heard without understanding, provide excellent distractors at an elementary level of discrimination.

14. Heterogeneous responses	The index of economic welfare is: a. square feet of housing space. b. per capita national income. c. rate of growth of industrialization. d. morbidity and mortality rates.	The responses to this item vary widely. Because of their wide differences, only an introductory knowledge of indices of economic welfare is required for a successful response.
15. Homogeneous responses (harder item)	Funds for occupational health programs were allocated to state and local health departments as a result of: a. Social Security Act. b. Clean Air Act. c. Community Health Centers Act. d. Occupational Health Act.	The homogeneity of the responses in this item requires a considerably high level of knowledge of public health acts and hence makes the item difficult in comparison to an item using heterogeneous options.
16. Multiple clues (easier item)	The amount estimated to eliminate poverty in our country is said to be which of the following: a. 2% of the gross national product and 1/5 of the cost for national defense. b. 3% of the gross national product and 1/6 of the cost for national defense. c. 4% of the gross national product and 1/4 of the cost for national defense. d. 5% of the gross national product and 1/3 of the cost for national defense.	The use of the values of two variables fitting the specification in the item stem makes it a fairly easy question. That is, the examinee need only know one of the values or know one in each of the three distractors to respond successfully.

Scaled Response

		A statement or question is presented and the respondents answer by marking the area on the scale that represents their answer. (See Nunnally, 1977, and Chapter 1 for additional discussion of rating scales.)
1. Number anchors	Rate your level of satisfaction with your present job using the following scale: 1 2 3 4 5 not very satisfied satisfied	The use of numerical anchors facilitates analysis of data by computer as well as serves to remind respondents of the meaning of the scale steps.

TABLE 4-7 Continued

Format	Example	Comments
2. Percentage anchors	Using the scale: A — None of the time B — 1–25% of the time C — 26–50% of the time D — 51–75% of the time E — 76–99% of the time F — all of the time rate each of the following actions performed by the nurse you observe administering medications on Ward B. Rating 1) washes hands prior to administering medications —— 2) selects correct medication to be given at designated time —— 3) checks patient's ID prior to administering medication —— 4) stays with patient until medication is taken —— 5) records administration of medication correctly ——	
3. Degrees of agreement/disagreement	Indicate your degree of agreement with the following statement: Antagonistic behavior on the part of a patient indicates a need on the patient's part for additional attention and time from the nurse. /1 /2 /3 /4 /5 /6 Completely Completely Agree Disagree	

4. Adjectives

Using the scale: A. No importance
                  B. Little importance
                  C. Some importance
                  D. Importance
                  E. A great deal of importance

rate the importance you place on each of the
following nursing faculty activities.

___ Conducting clinical   ___ Teaching graduate
      research   students
___ Consulting with   ___ Practicing clinically
      nursing service staff   ___ Pursuing professional
___ Teaching   development activities
      undergraduate
      students

See also Chapter 1 for the discussion of the semantic
differential, a special form of adjective rating scale.

5. Actual behavior

Observe the nurses intervening with the patients on
Ward C and then check the behavior that best
describes what you observed.

___ Does not adapt planned intervention to meet
      changes in patient situation.
___ Adapts implementation with guidance to
      accommodate changes in patient situation.
___ Adapts implementation independently to
      accommodate changes in patient situation.
___ Implements independently a preplanned alternate
      intervention to accommodate changes in patient
      situation.

6. Products

Here are four nursing care plans. Indicate the one
you believe to be the most reflective of good
principles and practices in gerontological nursing.

                  A. Care Plan X
                  B. Care Plan Y
                  C. Care Plan Z
                  D. Care Plan O

113

TABLE 4-7 Continued

Format	Example	Comments
Context-Dependent	Patients are given a series of pictures portraying behaviors usually observed in children of 2–3 years of age and asked to identify those observed in their own children.	In this case, the item has meaning to the subject only in relation to other material presented, e.g., scenario, picture, graph, table. Readers are referred to Wesman, 1971, for additional discussion. Visual presentation of material, especially pictures, permits the presentation of a problem or situation in a very clear and simple manner, thus eliminating confusion due to reading or inability to adequately describe a phenomenon.
Interpretation	ANOVA Table 1. How many treatments were studied in the above table? 2. How many subjects participated in the study?	Consists of introductory material followed by a series of questions calling for various interpretations, thus provides for measuring ability to interpret and evaluate materials. This type of item allows one to ask meaningful questions on relatively complex topics. Disadvantages stem from the fact that such items are time consuming to administer and difficult to construct. See Wesman, 1971, for more information.

ANOVA Table

Source	df	SS	MS	F
Between groups	9	72	24	1.5
Within groups	84	448	16	
Total	93	520		

1. How many treatments were studied in the above table?
   a. 2
   b. 3
   c. 4
   d. cannot answer from the table
2. How many subjects participated in the study?
   a. 84
   b. 92
   c. 93
   d. 94

*Adapted from Staropoli and Waltz, *Developing and Evaluating Educational Programs for Health Care Providers*. F.A. Davis, 1978, pp. 118–122, with permission.

5. In cases in which the purpose of the instrument is to serve a screening function, that is, to select a small percentage of the best, it should be a relatively difficult test for most subjects; or if it is designed to screen out the weakest or least appropriate, it should be a relatively easy test for most respondents (pp. 67–69).

It should be noted that the determination of item difficulty levels occurs at the time the measure is designed and constructed, and then the expected is compared with empirical findings via item analysis procedures (which are discussed in the next chapter).

Although the test blueprint specifies the number of items to be included on the measure during the planning stage, it is essential that test length be reconsidered during construction in light of subsequent decisions made regarding administration and item format. Although generally, the longer the test, the higher the probability of reliability and validity, there are situations in which length may become a liability. For example, if the setting in which the measure is to be given places time limits on administration, it may be necessary to reduce the number of items proportionally to accommodate the time limits. Equivalently, if the physical condition of the subjects precludes lengthy testing periods, the number of items may need to be reduced or subdivided and then administered on more than one occasion. Equivalently, if the most appropriate item format is also one that is time consuming and demanding, length may need to be traded for a format that better elicits the behavior to be assessed. The important point is that the ideal in terms of length may need to be compromised or modified because of conditions surrounding the measurement. When this occurs, it is important that the relative emphasis of the measurement be preserved by reducing the categories of items proportionally, according to the blueprint specifications.

SCORING. Generally, the more simple and direct the procedure used for obtaining raw scores for the norm-referenced measure, the better; that is, although a number of elaborate weighting schemes have been devised for assigning a raw score to a measure, it has been demonstrated empirically that the end result is usually consistent with that obtained by simply summing over items (Nunnally, 1967). For this reason, we recommend the use of summative scoring procedures, whenever it is appropriate, to obtain a total score or set of subscores for a measure.

To obtain a summative score, one assigns a score to each individual item according to a conceptual scheme and then sums over the individual item scores to obtain a total score. Usually, the conceptual scheme for assigning item scores derives from the conceptual model. If one designed a measure of faculty influence on nursing students' preferences for practice, using a theory of personal influence, items would be constructed to measure key influence variables, and item responses would be constructed in such a manner that high scores represent more amenability to influence and low scores less. For example, in *Theory of Personal Influence*, Bidwell (1973) suggests a number of conditions under which the teachers' interactions with students are more likely to influence students' attitudes toward the content. One such condition is when the student perceives a direct positive relationship (i.e., a link) between the teachers' attitudes and the content

TABLE 4-8 Illustrations of some of the more common pitfalls in the construction of multiple choice items*

Undesirable characteristic	Example	Comments
Uses citation of authority	John Sirjamiki believes that the application of a common set of cultural configurations to the study of the American family is valid if considered as an attempt to: a. strike an average pattern describing the present American family. b. describe a pattern that in time will characterize the entire American society. c. both a and b.	What a particular author has to say about this point is of less importance than what experts generally agree to be true. If there is no consensus among experts on the content addressed by a question, then the respondent should not be held responsible for knowing what one writer believes.
Admits no best answer	Family crises are built up by: a. one powerful inadequacy. b. weaknesses in family relationships. c. an initial cause that creates tension in other areas. d. social class conflicts.	Without a qualifier such as usually, most, etc., it would be difficult if not impossible to obtain agreement on a correct answer for this item. Also, it should be remembered that the importance of an event depends on the point of view of the judge and the context in which that judge is thinking of it. Unless experts can agree on a best answer, it should not be used as an item.
Deals with an incidental detail	The number of civilian nurses employed by U.S. federal government agencies in 1967 was: a. 25,000 b. 24,000 c. 23,000 d. 22,000	This item deals with the importance of nurse manpower and nurse utilization. This is an important consideration; however, it seems inappropriate to measure a respondent's recall of specific figures in order to assess understanding of nurse manpower and utilization.
Based on unique organization of subject	The second step in the nursing process is: a. assessment. b. planning. c. implementing. d. evaluating.	The only person capable of answering this question is one who has studied a particular book or article. This item shows an undesirably close tie-up with the particular organization advocated by a specific writer.

...the prospective type of study in community health may contribute valuable findings, many problems may be encountered. One of the greatest difficulties to manage is:

a. multiple variables.
b. complexity of human behavior.
c. mobile population groups.
d. agency permissions.

Too frequently the writer searches for one or two words that will convey his or her message. However, one word often does not convey all that is being asked by the item. Also, it is usually somewhat difficult to get good distractors for a one or two word correct response than for a phrase or sentence. When this is true, item discrimination may suffer.

Shows artificial inversion

According to the writer Edgar Sydensstricker, the survival curve of a society that had no deaths until the end of a fulfilled allocated living time would be:

a. a Descartes curve.
b. a normal curve.
c. a perpendicular curve.
d. an inverted curve.

This item was inverted to gain short responses. It would seem more useful to know how best to conceptualize the survival curve than to limit its description to curve labels whose meaning may not be remembered by the respondents.

Uses incomplete stem

A community may change:
a. as the population changes.
b. as needs change.
c. as political boundaries are crossed.
d. all of the above.

This item poses no specific question. A community change could occur for a variety of reasons and without a specific question that gives the respondent a context in which to respond, the item is useless. Without a qualifier or a context, this item would be just as inadequate if phrased as: When may a community change?

Uses a negative stem

Which of the following statements is *not* factual?
a. The first workmen's compensation law in the U.S. was enacted in 1908.
b. New York, California, Maryland, and Illinois were the first states to enact workmen's compensation laws.
c. In 1967, nineteen states had only partial workmen's health coverage.
d. In 1967, nine states still had no identifiable programs in occupational health.

Items that are negatively stated, i.e., require the respondent to pick an answer that is not true, tend to be somewhat confusing. Such questions in addition usually lack practical relevance in that such questions are usually not encountered in daily life.

Involves window dressing

†Nurse Harris was appointed to select the members of a special project committee. One of Nurse Harris's most important considerations would be that:

a. members are representative of the community as a whole.

The introductory sentence suggests that the item involves a practical question. Actually the question calls only for knowledge of selection principles in relation to specific project committees. Note also in this item that the longer distractor is the correct response and this

TABLE 4-8 Continued

Undesirable characteristic	Example	Comments
	b. members have special competence in the area of advisement. c. members have deliberative and leadership qualities. d. members who have time to devote, work well together, and are acceptable to the community.	may clue some respondents to select it even if they are unfamiliar with the content needed to answer it correctly.
Shows nonparallel construction	A plan of treatment for a community if it is to be effective must include: a. planning long range. b. giving first aid to immediate needs. c. pursuing continuing analysis of the present treatment. d. a strong leader.	The first three responses refer to actions, the fourth is a noun phrase.
Shows needless repetition in responses	Which is the best definition for a vein? a. a blood vessel carrying blood going to the heart. b. a blood vessel carrying blue blood. c. a blood vessel carrying impure blood. d. a blood vessel carrying blood away from the heart.	This item would be improved by using a statement in the stem that included the words "a blood vessel carrying."
Uses unnatural sequence of responses	According to the National Health Survey, more than half of the chronic invalids in the USA are: a. over 65 years. b. under 45 years. c. between 45 and 65 years. d. 50 years of age and older.	Whenever the responses for an item form a quantitative or qualitative scale, they normally should be arranged in magnitude from smallest to largest or largest to smallest. This may avoid some confusion on the part of the respondent and eliminate an irrelevant source of error.
Places response in a tandem	Chronic disease experts agree that there is at this time no certain method of primary prevention for which of the following: (a) alcoholism, arteriosclerosis; (b) cancer, diabetes; (c) multiple sclerosis, essential hypertension; (d) deafness, dental caries.	Responses in tandem save some space but are more difficult to compare in the process of selection than those placed in list form.

*Taken from Staropoli and Waltz, *Developing and Evaluating Programs for Health Care Providers.* F.A. Davis, Philadelphia, 1978, pp. 124–127, with permission.
†Taken from Staropoli and Waltz, *Developing and Evaluating Educational Programs for Health Care Providers;* Philadelphia: F.A. Davis, 1978, pp. 124–127, with permission.

TABLE 4-9 Supply-type item formats

Format	Example	Comments
Short Answer		
1. Question	What term is used to designate that portion of the infant's body that lies nearest the internal os? (presentation)	For cognitive tests this format tends to measure only facts. The respondents are presented with a question or incomplete statement written in such a way that it is clear to the respondents what is expected of them, followed by a blank space in which the respondents write what is called for by the directions. Preferably short answer questions should require an answer that is a single word, symbol, or formula. See Wesman, 1971.
2. Completion	Normal labor usually is divided into three stages: dilating, expulsive, placental.	
3. Identification/association	After each event indicate the stages of labor during which it usually occurs. a. effacement _____ b. dilatation of the cervix _____ c. fetal descent _____ d. placental separation _____	
Essay		
1. Multiple aspects of a single topic	An adolescent is being discharged from the hospital on insulin and a diabetic diet regimen. When you visit this home one week post discharge: (a) what observations will you make; (b) what information will you seek to elicit from the patient and his family and how; and (c) what type of evaluation will you expect to make on the basis of the observation and information you are able to obtain.	Essays lend themselves to measuring complex phenomena, especially the ability to organize and communicate information in an area of interest. Problems lie primarily in the area of (1) subjectivity in scoring (but this can be minimized if criteria for scoring are agreed upon prior to administration); (2) time required to respond; and (3) the limited number of questions that can be handled during a given administration, hence reducing the representativeness of the domain sampled. See Coffman, 1971.
2. Independent question	Describe your philosophy of nursing and the resulting implications it has for the delivery of nursing practice.	

taught. If one presumes that teachers' attitudes toward the content are reflected by their behavior in regard to it, then in operationalizing the theory one might choose to focus on the students' perception of the link between the content taught by the clinical instructors and the instructors' activities. More specifically, for illustrative purposes, suppose the key variable is defined as students' perceptions of their clinical faculty member's application of content to clinical performance. On the basis of the theory that the more students perceive a direct link—that is, the more they perceive that their faculty member applies the content taught to clinical performance—the more likely they are to be influenced, students are asked to rate from 1 (not at all) to 6 (very much) the extent to which they think their clinical faculty member is involved in each of the following activities:

1. Publishing materials that relate the content taught to clinical performance.

2. Speaking or in some manner presenting the content at professional meetings.

3. Consulting in the content area with practicing nurses in the agency where the faculty member has students.

4. Using the content in planning and/or developing programs for practicing nurses that deal with nursing and/or patient care.

5. Seeking continuing learning experiences that are relevant to the content taught.

6. Seeking continuing learning experiences that are relevant to patient care.

7. Participating in research regarding patient care and the content area.

8. Using the content in providing direct patient care.

Thus, the score for each of the 8 items is derived in such a manner that the higher the number selected by the respondent, the more amenable to faculty influence the respondent is expected to be, on the basis of the theory underlying the tool's development. Therefore, when individual item scores are summed to obtain a total score, scores can range from a low of 8 to a high of 48, with high scores reflecting students' very much perceiving a link between the faculty member's content and clinical performance and, hence, being more amenable to faculty influence, and low scores indicating less of a link and less amenability to influence. Since this is a norm-referenced measure, an individual respondent's score, that is, the respondent's amenability to faculty influence, would be interpreted on the basis of the scores of other respondents in the sample. To accomplish this, one would usually compute the arithmetic mean for the scores of all members of the sample and then use it to give specific meaning to the individual's score, for example, whether an individual is more or less amenable than other members of the sample, or whether a subject's score is above, below, or at the mean for the comparison group, which in this case is the sample.

Hence, in the norm-referenced case, an individual's score takes on meaning when compared with the scores of others in some well-defined referent group. The referent group might be other members of the same sample, or it might be subjects nationwide to whom the same measure was administered. In the latter case, the norm-referenced measure would most likely be a standardized test and the scores of the reference group would have been derived using an appropriate norming procedure for establishing national norms. Since standardized tests and norming procedures are discussed at length in Chapter 8, attention here will focus on those instances in which nurses construct norm-referenced measures for their own use rather than selecting and administering a standardized tool. It should be noted, however, that much of what is discussed here holds true in the case of standardized measures as well.

To facilitate the interpretation of norm-referenced scores, the distribution of raw scores is tabulated using a table, graph, or polygon. In each case, each score is paired with its frequency of occurrence in the set of scores. For example, if the same 10-item measure of ability was administered to 30 subjects, the distribution of their scores could be represented by a table as shown in Table 4-10. This table is called an *ungrouped frequency distribution* and is useful because it clearly displays how many subjects obtained each score. When there is a wide range of scores in a distribution or a number of scores are not received by subjects, it is more desirable and economical to group scores according to size in a *grouped frequency distribution*. Table 4-11 illustrates the use of a grouped frequency distribution to tabulate the scores of 30 subjects on a 100-item cognitive measure. Each group in Table 4-11 is called a score class, and the width of each score class interval in this case is 10. Although there are no fixed rules for when a grouped frequency distribution is preferred to an ungrouped one, Glass and Stanley (1970) suggest that the grouped frequency distribution be used when there is a large number of scores, 100 or more, and that it is usually best to construct not fewer than 12 nor more than 15 score classes. They state that with fewer than 12 classes one runs the risk of distorting the results, whereas with more than 15 classes the table produced is inconvenient to handle.

In lieu of a frequency distribution, one might opt to present scores using a graph such as that presented in Figure 4-4. The graph in Figure 4-4 is a histogram. It not only displays all the information in the frequency distribution, but it has the advantage of making information regarding the shape of the distribution more accessible to the reader (Glass and Stanley, 1970). The histogram is a series of columns, each having as its base one score or class and as its height the frequency or number of subjects in that class. A column is centered on the mid-point of the score/class interval.

TABLE 4-10 Ungrouped frequency distribution of scores on a 10-item measure of anxiety (n = 30)

Score	Number of Subjects
10	1
9	4
8	1
7	0
6	4
5	10
4	5
3	1
2	3
1	1

TABLE 4-11 Grouped frequency distribution of subjects' scores on a 150-item cognitive measure (n = 30)

Score	Number of Subjects
153–143	1
142–132	2
131–121	1
120–110	4
109– 99	3
98– 88	1
87– 77	1
76– 66	5
65– 55	3
54– 44	3
43– 33	1
32– 22	3
21– 11	1
10– 0	1

A frequency polygon is yet another way that one may choose to represent the scores. A polygon is very similar to a histogram. In the histogram, the top of each column is represented by a horizontal line, the length of one score or class placed at the proper height to represent the number of subjects in that class. In the polygon, a point is located above the midpoint of each score or class and at the height that represents the frequency at that score. These points are then joined by straight lines. Figure 4-5 illustrates a polygon for the data represented by the histogram in Figure 4-4. The main advantage of the polygon over the histogram is that it allows one to superimpose up to three distributions over each other with a minimum of crossing of lines (Glass and Stanley, 1970). Thus, the polygon facilitates making comparisons among distributions.

Standards for constructing tables, graphs, and polygons were first published in 1915 by Brinton and have changed little through the years. That report still covers most of the points required for the proper representation of data, thus the following rules are cited from it:

1. The general arrangement of a diagram should proceed from left to right.

2. The horizontal scale should usually read from left to right and the vertical scale from bottom to top.

3. Whenever practical, the vertical scale should be selected so that the zero line appears on the diagram.

4. In diagrams representing a series of observations, whenever possible the separate observations should be clearly indicated on the diagrams.

5. All lettering and figures on a diagram should be placed so they easily read from the base as the bottom, or from the right-hand edge of the diagram as the bottom.

6. The title of a diagram should be as clear and complete as possible (pp. 790–797).

Additional information regarding the tabulating of data can be found in Kelley (1947), Walker and Durost (1936), or Arkin and Colton (1936).

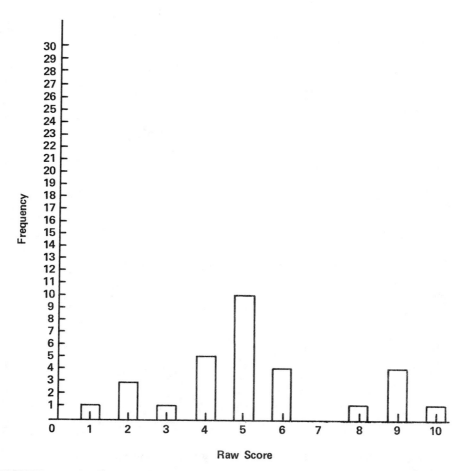

FIGURE 4-4. Distribution of scores on the anxiety measure represented by a histogram (n = 30).

Summary statistics, described in Chapter 3, are then employed to facilitate interpretation of an individual's score and to communicate information about the characteristics of the distribution of scores. Since the meaning of an individual's score is dependent upon how it compares with the scores of the other members of the referent group, it is necessary to obtain a measure of central tendency for the distribution of scores and then consider an individual's performance in light of it. The mean of the distribution represented in Figure 4-5 is 5.3, the mode is 5, and the median is approximately 5.5. Hence, one knows that an individual with a score of 3 is below the mean, received an anxiety score lower than most members of the group, and had an anxiety score falling in the lower half of the score distribution. Furthermore, by determining the variance and standard deviation for the distribution, interpretation of the individual's score can be enhanced by referring to how many standard deviations an individual's score lies above or below the mean.

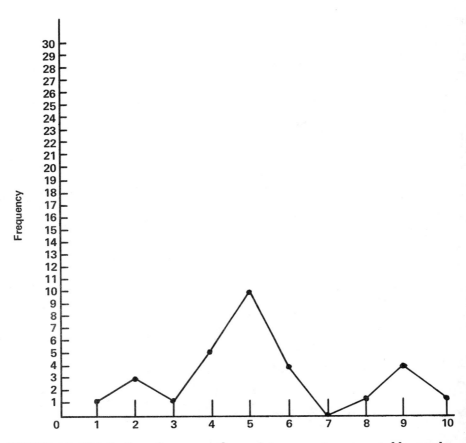

FIGURE 4-5. Distribution of scores on the anxiety measure represented by a polygon (n = 30).

If a norm-referenced measure performs in the intended manner, the resulting distribution of scores ought to display a wide range, large variance, and a shape resembling that of a normal distribution. The normal distribution (Fig. 4-6) is a symmetric distribution. Symmetric means the left half of the distribution is a perfect mirror image of the right half. The normal curve will always be symmetric around its mean; it is bell shaped, begins and ends near the baseline, but never quite touches it, and therefore is unbounded, meaning there is no beginning and no end. The normal curve is a mathematical construct first used as a model for distributions that closely approximate its characteristics or would if a very large sample were used. The distributions of scores on the anxiety measure in Figures 4-4 and 4-5 do in fact resemble a normal curve, and their measures of central tendency illustrate another important property, that is, in a normal distribution the mean, median, and mode are equal in value.

Because empirical distributions vary in terms of the extent to which they approximate the theoretical normal curve and because there are a number of normal curves, that is, as many different forms as there are combinations

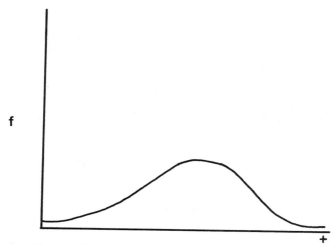

FIGURE 4-6. Shape of the normal curve.

of different means and standard deviations, the use of raw scores for the interpretation of norm-referenced measures can be very problematic. For example, if a tool were administered to two groups of 20 subjects and the distribution resulting from the first administration had a mean of 10 and a standard deviation of 5 and the distribution in the second case a mean of 20 and a standard deviation of 15, an individual with a score of 15 in the first group would be above average in his or her group, while a subject with a score of 15 in the second would be below average when compared with his or her group. Furthermore, because the standard deviation in the second group is considerably higher than that of the first, more error is present in the first set of scores and, hence, they are less accurate indications of subjects' true amount of the attribute being measured. Hence, it would be meaningless at best to attempt to compare subjects' scores across groups. For this reason, it is often useful on a norm-referenced measure to transform raw scores to a set of standard scores that allows comparison between different groups of subjects on the same measure as well as facilitates comparison within groups.

Standard scores* allow one to describe the position of a score in a set of scores by measuring its deviation from the mean of all scores in standard deviation units. This can be accomplished by converting the raw scores of each subject to a standard score. Any set of n scores with mean $\overline{X}$ and standard deviation σ_x can be transformed into a different set of scores with mean 0 and standard deviation 1, so that the transformed score immediately tells one the deviation of the original score from the mean measured in standard deviation units. This is accomplished by subtracting the mean ($\overline{X}$) from the score (X) and dividing the differences by σ_x. The resulting scores are Z scores.

---

*Portions of the material in this session are adapted from Waltz and Bausell with permission.

Formula 4-1 (Waltz and Bausell, 1981)

$$Z - \frac{X - \overline{X}}{\sigma_x}$$

Where:
    Z = a standard score
    X = the subject's raw score
    $\overline{X}$ = the mean of the raw score distribution
    σ_x = the standard deviation of the raw score distribution

Example: The mean and standard deviation of the scores 5, 10, and 18 are 11 and 5.11, respectively.

$$= \frac{5 - 11}{5.11}$$

$$= \frac{-6}{5.11}$$

$$= -1.17$$

$$= \frac{10 - 11}{5.11}$$

$$= \frac{-1}{5.11}$$

$$= -0.19$$

$$= \frac{18 - 11}{5.11}$$

$$= \frac{7}{5.11}$$

$$= 1.36$$

The resulting Z scores are -1.17, -0.19, and $+1.36$.

Aside from being a convenient means for communicating the position of a subject's score, Z scores are a step toward transforming a set of raw scores to an arbitrary scale with a convenient mean and standard deviation. There are many possible scales to which raw scores can be transformed (arbitrary means and standard deviations). For example, intelligence test scores are often transformed to a scale with mean 100 and standard deviation 15 or 16. Similarly, t scores with mean 50 and standard deviation of 10 are used widely.

Formula 4-2 To transform a Z score to any scale of measure:

$$\text{Transformed score} = (\sigma_{sm} \, Z_x) + \overline{X}_{sm}$$

where:

σ_{sm} = the desired standard deviation

Z_x = the Z score that results from $\dfrac{X - \overline{X}}{\sigma_x}$

$\overline{X}_{sm}$ = the desired mean

Example: To transform the Z score 1.36 to a t score with mean 50 and standard deviation 10:

$$\begin{aligned} t &= (10)\,(1.36) + 50 \\ &= 13.60 + 50 \\ &= 63.60 \end{aligned}$$

A distribution of Z scores is referred to as a unit normal curve, which is illustrated in Figure 4-7. It is referred to as the unit normal curve because the area under the curve is 1. Its mean and standard deviation are 0 and 1, respectively, and any other normal curve can be moved along the number scale and stretched or compressed by using a simple transformation.

As stated earlier there is an infinite number of normal curves, a different one for each different pair of values for the mean and standard deviation. The most important property they have in common is the amount of the area under the curve between any two points expressed in standard deviation units. In any normal distribution approximately:

1. 68 percent of the area under the curve lies within one standard deviation (σ) of the mean either way (that is, $\overline{X} \pm 1\sigma$).

2. 95 percent of the area under the curve lies within two σ's of the mean.

3. 99.7 percent of the area under the curve lies within three σ's of the mean.

It is useful if all references to normal distributions are in terms of deviations from the mean in standard deviation units; that is, when the normal

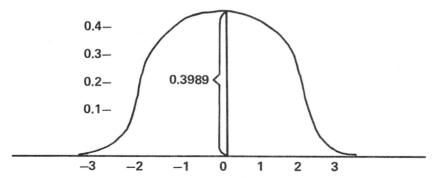

FIGURE 4-7. The unit normal curve (mean = 0; standard deviation = 1).

curve is employed, one wants to know how many standard deviations a score lies above or below the mean. The deviation of a score from its mean is $X - \overline{X}$; the number of standard deviations X lies from its mean is $\dfrac{X - \overline{X}}{\sigma_x}$ and is called the unit normal deviate. The shape of the normal curve does not change when one subtracts the mean and divides by the standard deviation.

Example: What proportion of the area lies to the left of a score of 30 in a normal distribution with mean 35 and standard deviation of 10?

It is the proportion of the area that lies to the left of $\dfrac{30 - 35}{10} = -0.5$ in the unit normal distribution.

Using a table of areas of the unit normal distribution found in most research and statistics books, one can further determine that the area that lies to the left of -0.5 in the unit normal distribution is 0.3085. A table of areas of the Unit Normal Distribution can be found in Waltz and Bausell, 1981, Appendix 1, pp. 338–340.

The Z score is sometimes referred to as a derived score. Two additional derived scores obtained from a raw score distribution using specific arithmetic operations are percentage scores and percentile ranks. Percentage scores are appropriate for criterion-referenced measures rather than norm-referenced; because they are frequently confused with the percentile rank, which is appropriate for norm-referenced measures, they will be briefly discussed here. A percentage score is the percentage of the total number of points available that have been earned by the subject.

The percentage score indicates where the individual's performance is in relation to the minimum and maximum possible values on the raw score scale. The percentage score is a measure of absolute performance; that is, the percentage score obtained by one subject is completely independent of the percentage scores of all other subjects in the group. Therefore, it is a useful measure of performance in a criterion-referenced context.

In contrast, the percentile rank of a particular raw score is the percentage of area in the histogram located to the left of the raw score in question. To determine the percentile rank:

1. Determine how many subjects obtained scores exactly equal to the subject's raw score value.

2. Divide the number obtained in Step 1 by half.

3. Count the number of subjects who obtained scores less than the subject's raw score value.

4. Add the results obtained in Steps 2 and 3.

5. Divide the result of Step 4 by the total number of scores in the distribution.

6. Multiply the resulting value by 100.

Example: Find the percentile rank of the raw score 2 in the following distribution:

Distribution

Raw Score	Frequency
5	0
4	3
3	2
2	4
1	1

1. Four subjects obtained scores exactly equal to 2.
2. One half of 4 is 2.
3. Exactly one subject had a raw score less than 2.
4. Adding the results from Steps 2 and 3, $2 + 1 = 3$.
5. Because there are 10 scores in the distribution, $\dfrac{3}{10} = 0.30$.
  6. Multiplying $0.30 \times 100 = 30$, indicating 30 percent of the area of the distribution is located to the left of the raw score 2.

The percentile rank is an indicator of relative performance. The percentile rank of a subject is totally dependent upon the quality of the subject's performance as compared with the performances of the other subjects in the group. Thus, it is an excellent measure in a norm-referenced context and totally inappropriate for use with criterion-referenced measures.

A percentile is simply a point on the raw score continuum. The Xth percentile is the point or value on the raw score scale that separates the leftmost X percent of the histogram area from the remainder of the graph. If a subject scored at the Xth percentile, the subject's performance was better than or equal to exactly X percent of the performances in the group.

Selected percentiles are sometimes referred to as quartiles. That is, the 25th percentile may be called the first quartile, the 50th percentile the second quartile, and the 75th percentile the third quartile. The first, second, and third quartiles are symbolically designated as Q_1, Q_2, Q_3, respectively. Q_2 is the median of the distribution. Quartiles are useful for summarizing data, because simply reporting that P_{50} is 10 and P_{25} is 15 tells the reader immediately that 50 percent of the observations are less than 10, and 25 percent of them lie between 10 and 15. For large groups of data, knowing the quartile values may enable the reader to readily envision the entire collection of observations.

Once the scores resulting from a norm-referenced measure have been transformed to sets of comparable values (e.g., standard scores), a *profile* chart can be plotted to demonstrate the comparability of two or more scores for the same subject or the comparability of two or more scores for groups of subjects. More specifically, profiles may be used to:

1. Obtain a visual representation of the relative performance of subjects in several different areas.
2. Compare the performance of a single group of subjects on several variables and with a set of norms (e.g., national norms).
3. Provide sample-by-sample comparisons in terms of common variables and with a set of norms (e.g., national norms).
4. Compare a subject's performance in successive years (Angoff, 1971). Usually a profile is constructed as a chart on which one axis represents the

tools and the other axis the scores as either standard scores, percentile ranks, or stanines. It must be emphasized that a profile must be based on the scores of subjects from the same or strictly comparable populations to whom the tools were administered at the same time. Because profiles are most often employed with standardized measures, which are a special type of norm-referenced measure, the development of profiles is discussed and illustrated in more depth in Chapter 8.

SUMMARY

The first step in the design of any nursing measurement is to clarify the purposes for the measurement. This is facilitated greatly when the measure is derived from a conceptual model. Objectives for the measure should be stated using good form. When taxonomies are employed in writing objectives, action verbs and critical behaviors to be observed are specified, hence, decreasing the possibility that the same behavior will be assessed differently by different people.

Specifications regarding the scope, emphasis, and length of the measure are explicated by the process of blueprinting. The blueprint facilitates the construction of items and the assessment of content validity of the resulting measure. The type of measure to be employed is a function of the conceptual model and subsequent operational definitions of key variables to be measured. Regardless of type, every measure has three components: (1) directions for administration; (2) a set of items; and (3) directions for obtaining and interpreting scores. Within the context of a given type of measure, there are a variety of specific item formats available, each with its own unique advantages and disadvantages in light of the specific purposes for and characteristics of the setting in which measurement is to occur. A variety of selection and supply type formats are presented and exemplified within the chapter.

Summative scoring procedures are advocated whenever it is appropriate to obtain a total score or set of subscores for a measure. A conceptual scheme should be employed for assigning scores and this scheme should derive from the conceptual model for operationalizing key variables. Various procedures for obtaining, tabulating, and summarizing norm-referenced scores are presented.

REFERENCES

ANGOFF, WH: "Scales, norms, and equivalent scores." In THORNDIKE, RL (ed): *Educational Measurement*, ed. 2. American Council on Education, Washington, DC, 1971, pp. 508–600.

ARKIN, H AND COLTON, RR: *Graphs: How to Make and Use Them*. New York, Harpern, 1936.

BIDWELL, CE: "The social psychology of teaching." In TRAVERS, R (ed): *Second Handbook of Research on Teaching*. Rand McNally, Chicago, 1973, pp. 414–429.

BLOOM, BS (ed): *Taxonomy of Educational Objectives. Handbook I, The Cognitive Domain*. David McKay, New York, 1956.

BORLICK, M, et al: *Nursing Examination Review Book, Vol. 9, Community Health Nursing*, ed. 2. Medical Examination Publishing Co., New York, 1974.

BRINTON, WC: "Preliminary Report by the Joint Committee on Standards of Graphic Representation." *Quarterly Publications of the American Statistical Association*, 14:790–797, 1915.

COFFMAN, WE: "Essay examinations." In THORNDIKE, RL (ed): *Educational Measurement*, ed. 2. American Council on Education, Washington, DC, 1971, pp. 271–302.

CLEMANS, WV: "Test administration." In THORNDIKE, RL (ed): *Educational Measurement*, ed. 2. American Council on Education, Washington, DC, 1971, pp. 188–201.

EBEL, RL: *Measuring Education Achievement*. Prentice-Hall, Englewood Cliffs, NJ, 1965

FITTS, PM: "Factors in complex skill learning." In GLASER, R (ed): *Training Research and Education*. University of Pittsburgh Press, Pittsburgh, PA, 1962, pp. 177–198.

FITTS, PM: "Perceptual—Motor skill learning." In METON, AW (ed): *Categories of Human Learning*. Academic Press, Inc., New York, 1964, pp. 224-285.

GLASS, GV AND STANLEY, JC: *Statistical Methods in Education and Psychology*. Prentice-Hall, Englewood Cliffs, NJ, 1970, pp. 28–29, 89, 91.

GRONLUND, NE: *Measurement and Evaluation in Teaching*. Macmillan, New York, 1965.

KELLEY, TL: *Fundamentals of Statistics*. Harvard University Press, Cambridge, MA, 1947.

KIBLER, RJ, et al: *Behavioral Objectives and Instruction*. Allyn and Bacon, Inc., Boston, 1970.

KING, EC: *Classroom Evaluation Strategies*. C.V. Mosby Co., St. Louis, 1979.

KRATHWOHL, DR, BLOOM, BS, AND MASIA, B: *Taxonomy of Educational Objectives. Handbook II. The Affective Domain*. David McKay, New York, 1964.

LORD, FM: "The relation of the reliability of multiple-choice tests to the distribution of item difficulties." *Psychometrika* 17:181–194, 1952.

MAGER, RF: *Preparing Instructional Objectives*. Fearon Publishers, Belmont, CA, 1962.

MARTUZA, VR: *Applying Norm-Referenced and Criterion-Referenced Measurement in Education*. Allyn and Bacon, Boston, 1977.

NUNNALLY, JC: *Psychometric Theory*. McGraw-Hill, New York, 1967.

STAROPOLI, C AND WALTZ, C: *Developing and Evaluating Educational Programs for Health Care Providers*. F.A. Davis, Philadelphia, 1978.

TINKELMAN, SN: "Planning the objective test." In THORNDIKE, RL (ed): *Educational Measurement*, ed. 2. American Council on Education, Washington, DC, 1971, pp. 46–80.

TYLER, RW: *Basic Principles of Curriculum and Instruction*. University of Chicago Press, Chicago, 1950.

WALKER, H AND DUROST, W: *Statistical Tables: Their Structure and Use*. Teachers College, Columbia University, New York, 1936.

WALTZ, CF AND BAUSELL, RB: *Nursing Research: Design, Statistics and Computer Analysis*. F.A. Davis Co., Philadelphia, 1981.

WESMAN, AG: "Writing the test item." In THORNDIKE, RL (ed): *Educational Measruement*, ed. 2. American Council on Education, Washington, DC, 1971, pp. 81–129.

5

RELIABILITY AND VALIDITY
OF NORM-REFERENCED MEASURES

Norm-referenced measures are derived from classical measurement theory. In Chapter 3, it was noted that in this view, every observed score (O) is composed of a true score (T) that represents the precise amount of the attribute possessed by the subject at measurement time and an error score (E). If a large number of subjects are measured on the attribute in question and their observed scores plotted, reliability would be conceptualized as the proportion of the variance in the observed score distribution that is due to true differences in subjects' possession of the attribute being measured. Unreliability would be conceptualized as the proportion of variance in the observed score distribution that is due to error. Hence, in this view every measurement involves some error that, although it can never be eliminated in total, can be reduced.

Measurement error may be random or systematic. If the nurse had only one thermometer and it was accurate, but she misread it while obtaining different measures, the error would be random. Random errors limit the degree of precision in estimating the true scores from observed scores and therefore lead to ambiguous measurement and decreased reliability of the measure. In practice, reliability concerns the extent to which measurements are repeatable by the same individual using different measures of the same attribute or by different individuals using the same measure of an attribute. Thus, nursing research and evaluation efforts are limited by the reliability of measuring instruments and/or the reliability with which they are employed. More specifically, sources of random error include but are not limited to imprecision in the measure itself, temporal factors, individual differences at measurement time, and/or imprecision in the administration or scoring of the measure.

If, in the foregoing example, the nurse employed the thermometer correctly, but the thermometer itself was inaccurate and always registered 0.5 points higher than it should, the error in the nurse's measurement would be systematic. This systematic or constant error would contribute to the mean score of all subjects equally and thus would become part of the true score of each individual. Since validity is defined as the extent to which an instrument measures what it purports to measure, systematic errors, because they affect the true scores of all subjects, would decrease the validity of the measure rather than its reliability.

In Chapter 3, it was also noted that reliability is a necessary but not sufficient condition for validity; that is, a measure that demonstrates reliability is not necessarily valid as well. The amount of random error places a limit on the validity that a measure can have, but even in the complete absence of random errors there is no guarantee of validity; that is, the correlations between a tool and an independent criterion can never be higher than the square root of the product of the reliability of the two and the reliability of the criterion variable (Isaac and Michaels, 1975, p. 87). Similarly, because random error may occur as a result of circumstances surrounding the administration of the measure and/or individual differences at measurement time, reliability and validity investigations conducted on one measurement occasion are not sufficient evidence for reliability and validity when measures are employed on other occasions or with different subjects. Thus, reliability and validity must be determined every time a given measure is employed.

CONCEPTUAL BASIS

The determination of reliability in the norm-referenced case will be conceptualized using the domain-sampling model. As noted in Chapter 3, this model views any particular measure as composed of a random sample of items from a hypothetical domain of items. For example, an adjective checklist designed to measure anxiety in presurgical patients would be thought of as containing a random sample of adjectives from all possible adjectives reflective of anxiety in that patient group. Obviously, the model does not hold strictly true empirically, because it is usually not practical or feasible to explicate all possible items defining a domain of interest, thus items are rarely actually randomly sampled for a specific measure. The model does however lead to principles and procedures for determining reliability that have much utility in practice.

On the basis of the domain-sampling model, the purpose for any measure is to estimate the measurement that would be obtained if all the items in the domain were employed. The score that any subject would obtain over the whole domain is his true score. To the extent that any sample of items on a given measure correlates highly with true scores, the sample of items is highly reliable. In other words, specific measures are viewed as randomly parallel tests that are assumed to differ somewhat from true scores in means, standard deviations, and correlations because of random errors in the sampling of items. Thus, in this view, the preferred way to estimate the reliability of a measure is to correlate one measure with a number of other measures from the same domain of content. Since in practice this is often impractical, usually one measure is correlated with only one other measure to obtain an *estimate* of reliability. The domain-sampling model suggests that the reliability of scores obtained on a sample of items from a domain increases with the number of items sampled. Thus, one item would be expected to have a small correlation with true scores, a 10-item measure a higher correlation, and a 100-item measure an even higher correlation.

NORM-REFERENCED RELIABILITY PROCEDURES

In the norm-referenced case, reliability is usually estimated by using a test-retest, parallel form, and/or internal consistency procedure.

The *test-retest* procedure is appropriate for determining the quality of measures and other devices designed to assess characteristics known to be relatively stable over the time period under investigation. For this reason, test-retest procedures are usually employed for determining the reliability of affective measures. Since cognitive measures assess characteristics that tend to change rapidly, this procedure is not usually appropriate for estimating their reliability.

When a test-retest procedure is employed, the concern is with the consistency of performance one measure elicits from one group of subjects on two separate measurement occasions. To estimate test-retest reliability for a given measure, the nurse would:

1. Administer the method or device under standardized conditions to a single group of subjects representative of the group for which the measure was designed.

2. Re-administer the same test under the same conditions to the same group of subjects. Usually the second administration occurs approximately two weeks after the first, although the time may vary slightly from setting to setting. It should be noted that it is important for the nurse to ascertain that no activities have occurred between the first and second administration that may have affected the stability of the characteristic being measured.

3. Determine the extent to which the two sets of scores are correlated. When data are measured at the interval level, the Pearson Product-Moment correlation coefficient (r_{xy}) is taken as the estimate of reliability. Computation of r_{xy} is discussed in Chapter 3. When data are measured at the nominal or ordinal level, a nonparametric measure of association, such as Chi Square-based procedures or Spearman Rho, is used. Discussion of the conditions under which specific correlational coefficients are appropriately used, as well as their computation, may be found in Waltz and Bausell (1981).

The value of the reliability coefficient resulting from a test-retest procedure reflects the extent to which the measure rank orders the performances of the subjects the same on the two separate measurement occasions. For this reason, it is often referred to as the coefficient of stability. The closer the coefficient is to 1.00, the more stable the measuring device is presumed to be.

Whenever two forms of an instrument can be generated, the preferred method for assessing reliability is the *parallel form* procedure. In parallel form reliability, the interest is in assessing the consistency of performance that alternate forms of a measure elicit from one group of subjects during one administration. Two measures are considered alternate or parallel if they (1) have been constructed using the same objectives and procedures: (2) have approximately equal means; (3) have equal correlations with any third variable; and (4) have equal standard deviations. To estimate parallel form reliability, the nurse would:

1. Administer two alternate forms of a measure to one representative group on the same occasion or on two separate occasions.

2. Determine the extent to which the two sets of scores are correlated, using an appropriate parametric or nonparametric correlation coefficient as an estimate of reliability.

If both forms of the measure are administered on the same occasion, the value of the resulting reliability coefficient reflects form equivalence only. If the measure is administered on two occasions, stability as well as form equivalence is reflected. Values above 0.80 are usually taken as evidence that the forms may be used interchangeably.

Internal consistency reliability is most frequently employed for cognitive measures when the concern is with the consistency of performance of one group of individuals across the items on a single measure. To estimate the internal consistency of a measure, the nurse would administer the measure under standardized conditions to a representative group on one occasion. The alpha coefficient KR 20 or KR 21 would be calculated as the estimate of reliability.

The *alpha* coefficient is the preferred index of internal consistency reliability because (1) it has a single value for any given set of data; and (2) it is equal in value to the mean of the distribution of all possible split-half coefficients associated with a particular set of test data. Alpha measures the extent to which performance on any one item on an instrument is a good indicator of performance on any other item in the same instrument. The formula for determining the alpha coefficient is:

Formula 5-1:

$$\text{alpha} = \left(\frac{K}{K-1}\right) \left[1 - \left(\frac{\Sigma \text{ Var Item}}{\text{Var test}}\right)\right]$$

Where K represents the number of items on the measure
Σ Var item = the sum of the individual item variances
Var test = the variance of the distribution of test scores
Example:

Five newly diagnosed diabetics are given a 10-item multiple choice test to assess their knowledge and understanding of diabetic food exchanges and the scores in Table 5-1 are obtained.
The alpha value for this test is calculated in the following manner:

1. K = 10, since there are ten items
2. Var test, the variance for the test score distribution is calculated in the usual manner using Formula 3-3 in Chapter 3.

TABLE 5–1 Scores obtained on a hypothetical test of diabetic food exchanges

Patient	Item										Total Test Score
	1	2	3	4	5	6	7	8	9	10	
A	1	1	1	1	1	1	1	1	1	1	10
B	0	1	1	1	1	1	1	1	1	0	8
C	0	0	1	1	1	1	1	1	1	1	8
D	1	0	0	0	1	1	1	1	1	1	7
E	0	1	0	0	0	0	1	1	1	1	5
Total	2	3	3	3	4	4	5	5	5	4	38
Mean	0.4	1	1	1	1	1	1	1	1	0.8	7.6
Variance	0.24	0.4	0.4	0.4	0.2	0.2	0	0	0	0.2	2.64

That is:

$$SS_x = (10 - 7.6)^2 + (8 - 7.6)^2 + (8 - 7.6)^2 + (7 - 7.6)^2 + (5 - 7.6)^2$$
$$= 13.20$$
$$\text{Var Test} = \frac{13.20}{5}$$
$$= 2.64$$

3. Var item, the variance for each item on the test is calculated in the same way using Formula 3-3 in Chapter 3. For example:

$$SS_{item1} = (1 - 0.4)^2 + (0 - 0.4)^2) + (0. - 0.4)^2 + (1 - 0.4)^2 + (0 - 0.4)^2$$
$$= 1.2$$
$$\text{Var}_{item1} = \frac{1.2}{5}$$
$$= 0.24$$

The variances for items 2 through 10 are calculated in the same manner and appear in Table 5-1.

4. Substituting in the formula for alpha

$$\text{alpha} = \left(\frac{10}{9}\right) \left[1 - \left(\frac{2.04}{2.64}\right)\right]$$
$$= (1.11) \ [1 - 0.77]$$
$$= (1.11) \ (0.23)$$
$$= 0.2553, \text{ rounded to } 0.26$$

The resulting alpha value of 0.26 indicates the test has a very low degree of internal consistency reliability, that is, that the item intercorrelations are low. As a result, performance on any one item is not a good predictor of performance on any other item. A high alpha value is usually taken as evidence that the test as a whole is measuring just one attribute, for example, knowledge of diabetic food exchanges, which in the example is not the case. In the case of tests designed to measure more than one attribute (e.g., those with subscales or components), alpha should be determined for each scale or subset of homogeneous items rather than for the test as a whole.

A number of factors surrounding the measurement situation may affect the alpha value obtained, and for this reason, it is wise to consider the following when alpha is employed:

1. Alpha is a function of test length. The longer the test, that is, the more items included, the higher the resulting alpha value.

2. A spuriously high alpha may be obtained in a situation in which it is not possible for most respondents to complete the test or measure. As a rule of thumb, Martuza (1977) suggests that if less than 85 percent of the subjects respond to all items on the test, alpha should not be used as an estimate of reliability. Equivalently, alpha should not be used when speeded tests are employed.

3. As with all reliability estimates, alpha should be determined each time a test is employed.

4. From the formula for alpha, it is apparent that alpha is dependent upon the total test variance, that is, the higher the value of the total test variance, the greater the alpha value obtained.

5. Alpha is dependent upon the shape of the resulting distribution of test scores. When a skewed test score distribution results, variance is usually less than that obtained when the distribution approximates a normal curve, and hence, alpha may be lower in value. Similarly, when alpha is employed with a group of subjects homogeneous in the attribute being measured, alpha will be lower than when a heterogeneous group is measured.

KR 20 and KR 21 are special cases of alpha used when data are dichotomously scored, that is, when each item in a test is scored 1 if correct and 0 if incorrect or missing. The formula for the determination of KR 20 is:

Formula 5-2
$$\text{KR 20} = \left(\frac{K}{K-1}\right) \left[1 - \left(\frac{pq}{\text{Var test}}\right)\right]$$

Where K is the number of items
p is the proportion of correct responses to an item
q is the proportion of incorrect or missing responses
Var test is the variance of the test score distribution
pq is the variance for each item

Example

Using the data in Table 5-1, KR 20 is calculated in the following manner:
1. K is equal to 10, since there are 10 items
2. pq, the variance for item 1, is obtained in the following manner:
p, the proportion of correct responses to item 1 is 2/5 or 0.4
q, the proportion of incorrect responses to item 1 is 3/5 or 0.6

$$pq = p \times q$$
$$= (0.4) \quad (0.6)$$
$$= 0.24$$

The variances for the remaining nine items are calculated in the same way and are 0.24, 0.24, 0.24, 0.16, 0.16, 0, 0, 0, 0.16, respectively.

3. The sum of the item variances is 1.44.
4. The variance for the test score distribution is determined using Formula 3-3 in Chapter 3 and is 2.64.
5. Substituting in the formula for KR 20,

$$KR\ 20 = \left(\frac{10}{9}\right) \left[1.00 - \left(\frac{1.44}{2.64}\right) \right]$$
$$= (1.11) \quad [1.00 - 0.54]$$
$$= (1.11) \quad (0.46)$$
$$= 0.51$$

If one can assume that the difficulty level of all items is the same, that is, p is the same for all items, then KR 21 may be employed. The formula for KR 21 is:

Formula 5-3

$$KR\ 21 = \left(\frac{K}{K-1}\right) \left[1.00 - \left(\frac{\text{test mean } (1 - \text{test mean}/K)}{\text{Var test}}\right) \right]$$

Where K is the number of items

Test mean is the mean of the test score distribution

Var test is the variance of the test score distribution

Since the p levels for the items in Table 5-1 are not the same, the computation of KR 21 is best exemplified using a different data set.

Example

A 20-item tool is used to assess six students' scores on a nursing research pretest. Items are scored 1 if correct, and 0 if incorrect. The mean of the resulting test score distribution is 15 and the variance is 25. KR 21 is obtained in the following manner:

1. k = 20, since there are 20 items on the tool
2. the mean of the test score distribution is 15
3. the variance of the test score distribution is 25
4. substituting in the formula for KR 21

$$KR\ 21 = \left(\frac{20}{19}\right) \left[1 - \left(\frac{15\ (1 - 15/20)}{25}\right) \right]$$
$$= (1.05) \left[1 - \left(\frac{15\ (1 - 0.75)}{25}\right) \right]$$
$$= (1.05) \left[1 - \left(\frac{(15)\ (0.25)}{25}\right) \right]$$
$$= (1.05) \left[1 - \left(\frac{3.75}{25}\right) \right]$$

$$
\begin{aligned}
&= (1.05) \quad (1 - 0.15) \\
&= (1.05) \ (0.85) \\
&= 0.897 \text{ or } 0.90 \text{ (rounded)}
\end{aligned}
$$

When a subjectively scored measure is employed, two types of reliability are important, interrater reliability and intrarater reliability.

Interrater reliability refers to the consistency of performance (i.e., the degree of agreement) among different raters or judges in assigning scores to the same objects or responses. Thus, interrater reliability is determined when two or more raters judge the performance of one group of subjects at the same point in time.

To determine interrater reliability, the nurse would:

1. Employ two or more competent raters to score the responses of one group of subjects to a set of subjective test items at the same point in time.

2. Use an appropriate correlation coefficient to determine the degree of agreement between the different raters in assigning the scores. If only two raters are used the Pearson Product-Moment correlation coefficient (r_{xy}) may be used as an index of agreement among them. When more than two raters are employed, coefficient alpha may be used, with the column headings representing the judges and the row headings representing the objects being rated. Table 5-2 presents an example of alpha employed for the determination of the interrater reliability of six judges of five subjects' performance on a subjective tool.

An interrater reliability coefficient of zero indicates complete lack of agreement between judges; a coefficient of 1.00 indicates complete agreement. It should be noted that agreement does not mean that the same scores were assigned by all raters, but rather that the relative ordering or ranking

TABLE 5–2 Example of alpha employed for the determination of interrater reliability for six judges' rating of five subjects' performances

Subjects	Judges						Total
	1	2	3	4	5	6	
A	10	5	4	5	10	8	42
B	8	4	4	3	9	7	35
C	10	5	5	4	8	10	42
D	10	4	5	4	10	10	43
E	9	5	5	5	10	8	42
Total	47	23	23	21	47	43	204
Mean	9.4	4.6	4.6	4.2	9.4	8.6	40.8
Variance	0.64	0.24	0.20	0.70	0.64	1.44	8.56

$$
\begin{aligned}
\text{Alpha} &= \frac{6}{5} \quad 1 - \left(\frac{3.86}{8.56} \right) \\
&= (1.2) \ (1 - 0.45) \\
&= (1.2) \ (0.55) \\
&= 0.66
\end{aligned}
$$

of scores assigned by one judge matches the relative order assigned by the other judges. Interrater reliability is especially important when observational measures are employed as well as when other subjective devices are used, such as free responses requiring categorization, essay, case study, and the like. Raters are often trained to a high degree of agreement in scoring subjective measures using the interrater reliability procedure to determine when the raters are using essentially the same criteria for scoring the responses.

Intrarater reliability refers to the consistency with which one rater assigns scores to a single set of responses on two occasions. To determine intrarater reliability:

1. A large number of subjects are asked to respond to the same subjective tool.
2. Scores are assigned to the responses using some predefined criteria.
3. Answers are not recorded on the respondents' answer sheets and anonymity of respondents is protected as much as possible.
4. Approximately two weeks after the first scoring, response sheets are shuffled and rescored a second time by the same rater who scored them on occasion one, using the same predefined criteria.
5. The Pearson correlation coefficient (r_{xy}) between the two sets of scores is determined as a measure of agreement.

A zero value for the resulting coefficient is interpreted as inconsistency, and a value of 1.00 is interpreted as complete consistency. Intrarater reliability is useful in determining the extent to which an individual applies the same criteria to rating responses on different occasions and should be employed for this purpose by those who use subjective measures. This technique, because of the time lapse between the first and second ratings, also allows one to determine to some extent the degree to which ratings are influenced by temporal factors.

NORM-REFERENCED VALIDITY PROCEDURES

Validity refers to the extent to which a measure achieves the purposes for which it was intended. Thus, the type of validity information to be obtained depends upon the aims or purposes for the measure rather than upon the type of measure per se. When the intent is to determine how an individual performs at present in a universe of situations that the measurement situation is claimed to represent, *content validity* is of import (APA, 1966).

Construct validity is assessed when the purpose is to infer the degree to which the individual possesses some hypothetical trait or quality presumed to be reflected by performance on the measure (APA, 1966). When the aim is to forecast an individual's future standing or to estimate present standing on some variable of particular significance that is different from the measure, *criterion-related validity* is investigated.

Content validity is important for all measures and is especially of interest for instruments designed to assess cognition. The focus is on determining whether or not the items sampled for inclusion on the tool adequately represent the domain of content addressed by the instrument. For this reason, content validity is largely a function of how an instrument is developed. When a domain is adequately defined, objectives are clearly explicated that represent that domain, an exhaustive set of items to measure each objective is constructed, and then a random sampling procedure is employed to select a subset of items from this larger pool for inclusion on the instrument, the probability that the instrument will have adequate content validity is high.

To determine content validity, the list of behavioral objectives that guided the construction of the tool and a separate list of items designed to specifically test the objectives are given to at least two experts in the area of content to be measured. These experts are then asked to (1) link each objective with its respective item; (2) assess the relevancy of the items to the content addressed by the objectives; and (3) judge if they believe the items on the tool adequately represent the content or behaviors in the domain of interest.

When only two judges are employed, the Index of Content Validity (CVI) is used to quantify the extent of agreement between the experts. To compute the CVI, two content specialists are given the objectives and items and are asked to independently rate the relevance of each item to the objective(s) using a four-point rating scale: (1) not relevant, (2) somewhat relevant, (3) quite relevant, and (4) very relevant. The CVI is defined as the proportion of items given a rating of quite/very relevant by both raters involved. For example, suppose the relevance of each of 10 items on an instrument to a particular objective is independently rated by two experts using the four-point scale, and the results are those displayed in Table 5-3. Using the information from the table, the CVI = the proportion of items given a rating of 3 or 4 by both judges or:

$$CVI = 8/10$$
$$= 0.80$$

If all items are given ratings of 3 or 4 by both raters, interrater agreement will be perfect and the value of the CVI will be 1.00. If one half of the items are jointly classified as 1 or 2, while the others are jointly classified as 3 or 4, the CVI will be 0.50 indicating an unacceptable level of content validity (Martuza, 1977).

It should be noted that content validity judgments require subject matter expertise and are different from the judgments referred to in determining face validity. Face validity is not validity in the true sense and refers only to the appearance of the instrument to the layman, that is, if upon cursory inspection an instrument appears to measure what the test constructor claims it measures, it is said to have face validity. If an instrument has face validity, the layman is more apt to be motivated to respond, thus its presence may serve as a factor in increasing response rate. Face validity, when it is present, however, does not provide evidence for validity, that is, that the instrument measures what it purports to measure.

TABLE 5-3 Two judges' ratings of ten items

Judge 1

Judge 2	1 or 2 not/somewhat relevant	3 or 4 quite/very relevant	Total
1 or 2 not/somewhat relevant	2	0	2
3 or 4 quite/very relevant	0	8	8
Total	2	8	10

CONSTRUCT VALIDITY. This type of validity is especially important for measures of affect. Construct validity is usually determined using: (1) the contrasted groups approach; (2) experimental manipulation approach; and/or (3) the multitrait-multimethod approach (Martuza, 1977).

In the *constrasted groups approach*, the investigator identifies two groups of individuals who are known to be extremely high and extremely low in the characteristic being measured by the instrument. The instrument is then administered to both the high and low group, and the differences in the scores obtained by each are examined. If the instrument is sensitive to individual differences in the trait being measured, then the mean performance of these two groups should differ significantly. Whether or not the two groups differ is assessed using an appropriate statistical procedure such as the t test, or an analysis of variance test. For example, to examine the validity of a measure designed to quantify venous access, the nurse might ask a group of clinical specialists on a given unit to identify a group of patients known to have good venous access and a group known to have very poor access. The nurse would then employ the measure with both groups, obtain a mean for each group, and then compare the differences between the two means using a t test or other appropriate statistic. If a significant difference is found between the mean scores of the two groups, the investigator may claim some evidence for construct validity, that is, that the instrument measures the attribute of interest. Since the two groups may differ in many ways in addition to varying in the characteristic of interest, the mean difference in scores on the instrument may be due to group noncomparability on some other variable that was not measured. Hence, a claim for validity using the contrasted groups approach must be offered in light of this possibility. If no significant difference is found between the means of the high and low group, three possibilities exist: (1) the test is unreliable; (2) the test is reliable, but not a valid measure of the characteristic; or (3) the constructor's conception of the construct of interest is faulty and needs reformulation.

When the *experimental manipulation approach* is employed, the investigator uses the theory or conceptual framework underlying the measure's design to state hypotheses regarding the behavior of individuals with varying scores on the measure, gathers data to test the hypotheses, and makes inferences on the basis of the findings regarding whether or not the rationale underlying the instrument's construction is adequate to explain the data collected. If the theory or conceptual framework fails to account for the data, it is necessary to (1) revise the measure; (2) reformulate the rationale; or (3) reject the rationale altogether.

For example, Bidwell (1973) in his Theory of Personal Influence suggests a set of conditions under which a faculty member's interactions with students are more likely to affect or influence students' attitudes toward the content. One such condition is that a faculty member will positively affect students' attitudes toward the content when the student perceives a direct positive relationship or link between the teacher's attitudes and the content taught. This theory and more specifically the set of conditions are used as a conceptual framework for identifying variables that may explain variation in students' attitudes toward the content at the completion of a course in clinical nursing. The condition regarding the link is operationalized into a set of questionnaire items that assesses students' perceptions of the link between the content taught and faculty activities. For example, students rate from 1 (not at all) to 6 (very much) how much they thought their clinical faculty member or members were involved in the following activities:

—Applying the content they teach to their own clinical performance
—Speaking or in some manner presenting the content at professional meetings
—Consulting with nurses in the agency where they have students, regarding nursing and/or patient care problems in the content area
—Planning and/or developing programs for other nurses that deal with nursing and/or patient care in the content area
—Seeking continuing learning experiences that are relevant to the content they are teaching
—Participating in research in their content area.

It is hypothesized that students who respond to the questionnaire items in a manner that indicates that they are aware of a positive link (i.e., obtain higher scores) will demonstrate more positive attitudes toward the clinical content upon completion of the course than will students who respond to the items in a manner that indicates they do not perceive a positive link between faculty activities and the content (i.e., obtain lower scores). To test this hypothesis a random sample of students is selected from the available population of students and administered the questionnaire and a second measure to assess their attitudes toward the clinical content upon completion of the course. The significance of the differences in attitudes between those students who perceive a positive link and those who do not is assessed using an appropriate statistical technique. If a significant difference is found in the expected direction (i.e., high scores on the questionnaire obtain high scores on the attitude measure and vice versa), one can say some evidence has been obtained for the construct validity of the measure. It should be noted that this is a simplified example and that in actually designing such a study it would be necessary to control variables such as students' past exposure to faculty and the like in order to test the research hypothesis more precisely.

The *multitrait-multimethod approach* (Campbell and Fiske, 1956) is appropriately employed whenever it is feasible to:

(1) measure two or more different constructs

(2) use two or more different methodologies to measure each construct

(3) administer all instruments to every subject at the same point in time

(4) assume that performance on each instrument employed is independent, that is, not influenced by, biased by, or a function of performance on any other instrument.

Whenever these conditions can be met, the multitrait-multimethod approach to instrument validation is preferred, because it produces more data with more efficiency than other available techniques.

Two basic premises underlying the multitrait-multimethod approach are (1) that different measures of the same construct should correlate highly with each other (the *convergent validity principle*) and (2) that measures of different constructs should have a low correlation with each other (the *discriminant validity principle*). An inherent aspect of the approach and one that accounts for its popularity over other approaches is the ability to separate trait from method variance. *Trait variance* is the variability in a set of scores resulting from individual differences in the trait being measured. *Method variance* is variance resulting from individual differences in a subject's ability to respond appropriately to the type of measure used. The size of the correlation between any two measures is a function of both trait and method variance. Validity techniques that focus only on the size of the correlation between two measures are not able to account for the extent to which each of these types of variance are represented in their result. When validity is evident the correlation between two measures of the same construct will be more a function of trait than method variance. In order to assess that this is so, it is necessary to focus not only on the size of the correlation but also on the patterns of the relationships between correlations of measures of the same and different constructs using common and different methods as well.

The multitrait-multimethod approach is best illustrated via example. In the simplest case, suppose a nurse had two instruments designed to measure the construct, maternal-infant bonding, and two instruments designed to measure the mother's incorporation of prenatal learnings into her perinatal infant care (a second construct). Also, suppose that the format for one measure of each construct consists of a series of behaviors rated on a five-point scale. Each rating indicates the consistency with which a particular behavior is performed. The second measure of each construct is in the form of a performance checklist, that is, all of the behaviors on a standard list that describe subjects' performance are checked.

Each of these four instruments (1) maternal-infant bonding rating scale; (2) maternal-infant bonding checklist; (3) perinatal care rating scale; and (4) perinatal care checklist is administered to every member of the validation sample at the same point in time. The reliability of each instrument is then determined using an index of internal consistency (alpha/KR 20/KR

21), and the correlation (r_{xy}) between each pair of forms is computed. A multitrait-multimethod matrix is constructed and the correlations are entered in the following manner.

The reliability estimate for each form is entered as in Figure 5-1 to form what is referred to as the *reliability diagonal*. If these values are sufficiently high, the procedure continues; if not, the procedure terminates because reliability is a prerequisite for validity. The values of the reliability estimates in Figure 5-1 range from 0.81 to 0.91, indicating sufficient evidence for reliability and thus the analysis may continue.

Convergent validity is examined by entering in the lower left block of the matrix in Figure 5-2 the correlation between the two measures of each construct assessed using different methods to form the *validity diagonal*. The values entered are 0.75 and 0.70, high enough to provide evidence for convergent validity.

The correlation between measures of different constructs employing a rating scale is entered in the upper block of Figure 5-3, and the correlation between measures of different constructs using a checklist is entered in the lower right block of the matrix. These coefficients indicate the relationship between measures of different constructs that use the same method of measurement and thus are a function of the relationship existing between the two constructs and the use of a common method. The size of these *heterotrait-monomethod coefficients* will be lower than the values on the validity diagonal if variability is more a function of trait than method variance. Since the values in Figure 5-3 follow this pattern, they provide evidence for *construct validity*.

The remaining correlations between measures of different constructs measured by different methods are entered in the lower block in the left of the matrix as shown in Figure 5-4. The values of these *heterotrait-heteromethod coefficients* should be lower than the values in the validity diagonal and the corresponding values of the heterotrait-monomethod coefficients. Since this pattern is apparent in Figure 5-4, evidence is present for *discriminant validity*.

In summary, if the information in Figure 5-4 resulted from an actual study, it would provide evidence for reliability, convergent validity, con-

| | | Method 1 (Rating Scale) | | Method 2 (Checklist) | |
		Bonding	Perinatal Care	Bonding	Perinatal Care
Rating Scale	Bonding	0.85			
	Perinatal Care		0.88		
Checklist	Bonding			0.81	
	Perinatal Care				0.91

FIGURE 5–1. Reliability diagnosis in constructing a multitrait-multimethod matrix.

146

		Method 1 (Rating Scale) Bonding	Method 1 (Rating Scale) Perinatal Care	Method 2 (Checklist) Bonding	Method 2 (Checklist) Perinatal Care
Rating Scale	Bonding	0.85			
	Perinatal Care		0.88		
Checklist	Bonding	0.75		0.81	
	Perinatal Care		0.70		0.91

FIGURE 5–2. Validity diagonal in constructing a multitrait-multimethod matrix.

struct validity, and discriminant validity, that is, more data more efficiently and economically than those obtained using other approaches.

Figure 5-5 presents an extension of the example in which a multitrait-multimethod matrix is employed for the analysis of three constructs: bonding, perinatal care, and anxiety; each measured using two different methods, a rating scale and checklist. As in the simplest case both the size and patterns of the relationships are examined.

1. The reliability diagonal is examined first and correlations are found to range from 0.81 and 0.90, indicating sufficient reliability for the analysis to proceed.

2. The validity diagonals (in the lower left block of the matrix) indicate that the relationships between measures of the same construct using different methods range from 0.70 to 0.75, high enough to provide evidence for convergent validity.

3. Correlations between measures of different constructs employing a rating scale (upper left block solid line triangle) and the correlations between measures of different constructs using a checklist (lower block solid line triangle) are examined in light of the values in the validity diagonal. The values in the heterotrait-monomethod triangle are lower than those in the validity diagonal and hence provide evidence for construct validity.

		Method 1 (Rating Scale) Bonding	Method 1 (Rating Scale) Perinatal Care	Method 2 (Checklist) Bonding	Method 2 (Checklist) Perinatal Care
Rating Scale	Bonding	0.85			
	Perinatal Care	0.40	0.88		
Checklist	Bonding	0.75		0.81	
	Perinatal Care		0.70	0.35	0.91

FIGURE 5–3. Heterotrait-monomethod correlations in constructing a multitrait-multimethod matrix.

| | Method 1 (Rating Scale) | | Method 2 (Checklist) | |
	Bonding	Perinatal Care	Bonding	Perinatal Care
Rating Scale Bonding	0.85			
Perinatal Care	0.40	0.88		
Checklist Bonding	0.75	0.18	0.81	
Perinatal Care	0.15	0.70	0.35	0.91

FIGURE 5–4. Heterotrait-heteromethod correlations in constructing a multitrait-multimethod matrix.

4. The correlations between measures of different constructs measured by different methods (lower block broken line triangles) are examined in regard to the values in the validity diagonal and the heterotrait-monomethod triangles. Since the values in the heterotrait-heteromethod triangles are lower than those in the heterotrait-monomethod triangle which, in turn, are lower than those on the validity diagonal, evidence for discriminant validity is present. Hence, from Figure 5-5, it can be seen that extension of the multitrait-multimethod approach from the simplest case to those employing more than two constructs is straightforward.

A word of caution is in order regarding the considerations to be made before employing the multitrait-multimethod approach. One disadvantage of this approach results from the demands it may place on subjects who must respond to multiple instruments at one point in time. Such a request not only has the potential for decreasing respondents' willingness to participate, hence reducing the response rate, but also introduces the potential for more errors of measurement as a result of respondent fatigue. For this reason, it is important, especially in measuring clinical variables, to carefully consider the appropriateness of using the method in light of the setting as well as the respondents' other needs. A second disadvantage may

| | Method 1 (Rating Scale) | | | Method 2 (Checklist) | | |
	Bonding	Perinatal Care	Anxiety	Bonding	Perinatal Care	Anxiety
Rating Scale Bonding	0.85					
Perinatal Care	0.40	0.88				
Anxiety	0.50	0.30	0.90			
Checklist Bonding	0.75	0.18	0.11	0.81		
Perinatal Care	0.15	0.70	0.15	0.35	0.91	
Anxiety	0.10	0.13	0.73	0.30	0.35	0.83

FIGURE 5–5. Example of a multitrait-multimethod matrix employed for analysis of three constructs using two methods.

stem from the cost in time and money necessary to employ the method. One way to reduce the potential cost is to select or design individual measures that are economical and efficient themselves.

CRITERION-RELATED VALIDITY. When one wishes to infer from a measure an individual's probable standing on some other variable or criterion, criterion-related validity is of concern. It is important to distinguish between two types of criterion-related validity: predictive validity and concurrent validity. *Predictive validity* indicates the extent to which an individual's future level of performance on the criterion can be predicted from knowledge of performance on a prior measure. *Concurrent validity* refers to the extent to which a measure may be used to estimate an individual's present standing on the criterion. Predictive validity, unlike concurrent validity, involves a time interval during which events may occur, for example, people may gain experience or be subjected to some type of learning experience (APA, 1966, p. 26).

In both cases, predictive and concurrent, the nurse wants to determine the extent to which performance on an important or significant criterion variable can be estimated using information on a measure that is usually more economical and/or accessible. For example, if the score on a confidence in nursing practice measure administered at the completion of a continuing education learning experience is found via criterion-related validity studies to be a good predictor of participants' later incorporation of learnings into nursing practice, use of the confidence measure on an ongoing basis would be a cost-effective way for continuing education staff to assess incorporation at a time when they might intervene to improve the expected outcome. Similarly, a confidence measure is far more economical than an ongoing longitudinal study of incorporation into practice using as subjects all who complete the learning experience.

To assess criterion-related validity, a target population is identified, a representative sample of the population is measured on both the predictor and criterion variables, and the linear correlation (e.g., r_{xy}) between scores on the two measures is determined. The value of the resulting correlation coefficient provides a measure of the usefulness of that predictor for estimating performance on the criterion in that target population. It should be noted that results may not be generalized, but rather provide information about the predictor-criterion relationship only in the target population studied.

The results of criterion-related studies must be carefully evaluated in light of several factors. Factors to be considered in planning and interpreting criterion-related studies relate to: (1) the target population; (2) the sample; (3) the criterion; (4) measurement reliability; and (5) the need for cross validation (Martuza, 1977). More specifically, it should be noted that:
1. Criterion-related validity coefficients obtained at one point in time must be interpreted in light of other events occurring within the target population at the same point in time and later, and in most cases will have little or no value at later points in time.

An assumption underlying criterion-related validity procedures is that the nature of the target population is relatively static and unchanging. In reality, however, the relationship between any two variables within a particular population is more apt to change than to remain static, rendering the value of most validity coefficients short-lived.

2. Validity coefficients obtained when procedures for sampling the target population are inadequate frequently underestimate the true validity of the predictor in question.

The sampling procedure used in criterion-related validity studies must be such that it provides a sample representative of the target population in general and gives each potential subject an equal chance of being selected for inclusion in the sample. Similarly, during the conduct of the study, careful attention must be directed toward assessing the presence of attrition and its potential influence on study results. Selection bias and attrition when present may reduce score variability, that is, restrict the range of scores on the predictor and/or criterion variables, thus lowering the value of the resulting correlation coefficient and providing an inaccurate estimate of the true validity of the predictor in question.

3. A given criterion-related validity coefficient is interpretable only in terms of how the criterion is defined in that study.

Important criteria are usually difficult to define and measure in a universally acceptable manner. Occasionally this fact leads to compromise and results in the selection of a criterion variable that is expedient, convenient, or agreeable to those involved, rather than a criterion that is appropriate and of sufficient quality. For example, in nursing, because of the long amount of time often required to collect information (e.g., to assess the incorporation of learning into practice may involve years of costly data collection), it is tempting to use some substitute criterion rather than to wait until the desired criterion is available. However, the substitute criterion used may not typically bear the same relevance to the predictors as the desired criterion. In criterion-related validity studies this possibility must be given careful consideration and expediency alone should not rule the conduct of the study.

4. A spurious increase in the validity coefficient may result from criterion contamination.

If criterion contamination is to be avoided, measures of the predictor and criterion variables must be independently obtained and free of bias. Whenever criterion-related studies employ a rating or judging procedure, the probability of criterion contamination is present; that is, if the raters have knowledge of how members of the sample performed on the predictor, this knowledge may influence their rating on the criterion—high scorers on the predictor tend to be rated high on the criterion and vice versa. The result is an erroneous increase in the correlation between predictor and criterion, providing evidence that the predictor is more effective than it actually is.

5. A reduced validity coefficient may result when the predictor and/or criterion measures have not demonstrated sufficient reliability.

Reliability is a necessary prerequisite for validity. Prior to employing predictor and criterion measures in criterion-related validity studies, each should have been examined for and demonstrated sufficient evidence for reliability. Although there is a formula that exists for estimating the attenuation of a correlation resulting from measurement error (Nunnally, 1967, pp. 217–220), its general use is not recommended. In most practical situations, it is preferable to employ the most reliable predictor and criterion measures one can and then live with the results obtained in that manner, rather than attempting to estimate what might be given an error free world, that is, to estimate the correlation that would be obtained if infallible measurement techniques were ever available.

6. Correlation coefficients resulting from criterion-related validity studies tend to overestimate the strength of the predictor-criterion relationship.

In criterion-related validity studies, the validity of a given predictor-criterion relationship in a specific population is simply the linear correlation between the predictor and the criterion in that specific population. As a result, the correlation coefficient tends to overestimate the true predictor-criterion relationship. To obtain a more realistic estimate of the relationship, a cross validation procedure should be employed whenever possible.

Ideally, two separate and independent samples from the same population should be employed in a cross validation procedure. In those instances in which it is not feasible to obtain two samples, it is better to randomly split the existing sample into two subsamples rather than to opt not to cross validate at all. Given two samples, cross validation proceeds in the following manner. First, a prediction equation is calculated using data from the first sample. Then the predictor measure is administered to the second sample. The prediction equation obtained for the first sample is used to estimate the criterion performance for each of the individuals in the second sample (C'). Then, r_{xy} is used to determine the linear correlation between the criterion scores predicted using the second sample (C') and the actual criterion scores (C) obtained for the members of the second sample. This correlation $r_{c'c}$ is then taken as a more precise estimate of the true correlation between the predictor and the criterion in the population of interest.

NORM-REFERENCED ITEM ANALYSIS PROCEDURES

Item analysis is a procedure used to increase the reliability and validity of a measuring device by separately evaluating each item to determine whether or not that item discriminates in the same manner in which the overall measure is intended to discriminate (Issac and Michaels, 1975, p. 80). Three-item analysis procedures are of interest in the norm-referenced case: (1) item p level, (2) discrimination index, and (3) item response chart.

ITEM P LEVEL. The p level (also referred to as the difficulty level) of an item is the proportion of correct responses to that item. It is determined by counting the number of subjects selecting the correct or desired response to a particular item and then dividing this number by the total number of subjects.

Example

A ten-item performance measure is employed to observe the behaviors of 20 nurses working on a medical-surgical nursing unit. It is determined that 10 subjects performed correctly in response to item 1; the remaining subjects did not. Thus, the p level for this item is 10/20 or 0.50. P levels range from 0 to 1.00. The closer the value of p is to 1.00, the easier the item; the closer p is to zero, the more difficult the item. When norm-referenced measures are employed, p levels between 0.30 and 0.70 are desirable, because extremely easy or extremely difficult items have very little power to discriminate or differentiate among subjects (Martuza, 1975, p. 17–2).

DISCRIMINATION INDEX. D assesses an item's ability to discriminate; that is, if performance on a given item is a good predictor of performance on the overall measure, the item is said to be a good discriminator. To determine the D value for a given item:

1. Rank all subjects' performance on the measure by using total scores from high to low.
2. Identify those individuals who ranked in the upper 25 percent.
3. Identify those individuals who ranked in the lowest 25 percent.
4. Place the remaining scores aside.
5. Determine the proportion of respondents in the top 25 percent who answered the item correctly (P_u).
6. Determine the proportion of respondents in the lower 25 percent who answered the item correctly (P_L).
7. Calculate D by subtracting P_L from P_u (i.e., $D = P_u - P_L$)
8. Repeat steps 5 through 7 for each item on the measure.

D ranges from –1.00 to +1.00. D values greater than +0.20 are desirable for a norm-referenced measure (Martuza, 1975, p. 17–2). A positive D value is desirable and indicates that the item is discriminating in the same manner as the total test, that is, those who score high on the test tend to respond correctly to the item, while those who score low do not. A negative D value suggests that the item is not discriminating like the total test, that is, respondents who obtain low scores on the total measures tend to get the item correct, while those who score high on the measure tend to respond incorrectly to the item. A negative D value usually indicates that an item is faulty and needs improvement. Possible explanations for a negative D value are that the item provides a clue to the lower scoring subjects that enables them to guess the correct response or that the item is misinterpreted by the high scorers.

ITEM RESPONSE CHART. Like D, the item response chart assesses an item's discriminatory power. The respondents ranking in the upper and lower 25 percent are identified as in steps 1 through 4 for determining D. A fourfold table like the one in Figure 5–6 is then constructed using the two categories, high/low scorers and correct/incorrect for a given item.

Using the information in Figure 5–6, one first calculates the Chi square (χ^2) value of the resulting proportions.

Formula 5–4

$$\chi^2 = \frac{N (AD - BC)^2}{(A + B) (C + D) (A + C) (B + D)}$$

$$df = (r - 1) (c - 1)$$

		Response		Totals
		Incorrect	Correct	
		B	A	A+B
Score	High	1	10	11
		D	C	C+D
	Low	8	1	9
		B + D	A + C	N
	Totals	9	11	20

FIGURE 5–6. Item response chart for a true/false or multiple choice measure (n = 20).

Where N represents the total number of subjects
A, B, C, D, represent the values in the cells as labeled in the figure
r is the number of rows
c is the number of columns

Example   Using the information in Figure 5–6:

$$\chi^2 = \frac{20 \ (80 - 1)^2}{(11) \ (9) \ (11) \ (9)}$$
$$= \frac{20 \ (79)^2}{(11) \ (9) \ (11) \ (9)}$$
$$= \frac{124820}{9801}$$
$$= 12.7$$

$df = (1) \ (1)$
$= 1$

Using a table of critical values of the Chi Square statistic that can be found in most research and statistics books, including the one by Waltz and Bausell (1981), a value as large as or larger than 1.84 for a Chi Square with one degree of freedom is significant at the 0.05 level. A significant Chi square value as in the example (12.7) indicates that a significant difference exists in the proportion of high and low scorers who gave correct responses. Items that meet this criterion should be retained, while those that do not should be discarded or modified to improve their ability to discriminate.

Next, one inspects the total response pattern in the item response chart to identify problems with distractors. Examination of the chart in Figure 5–7 suggests that the item does not discriminate well. The incorrect option was selected by only ten percent of the subjects. It would therefore be prudent to examine the item to determine if these results are due to some item defect and to revise the item accordingly. Potential problems are that the correct option contains a clue that is used by many of the lower group in

Response

Score		Incorrect	Correct	Total
High		5	80	85
Low		5	10	15
Total		10	90	100

FIGURE 5-7. Example of an item response chart indicating an item without discriminatory power resulting from a faulty distractor.

responding; or that the incorrect option is grammatically inconsistent with the stem thus cluing subjects not to select it. If the item appeared sound as constructed, it would be useful to analyze the content and procedures to which this item relates for the purpose of determining why the item's discriminating power is marginal.

In addition to its utility in analyzing true/false or multiple choice measures, the item response chart is also useful in situations in which affective measures with more than two choices are employed in an attempt to distinguish between the attitudes, values, or preferences of two groups of subjects on a given measure.

For example, one would use an item response chart in the following manner to assess an item's ability to distinguish between clinical specialists' and educators' preferences for involvement in a particular type of nursing practice.

Example
    Item
        I prefer working directly with patients to working with students in the clinical area.
    Options
        A agree (desired response by clinical specialists)
        U undecided
        D disagree (desired response by educators)
    Item Response Analysis
        1. Data are divided into two groups—educators and clinical specialists.
        2. A 2×3 table is constructed as in Figure 5–8.
        3. Chi square is determined using the formula.

Formula 5-5

$$\chi^2 = \frac{(O - E)^2}{E}$$

$df = (r - 1)(c - 1)$

154

Group	Disagree	Undecided	Agree	Total
Clinical Specialists	10	5	35	50
Educators	20	5	25	50
Total	30	10	60	100

FIGURE 5–8. Item response table for an affective measure with more than two responses.

where O represents the observed frequencies of responses
E represents the expected frequencies of responses and is determined by multiplying the column total times the row total for each cell in the table and dividing the resulting product by N
r = the number of rows
c = the number of columns

Group	Disagree	Undecided	Agree	Row total
Clinical Specialists	10 (15)	5 (5)	35 (30)	50
Educators	20 (15)	5 (5)	25 (30)	50
Column total	30	10	60	100

O	E	O − E	$(O-E)^2$	$\frac{(O-E)^2}{E}$
10	15	−5	25	1.66
20	15	5	25	1.66
5	5	0	0	0
5	5	0	0	0
35	30	5	25	0.83
25	30	−5	25	0.83

$$\chi^2 = 4.98$$
$$df = 2$$

A Chi Square with 2 df is significant at the 0.05 level when the Chi Square value is 5.99 or larger (Waltz and Bausell, 1981, p. 341). In the example the obtained value of Chi Square (4.98) does not meet or exceed the critical value and is therefore not significant. Hence, it cannot be concluded that a difference exists in the proportion of clinical specialists and educators who answered as expected, that is, it was expected that clinical specialists would agree with the statement, "I prefer working directly with patients to working with students in the clinical area" and that educators would disagree. If Chi Square had been significant the item would be discriminating as expected and would be retained. The item as it stands however needs revision or should be eliminated and replaced by an item with more power to discriminate between clinical specialists' preferences and educators' preferences for nursing care.

ESTIMATING THE RELIABILITY AND VALIDITY OF CHANGES IN TEST LENGTH

In many instances, as a result of item analysis, it appears that a measure might be improved either by shortening its length by eliminating faulty items or by adding more items. Similarly, when a measure is being developed and tested, the test constructor often will include more items than the number desired for the final form in order to assess via item analysis the performance of individual items with the intent to retain the best items and eliminate faulty items. In these cases it is important to remember that reliability is a function of test length, that is, a longer test tends to demonstrate a higher reliability than a shorter test and vice versa. For this reason, following an item analysis, it is often useful to estimate what the reliability of the measure would be if test length were also varied from the form tested.

The Spearman-Brown formula permits one to estimate the reliability of a shortened or lengthened measure with known reliability. The assumption, when this formula is used, is that while test length is changed, the nature of the test is not.

An original 100-item measure has a known reliability of 0.80 and as a result of item analysis is to be reduced to half its original length or 50 items. The reliability of the shortened version is estimated in the following manner:

Formula 5–6 Spearman-Brown formula for estimating the reliability of a shortened test or measure.

$$r_{1/2} = \frac{1/2\ r}{1 + (1/2 - 1)\ r}$$

Where   r is the original reliability
      $1/2$ is the length of the shortened test
      $r_{1/2}$ is the reliability of the shortened test

Example

$$
\begin{aligned}
r_{1/2} &= \frac{1/2\ (0.80)}{1 + (1/2 - 1)\ (0.80)} \\
&= \frac{0.40}{1 + 1/2\ (0.80)} \\
&= \frac{0.40}{1 - (0.40)} \\
&= \frac{0.40}{0.60} \\
&= 0.66
\end{aligned}
$$

The reliability of the shortened version is estimated to be 0.66.

Formula 5–7 To estimate the reliability of a lengthened test using Spearman-Brown formula

$$r_n = \frac{nr}{1 + (n - 1)\, r}$$

Where r is the original reliability
r_n is the reliability of the test n times as long

Example To estimate the reliability of a measure three times as long as the original measure, n in the formula would equal 3. If the original test reliability is known to be 0.20:

$$
\begin{aligned}
r_3 &= \frac{3\,(0.20)}{1 + (3 - 1)\, 0.20} \\
&= \frac{0.60}{1 + 0.40} \\
&= \frac{0.60}{1.40} \\
&= 0.42
\end{aligned}
$$

The reliability of the lengthened test is estimated to be 0.42.

It should be noted that whenever a test is to be lengthened, it is important to consider the potential negative effects of increased test length; that is, extreme increases in test length may introduce unwanted factors such as boredom, fatigue, diminished response rate, and other variables that may actually serve to decrease rather than increase test reliability.

SUMMARY

Every norm-referenced measurement involves some error that cannot be eliminated but can be reduced via the use of sound approaches to measurement. Random errors of measurement affect reliability, while systematic errors decrease validity. Reliability and validity must be assessed every time a given measure is employed. The domain-sampling model is the conceptual basis of choice for the determination of reliability in the norm-referenced case. Reliability is usually estimated using a test-retest, parallel form, and/or internal consistency procedure. In addition, when a subjectively scored measure is used it is important to consider interrater and/or intrarater reliability as well. Three types of validity are of concern with norm-referenced measures: content, construct, or criterion-related validity. Item analysis procedures contribute to reliability and validity by separately evaluating each item on a measure to determine whether or not that item discriminates in the same manner as the overall measure is intended to discriminate. Three-item analysis procedures are used in the norm-referenced case: item p level, the discrimination index, and item response charts. When variations in the length of a measure result from item analysis, estimations of reliability using the Spearman-Brown formula should be considered prior to actually making such modifications.

REFERENCES

BIDWELL, CE: "The social psychology of teaching." In TRAVERS, R (ed): *Second Handbook of Research on Teaching.* Rand McNally, Chicago, 1973.

CAMPBELL, DT AND FISKE, DW: "Convergent and discriminant validity by multitrait-multimethod matrix." *Psychological Bulletin* 56:81, 1959.

ISSAC, S AND MICHAEL, WB: *Handbook in Research and Evaluation.* Edits Publishers, California, 1975.

MARTUZA, VR et al: "EDF 660 tests and measurements course manual, 4th revision." University of Delaware, College of Education, 1975.

MARTUZA, VR: *Applying Norm-Referenced and Criterion-Referenced Measurement in Education.* Allyn and Bacon, Inc., Boston, 1977.

NUNNALLY, JC: *Psychometric Theory.* McGraw-Hill Book Co., New York, 1967. *Standards for Educational and Psychological Tests.* American Psychological Association, Washington, DC, 1966.

WALTZ, CF AND BAUSELL, RB: *Nursing Research: Design, Statistics, and Computer Analysis.* F.A. Davis, Philadelphia, 1981.

6

CRITERION-REFERENCED MEASUREMENT

In Chapters 4 and 5 the development and testing of norm-referenced measures were discussed. Attention now turns to another type of measurement framework used in nursing: criterion-referenced measurement.

For illustrative purposes, suppose that a nursing instructor wants to know if a student can apply the principles of sterile technique while catheterizing a patient. This is quite a different concern from how well the student can perform this task when compared with classmates. The former concern has a criterion-referenced measurement focus and the latter is an example of the focus of norm-referenced measurement. In criterion-referenced testing the emphasis is clearly on determining what a person can or cannot do or knows or does not know, not on how the person compares with others.

Criterion-referenced measures are used to determine an object's status, usually with respect to some predetermined criterion or performance standard. The emphasis is on the determination of the object's domain status and the objective of the test or measure specifies the domain that is being measured. In the example cited above the criterion or performance standards guide the instructor in determining whether the student can perform the expected set of target behaviors. When the criterion-referenced framework is applied to a testing situation, whether an individual passes or fails the test would be defined by a preset standard of performance or cut score. If the student scores above the cut score, the student would pass the test regardless of how many peers scored above or below the cut score.

Use of criterion-referenced measurement is not limited to testing achievement, skills, or other similar behaviors, but it also is used to determine an object's status in relation to some designated attribute or property. The criterion-referenced measurement framework is applied in the classification of individuals by sex or social class. It also is used in the specification of fetal position during labor. These are some examples of nominal level use of criterion-referenced measurement, since the results will serve to simply classify an object in relation to a specified attribute rather than imply quantitative value. In this type of criterion-referenced measurement an object's domain status is predetermined by distinguishing characteristics or features that have been clearly identified and explicated in terms of the nature of the domain. Such predetermined distinguishing characteristics serve as the criterion or standard(s) for measurement.

The distinguishing feature of criterion-referenced measurement is that an interpretive frame of reference is used that is based on a specified domain rather than a specified population or group (Popham, 1978). The principal difference between criterion-referenced and norm-referenced measurement lies in the standard used as a reference for interpretation of results (Glaser, 1963; Maruza, 1977). In contrast to norm-referenced measurement in which results are interpreted in terms of those obtained by others on the same measuring device, interpretation of criterion-referenced measurements is based on a predetermined criterion or standard of performance, that is, specific task or performance behaviors.

UTILITY IN NURSING

The use of criterion-referenced measurement in nursing has been increasing within the last decade. This trend is related to several factors such as the emphasis on mastery learning, the development of computer-assisted instruction to aid individualized teaching and learning, and an increasing emphasis on the construction of tools useful for measuring behaviors and other phenomena for the purposes of clinical nursing practice and nursing research.

Criterion-referenced measures are particularly useful when the purpose of testing is to ascertain whether an individual has attained minimum requirements, such as for practice or for admission to a specific educational program or course. The Nursing State Board Test Pool Examination is probably the most commonly used criterion-referenced test in nursing. A cut score is set and each individual must score at that level or above in order to be considered safe to practice and to receive nursing licensure. The American Nurses Association Certification Examination is still another example of the use of criterion-referenced testing in nursing on a wide-scale basis.

The application of criterion-referenced measurement is usually best suited for testing basic skills (Anastasi, 1976), such as the ability to do manipulative procedures or to demonstrate simple cognitive skills. However, this should not be taken to de-emphasize the importance and usefulness of criterion-referenced measurement in testing domains that include advanced levels of knowledge. Clearly, it is the intended use of test results that should determine whether a criterion-referenced measure should be used rather than the complexity of the content domain.

NURSING RESEARCH

Criterion-referenced measurement is amenable for use in the measurement of variables in nursing research, and in many instances, it may be the most appropriate measurement framework to use in the operationalization of concepts. Suppose a nurse researcher is conducting a study to determine if adjustment to the parental role by parents who have a child with meningomyelocele is related to their acceptance of the child's condition. In this example both the independent variable (adjustment to the parental role) and the dependent variable (acceptance of the child's condition) can be conceptualized so that the criterion-referenced measurement framework would be the more appropriate framework to use for measurement of the variables. If the conceptualization of the variables indicates that parents either adjust to their role or do not adjust and the parents either accept their child's condition or do not accept it, then the criterion-referenced framework is the better framework to use in the measurement of the variables. This is the case because the variables are conceptualized in a criterion-referenced manner. Crucial in the measurement of the variables would be the specification of critical behaviors that each parent must exhibit in order for the researcher to make the determination that adjustment to the parental role had occurred or not occurred or that acceptance of the child's condition had occurred or not.

Whether a nurse researcher should choose a measuring tool that uses the criterion-referenced measurement framework depends on the conceptualization of the variables under study and the nature of the research questions addressed. However, some researchers have a bias toward using norm-referenced measurement when operationalizing variables, because criterion-referenced measures usually yield nominal and ordinal data. Many variables are best operationalized through the use of criterion-referenced measurement. A number of the measures that have been developed for use in clinical nursing practice and in nursing education also are used in nursing research. In some instances norm-referenced measures would be neither appropriate nor practical for operationalizing a variable in a specific research study.

CLINICAL PRACTICE

In the clinical practice setting criterion-referenced measures are sometimes used to determine client ability to perform specific tasks and skills. The Denver Developmental Screening Test (Frankenburg, Dodds, and Fandel, 1970) is an example of such a measure. This tool is designed to classify a child's development in each of several areas as either normal or abnormal for his age, thereby facilitating the nurse clinician's ability to identify children with problems in development and behavior. The criterion-referenced measurement framework also is used to classify attributes related to client conditions that may be assessed through direct clinical observation or by laboratory tests. For example, the results of pregnancy tests are interpreted as either positive or negative; the intensity of a heart murmur may be classified as Grade 1,2,3,4,5, or 6; the measurement of reflexes during a neurological exam may be recorded as 0, 1+, 2+, 3+, or 4+; and a test of the presence of albumin in the urine may be interpreted as either negative, trace, or 1+, 2+, or 3+. Such criterion-referenced measurements are used on numerous occasions daily in the clinical setting. In most cases, criterion-referenced measures that are used in the clinical milieu provide a means for classifying data for descriptive purposes. The criterion standards that are applied during the classification process have been explicated and incorporated into these procedures so that results will be as accurate as possible. Figure 6-1 is illustrative of the use of the criterion-referenced framework for the classification of primary skin lesions. Types or classes of lesions have been specified and defined in descriptive terms so that the approach to classification is clear and unambiguous. These criterion standards guide the classification process by the examiner.

NURSING EDUCATION

In nursing education criterion-referenced measurement is best applied when there is a need for tests to examine student progress toward the attainment of a designated skill or knowledge level. Criterion-referenced measurement is better suited for such functions than norm-referenced measures (Martuza, 1977, p. 333). Instruction and evaluation of nursing students in the clinical setting is highly amenable to the use of criterion-referenced measures because of the emphasis placed on the application of knowledge and skills. Clearly the focus of evaluation in the assessment of clinical skills in nursing should be on what a person is able to do rather than on how the person compares with others. The application of criterion-referenced measurement for ascertaining clinical skills would require each student to demonstrate critical behaviors before performance would be considered satisfactory.

The increased use of mastery learning theory concepts (Block and Burns, 1976; Bloom, 1968; Carroll, 1963; 1970; May, 1970) by nurse educators has increased the acceptance and application of criterion-referenced measurement for instruction in nursing programs. This type of criterion-referenced test is used to classify students as masters or nonmasters of a single learning objective. Mastery testing yields an all-or-none score (i.e., pass or fail) that indicates whether a person has attained the predetermined level of skills or knowledge. When basic skills are tested, it is not unusual for nearly complete mastery to be expected. Items on the mastery test should be highly instructionally sensitive and discriminate between those who do and do not master the objective tested. Scores are reported in terms of the student's performance in relation to each objective. The methods for setting performance standards or cut scores for mastery are particularly important and involve the identification of critical behaviors.

In mastery testing, individual differences in performance are of little importance. The emphasis is on checking and rewarding student learning based on the attainment of criterion performance for each instructional objective. Some advocates of mastery learning argue that nearly everyone can master a selected set of instructional objectives if given the time and proper

Type of Lesion	Criterion or standard for classification
Macule	Circumscribed, flat discoloration of the skin that is less than 1 cm in size. Occurs in various shapes and colors.
Patch	Circumscribed, flat discoloration of the skin that is larger than 1 cm in size. Occurs in various shapes and colors.
Papule	Circumscribed, elevated, superficial solid lesion that is less than 1 cm in size. Border and top may assume various forms.
Wheal	Circumscribed, irregular, relatively flat edematous lesion. Color varies from red to pale. Varies in size.
Plaque	Circumscribed, elevated, superficial solid lesion larger than 1 cm in size. Border may assume various forms.
Nodule	Solid, elevated skin lesion that extends below the dermis that is up to 1 cm in size. Borders may assume various shapes.
Tumor	Solid, elevated skin lesion that extends below the dermis that is larger than 1 cm in size. Border may assume various shapes.
Vesicle	Circumscribed elevation of the skin with an accumulation of serous fluid between the upper layers of the skin. Covered by a translucent epithelium, less than 1 cm in size. Occurs in various shapes.
Bulla	Circumscribed elevation of the skin with an accumulation of serous fluid between the upper layers of the skin. Covered by a translucent epithelium, larger than 1 cm in size. Occurs in various shapes.
Pustule	Circumscribed elevation of the skin with an accumulation of purulent fluid between the upper layers of the skin. Covered by a translucent epithelium. Contents appear milky, orange, yellow, or green. Occurs in various shapes and sizes.

FIGURE 6-1. Classification of primary skin lesions. (Adapted from: DeGowin, E.L. and DeGowin, R.L.: *Bedside Diagnostic Examination,* ed 2. Macmillan, New York, 1969; and Delp, M.H. and Manning, R.T.: *Major's Physical Diagnosis,* ed 7. W.B. Saunders, Philadelphia, 1968.)

instructional strategies (Bloom, 1968; Carroll, 1963, 1970; Gagne, 1965). Numerous issues about the nature, application, practicality, and definition of mastery learning have been raised. These controversies have been given attention in Nunnally (1976).

One of the major issues raised in regard to mastery testing is that it often is insufficient beyond testing for basic skills (Anastasi, 1976). Achievement is open-ended in more advanced and less structured content areas, and a person's learning can advance almost without limits. Under such conditions complete mastery of content becomes almost impossible and unnecessary. When advanced content is tested, it is virtually impossible to set the cut score or level of mastery completely in terms of critical requisite skills, but this often must be done partly in a normative manner. The mastery level is often determined in a normative manner by performance of previous groups or through the judgment of the instructor who is teaching the course. The application of mastery testing in instances in which cut scores are determined in a normative manner is questionable.

CRITERION-REFERENCED
AND DOMAIN-REFERENCED MEASURES

A criterion-referenced measure is used to ascertain an object's status in terms of a clearly specified domain. Because criterion-referenced measures test a well-defined domain they are often referred to as domain-referenced (Berk, 1980). However, Martuza (1977) carefully points out that criterion-referenced and domain-referenced are not conceptually synonymous. As indicated earlier, criterion-referenced refers to the way in which test scores are interpreted (i.e., an object's domain status, usually in regard to some criterion or performance standard). On the other hand, domain-referenced refers to the representativeness between a set of items that make up a measure and the specified domain that the items are supposed to measure. Therefore, criterion-referenced tests should be domain-referenced; however, not all domain-referenced tests are used in the criterion-referenced sense. Domain-referenced tests can be interpreted either in the norm-referenced or criterion-referenced sense.

Some domain-referenced measures have been developed to be used in either a norm-referenced or criterion-referenced manner. For example, a test may be constructed so that a domain score and a percentile score will result on the same test. The domain score would represent the person's knowledge or skill in relation to the specified content domain tested, and an estimate of the person's domain status would be the proportion or percentage of items or tasks on the measure to which he is able to respond correctly.

Although some domain-referenced measures have been constructed to be used in the criterion-referenced or norm-referenced manner, this should not be taken to imply that norm-referenced measures can be readily adapted and used as criterion-referenced measures and vice versa. Whenever an individual chooses to use a measure there should be clarity about what is being measured and whether it is constructed to be used in a criterion- or norm-referenced manner. A measure should be used and interpreted only in the way that it is designed to be used. In most instances, the construction of a measure for optimization of one type of interpretation will tend to diminish its usefulness for the other type (Martuza, 1977; Millman, 1974). For example, one method of constructing a norm-referenced test to maximize its discrimination power is to eliminate the easy and difficult items. When this is done the measure's utility for criterion-referenced measurement is reduced because this destroys the representativeness of the domain it was originally constructed to represent. Use of the measure would not effectively ascertain a person's domain status, because simple and complex aspects of the domain would not be adequately measured.

DEVELOPING CRITERION-REFERENCED MEASURES

The primary goal of criterion-referenced measurement is to accurately determine the status of some object in terms of a well-defined domain. When one considers this goal, two major assumptions regarding a criterion-referenced measure become apparent. First, the items included in the measure sample the specified content domain carefully. Second, the preset criteria or standards of performance estimate the object's domain status. These assumptions encourage one to consider several key points that are crucial for the development of criterion-referenced measures, among which are the need for (1) a clear definition or explication of the content domain tested; (2) the inclusion of a relatively homogeneous collection of items or tasks that accurately assess the content domain that is the focus of measurement; and (3) the determination of criteria or performance standards that define an object's domain status. Figure 6-2 presents the various steps for developing and validating criterion-referenced measures. Attention for the remainder of this chapter is concentrated on steps 2 through 5, which focus on the construction of criterion-referenced measures. The need to delineate a conceptual model as a basis for tool development is discussed in Chapters 1 and 2. Concerns related to establishing reliability and validity will be discussed in detail in Chapter 7.

EXPLICATING OBJECTIVES OR DOMAIN DEFINITION

A precise and rigorous domain definition is necessary to maximize the interpretability of the results of measurements. As indicated in Chapter 4, the conceptual model that serves as the basis for the development of the measure helps to clarify its purpose and guides the manner in which it is developed. However, it is the objective of the measure that defines and specifies the domain that is to be assessed. The objective for the measure, therefore, must be explicated prior to its construction. A well-formed objective for a criterion-referenced measure is best stated in terms of the approach purported by Mager (1962). Methods for stating behavioral objectives were discussed in Chapter 4; however, a brief review and example of Mager's approach seem useful at this point. The objective should contain (a) a description of the respondent; (b) a clear specification of the expected (target) behavior; (c) a description of the criterion or standard of acceptable

---

1. Specify conceptual model.
2. Explicate objective(s) or domain definition.
3. Prepare test specifications including:
   (a) Type of test items and how they will be created
   (b) Method of administration
   (c) Test restrictions and givens
   (d) Scoring rules and procedures
4. Construct the measure including:
   (a) Developing items or tasks matched to objective(s)
   (b) Determining content validity of items or tasks, and edit or delete items as indicated
   (c) Assembling test (including item selection, preparation of directions, preparation of scoring keys, answer sheets, etc.)
5. Set standards for interpreting results.
6. Administer the test or measure.
7. Assess reliability and validity of measure.

FIGURE 6-2. Stages in the development and validation of criterion-referenced measures.

performance; and (d) a description of the conditions under which the expected behavior will be demonstrated.

The clear specification of the behavior that the respondent will exhibit to demonstrate accomplishment of the objective is the most important element of the objective. It is this aspect of the objective that sets the boundaries on the domain that the measure will assess. The behavior identified should be observable, and hence, provide a basis for measurement. Action verbs, such as will rate, will check, will select, or will demonstrate clarify the expected target behaviors. For example, suppose a nursing instructor desires to test a student's ability to insert a nasogastric tube and wants to develop a measure to assess the student's skill in this area. The objective for the measure then is: "Given a conscious adult, the student will insert a nasogastric tube. All necessary actions for safe insertion as specified in the procedure manual must be performed." Analysis of this objective follows.

Description of the respondent: Student
Target Behavior: Will insert a nasogastric tube.
Performance Standard: All necessary actions for safe insertion as specified in the procedure manual must be performed.

The objective of the measure not only defines the domain, but it often serves as a guide to the test constructor as to the type of items or tasks that will be best for measurement of the objective and the mode of administration that is most appropriately employed. In the example cited, it would be totally inappropriate to expect to test the student by any other means, except by having the student perform the target behavior. In addition, the objective indicates that items or tasks to be included in the test are all actions that are requisite for the correct and safe insertion of a nasogastric tube. An example of a measure that could result from the objective cited above is presented in Figure 6-3.

When developing a criterion-referenced measure, an objective that is formulated to specify the domain should be neither too broad nor too narrow. The goal should be to make the objective specific enough to clearly communicate the limits of the domain. At the same time, the objective should be broad enough to include the necessary scope for suitable operationalization of the concept or skill to be measured. One can use taxonomies of the cognitive (Bloom, 1956) and affective (Krathwohl, Bloom, and Masia, 1964) domains to facilitate the development of objectives with appropriate scope.

PREPARATION OF TEST SPECIFICATIONS

It has been noted previously that the objective of a measure defines the content domain that is the focus of measurement. However, the objective, in most instances, is not sufficiently constraining to guide the specifics of the construction of the measure such as test item format, test restrictions, or test scoring. That is the purpose of test specifications. When the test constructor has provided a description of what items on the measure are supposed to be like, has set forth the rules that govern how items will be created, and has spelled out the givens and restrictions associated with

Case No. _____   Name of Subject _____

Date _____   Name of Rater _____

Behaviors (steps)	Correct	Incorrect
1. Gathers necessary equipment. (i.e., Levine type lumen tube, large 30 cc syringe and stethoscope, cup of drinking water).		
2. Marks distance on tube as measured from the tip of the nose, around the ear, to the xiphoid.		
3. Places client in a sitting position (or as near to sitting as possible).		
4. Maintains position throughout procedure.		
5. Advances tube firmly but gently through the client's nostril to the pharynx.		
6. Has the patient swallow sips of water to carry the tube down the esophagus until tube is in the predetermined distance (see step 2). NOTE: Removes tube and begins again if coughing or cyanosis occurs during insertion.		
7. Checks to determine if tube is in the stomach by aspirating gastric juices up the tube. —OR— Putting 20 ml of air into the tube by syringe while listening with a stethoscope over the stomach for a gurgling noise.		

Scoring Key:
Pass = Correctly performs all steps (1–7) in procedure.
Fail = Incorrectly performs at least one step in the procedure.

FIGURE 6-3. A measure of skill for inserting a nasogastric tube.

administration of the measure, then a set of test specifications has been explicated.

It is not only possible but likely that the approach used to collect the data for a criterion-referenced measure will influence the results. Some individuals perform better on true-false items than on multiple-choice items. Others may perform better on nonverbal rather than verbal measures of specific attributes. The same is true of the manner in which data are collected. For example, one might expect quite different findings if attachment of a mother to her infant were measured through observation of the mother with her infant than if it were measured by maternal self-report. Therefore, the form of the items and method of data collection must be clarified and be consistent with the conceptual framework and objective for the measure. If an individual conceptualizes attachment as an emotional tie or bond that one person feels for another, then it is conceptualized as an affective subjective phenomenon, and measurement of the concept would best use an affective-subjective approach. Similarly, if an individual is interested in determining if a nurse has the skill to perform a physical examination, it would be neither logical nor appropriate to use a paper-and-pencil test, which assesses cognitive rather than psychomotor skills. Only through observation of the nurse's performance could a reasonable assessment and judgment of the desired skill be made. The point is that test items, form, and method of administration must be congruent and consistent with the conceptual framework and objective for the measure in order for accurate interpretations to be made of the results. These are included in test specifications, which should facilitate congruence between these aspects of a measure.

The restrictions and givens of the test conditions should be spelled out. Often these are incorporated into the statement of the objective. Restrictions may be placed on resources or aids that can be employed or on the amount of time that may be taken to perform a task or behavior. In some instances time may be an important indicator of the quality of performance, such as in the administering of medications or certain treatments. For example, the time specification in the objective, "The student administers medications within 30 minutes of the scheduled time of administration," is strongly related to quality of performance. However, in most situations, time is not usually an important indicator of the quality of performance. Time restrictions may be placed on some skill or achievement tests. Such restrictions should include a long enough period of time to allow those who normally would have mastered the domain to have a sufficient opportunity to exhibit mastery. In addition to resources that a subject may be prohibited from using there may be a variety of resources that the subject may use during a testing period. Such resources are referred to as givens. Any givens or restrictions in resources, aids, or time used during the testing period should be clearly communicated.

Popham (1978; 1980) suggests that a set of test specifications generally consist of: (a) a general description; (b) a sample item; (c) stimulus attributes (item characteristics); and (d) response attributes. The *general description* specifies what it is that the test measures through a succinct overview of the set of target behaviors. In most criterion-referenced test specifications this is the test objective. Although succinct, the general description provides information about the form of the test and approach to administration of the measure. The following is illustrative of the general description for a measure of knowledge of fluid and electrolyte balance.

General Description:
  Given a written test of knowledge relevant to the care of clients at risk for fluid and electrolyte imbalance, the student will respond to at least 80 percent of the items correctly.

A *sample item*, similar to those offered in the measure, is provided along with complete directions to the examinee or respondent. Usually, it is rather simple to provide a sample item, because most measures consist of relatively short items. Sometimes it becomes difficult to supply a sample item if items are lengthy and complicated. In any case, an illustrative item is provided for two reasons. First, for many measures the general description statement along with the illustrative item can provide enough information about the test to clarify the purpose, scope, and intended use for the measure. The second reason is that the illustrative item can provide format cues for those who will assist in the generation of items that will constitute the test. It should be noted that criterion-referenced test items may consist of most of the item forms discussed in Chapter 4. Below is an example of a sample item that is compatible with the general description provided above.

Sample Item:

    Directions: This test presents situations that are followed by sets of related test items. Read each situation carefully and answer the multiple choice items that follow it, based on the information in the situation. Select only one answer. Write the letter of the answer you select in the designated space on the answer sheet provided.

    Situation: Mr. Johnson is a 65-year-old retired farmer who has come to the Rural Health Clinic complaining of weakness, frequent episodes of diarrhea of 5 days duration, and abdominal pains. He says he has not been able to eat and drink fluids well because they "make my stomach hurt." Mr. Johnson has a temperature of 102°F, a thready pulse of 92, and a respiratory rate of 18. His blood pressure is 124/70. Mr. Johnson's skin is dry with poor turgor. There have been no episodes of vomiting.

1. In addition to a deficit of water (fluids), which of the following problems should the nurse be most concerned about in observing Mr. Johnson?

    A. Sodium deficit   C. Potassium deficit
    B. Chloride deficit   D. Bicarbonate deficit

    Stimulus attributes (item characteristics) are the factors that constrain or limit the composition of the set of items included in the measure. Generally, the items within a measure are designed to yield a response that is used in the measurement of the phenomenon of interest. Therefore, the attributes of the stimulus materials (i.e., the items) are set forth and described. This means that careful thought must be given to the nature of items in an attempt to identify significant factors associated with the desired item characteristics. Attention must be focused upon content considerations that may influence item characteristics. A decision must be made about how the range of eligible content can be most effectively circumscribed through test items. The following is illustrative of stimulus attributes that might be developed for a nursing test that is to measure knowledge requisite for the care of clients at risk for fluid and electrolyte imbalance and that is to consist of multiple-choice items.

Stimulus Attributes:
    1. Each multiple-choice item will relate to a nursing situation that describes a client at risk for fluid and electrolyte imbalance. The client's diagnosis, pertinent lab results, physical condition, treatment regimen, and significant history will be presented in each situation.
    2. Each item will focus on prevention, assessment, or treatment/care related to clients at risk for fluid and electrolyte imbalance.

3. The item stem will not include irrelevant material. Neither should a negatively stated stem be included, except when significant learning outcomes require it. Item stems will consist of complete sentences.

Response attributes make up the final component of a set of test specifications and focus on the nature of the examinee's or subject's response to items within the measure. Two types of response are possible. The subject may either select from a collection of response options presented in the measure (e.g., in multiple-choice or true-false questions), or the respondent may construct a response (e.g., in oral presentations, essay items, short-answer items, or behavioral skills tests). It is within the response-attributes section of the test specifications that rules regarding the two response possibilities are specified.

If the response attribute is the selected response, then specific rules are provided that determine the nature of the correct response and also the nature of the incorrect options. For example, if multiple-choice items are to be used in the measure, guidelines for creating not only the correct response but also the wrong answer options must be carefully explicated. Incorrect responses usually reflect common errors encountered in meeting the objective. Hence, by looking at the wrong answers, diagnostic information may be obtained. Illustrated below are a set of response attributes that are complementary to the set of stimulus attributes.

Response Attributes:
1. A set of four short one- or two-word responses or single-sentence response alternatives will follow each item stem. All responses within an item should be approximately of the same length and must plausibly relate to the item stem.
2. An item will contain only one correct or clearly best answer. All response alternatives will be grammatically consistent with the stem of the item.
3. The three incorrect response alternatives will lack accuracy or appropriate scope.
4. An incorrect response alternative exemplifies a lack of accuracy when it makes a statement contradicted by information in the textbook or makes a statement incapable of verification.
5. An incorrect response alternative exemplifies the lack of appropriate scope when it does not include all of the important details to fully answer the item stem; or it is too general to account for all of the important details needed to clearly answer the item stem.
6. The correct response alternative must be entirely accurate and have appropriate scope, in that it includes all the important information to answer the stem and is verifiable by agreement of experts in the area.

When the respondent is required to construct a response, the response attributes should explain the criteria that will be used to ascertain a reliable judgment of the adequacy of the constructed responses. These response attributes should be so well formulated that determination of the acceptability of any constructed responses would be a rather simple matter. In reality, depending upon the nature of the measure, this ideal may not be easily approximated. In Figure 6-4, an illustrative set of criterion-referenced test specifications is presented for a Measure of Skill for Inserting a Nasogastric Tube, which was provided in Figure 6-3. This example presents an illustration of response attributes for the constructed response required in this situation.

Finally, in some cases the nature of the content domain or items may be such that a full description of stimulus attributes or response attributes may be too voluminous to include in a focused presentation of the test specifications. In such cases, key statements could be emphasized within an abbreviated description for these sections, and the detailed specifications would be included in a supplement or appendix. This approach should be taken when lengthy content citations might distract the reader from focusing on important specification statements.

In summary, the purpose of test specifications is to communicate the specifics related to the construction of the measure. This includes explication of not only what the items on the measure will assess but also the rules that govern the creation and administration of the measure. The goals of the developer of test specifications are to be sufficiently specific to communicate the scope and constraints to potential users of the measure; and to be sufficiently targeted and explicit to guide those who might be involved in the construction and development of the measure.

Clearly, one of the major purposes of test specifications is to facilitate the creation of a measure with items that are homogeneous. Since criterion-ref-

---

General Description
Given a conscious adult, the nurse will insert a nasogastric tube. All necessary actions for safe insertion must be performed.

Sample Item
Directions: You are to insert a nasogastric tube from the nostrils into the stomach of an adult client. You must employ the necessary materials and proceed sequentially through each requisite step of the procedure.
Step 1. Gather necessary equipment. (i.e., Levine type lumen tube, large 30 cc syringe and stethoscope, cup of drinking water)

Stimulus Attributes or Item Characteristics
1. Each item will consist of a necessary step in the procedure and describe the behaviors required of the nurse to complete the step. Each item will be stated in behavioral terms.
2. Each item should be listed sequentially (i.e., will follow the item that should be completed immediately prior to it).
3. Where appropriate, more than one descriptive behavior will be included in an item (step), if either may be correctly employed for the completion of that item.

Response Attributes
1. A correct response to an item occurs if both of the following are observed:
   a. The nurse performs the behaviors as described in the item.
   b. The nurse performs the item in its proper sequence.
2. An incorrect response to an item occurs if any one of the following is observed:
   a. Nurse's behavior is not consistent with behaviors described in the item.
   b. Nurse does not perform the item in its proper sequence.
   c. Nurse omits the item.

FIGURE 6-4. An illustrative set of criterion-referenced test specifications for a measure of skill for inserting a nasogastric tube.

erenced measures are supposed to assess one content domain, then homogeneity of items within a measure is an important indicator of this desirable characteristic. The more homogeneous the items, the more likely it is that the items within the measure are representative of one domain. On the other hand, the more heterogeneous the items, the greater is the likelihood that the measure taps factors outside the domain. Precise and rigorous test specifications help to delimit the domain and thereby facilitate the inclusion of homogeneous items that tap the same domain, even though items may be of various levels of difficulty. However, ambiguous and fuzzy test specifications most often lead to incongruent and heterogeneous test items, which reduce the interpretability and, hence, the validity of results.

If test specifications are clearly and rigorously prepared, they will be useful and effective for the construction of a criterion-referenced test with high validity. The approach to test specifications presented above can be written to structure almost any type of criterion-referenced measure and to specify any domain. Therefore, this approach can not only facilitate the construction of a reliable and valid criterion-referenced test but also has the flexibility for broad application.

The test specification approach represents an evolution of and further development of the amplified objectives approach (Popham and Baker, 1973), which was advocated earlier by Popham and his associates. Unlike test specifications, amplified objectives did not include an item-writing recipe that could be used to generate content valid items, nor did the approach clearly specify response criteria.

OTHER ITEM GENERATION AND TEST SPECIFICATION STRATEGIES

In the previous section, a rather flexible approach to preparing test specifications that has been suggested by Popham (1978; 1980) was presented. However, several other approaches to the construction of homogeneous test items exist. In this section attention is given to a brief discussion of several of these strategies: (1) the facet design approach; (2) the item form/item frame approach; and (3) linguistic transformation. Each of these strategies has its strengths and limitations in terms of its utility for criterion-referenced test construction. There is no known approach that is best for constructing criterion-referenced measures in all situations. In some instances it may be best to employ a combination of approaches. The approaches in this section can be considered as potentially complementary and supplemental to the test specifications approach discussed above.

THE FACET DESIGN APPROACH. The facet design approach was originally developed by Guttman (1969) to specify and map out a research domain but has since been applied in the generation of items and for domain specification in domain-referenced measures. The test developer must first analyze the content to ascertain whether it is amenable to item faceting. In this approach it must be possible to conceive both fixed and variable aspects within a content domain. Fixed categories for facets within a content domain are identified initially and are linked by what is called a mapping sentence. Variable elements within each category or facet are then identified. By using the overall mapping sentence, it is quite easy to generate a number of items rather mechanically by changing the elements in one or more of the fixed categories or facets. To illustrate this approach, assume that a test is being constructed to test one's understanding of the transmission of dominant and recessive genetic disorders. The test developer would first identify pertinent fixed categories of content that would have to be understood in order to demonstrate knowledge of transmission of dominant and recessive genetic disorders. In this situation, maternal genotype, paternal genotype, type of genetic disorder, and the potential hereditary patterns that can occur are fixed categories or facets that might be linked by a mapping sentence to generate relevant items. Elements of each of these facets also can be readily specified. An illustration of a mapping sentence for this example, along with elements within each facet, is given in Figure 6-5. The facets are identified by the letters beside them, and elements are the numbered portions of each facet. In this example, the overall mapping sentence is as follows:

Given a mother that is (specified maternal genotype) and a father that is (specified paternal genotype) for the same (specified type of genetic disorder), the student will determine the probability of (specified hereditary pattern) of defective gene in their child.

If each of the first elements within each facet was selected (i.e., A-1, B-1, C-1, and D-1), the following item would be generated:

Given a mother that is a homozygous noncarrier and a father that is a homozygous noncarrier for a dominant genetic disorder, the student will determine the probability of transmission of a defective gene to their child.

If the last element in each facet was selected (i.e., A-3, B-3, C-2, and D-2), the item would then be:

Given a mother that is	A. Maternal Genotype 1. Homozygous noncarrier 2. Homozygous carrier 3. Heterozygous	and a father that is
B. Paternal Genotype 1. Homozygous noncarrier 2. Homozygous carrier 3. Heterozygous	for the same	C. Type of Genetic Disorder 1. Dominant disorder 2. Recessive disorder
the student will determine the probability of	D. Hereditary Pattern 1. Transmission 2. Expression	of defective gene in their child.

Generation of Items
A-1 B-1 C-1 D-1
A-1 B-2 C-1 D-2
A-1 B-1 C-2 D-1
A-1 B-2 C-1 D-1
A-1 B-2 C-1 D-2
A-1 B-2 C-2 D-1
etc.

FIGURE 6-5. Example of mapping sentence.

Given a mother that is heterozygous and a father that is heterozygous for the same recessive genetic disorder, the student will determine the probability of expression of the defective gene in their child.

Any of the elements may be selected from each facet and placed within the context of the mapping sentence to generate items. One advantage of this approach is the possibility for the generation of a large number of items with systematic differences between them which can be easily described. The combination of all possible items that might result is the content domain for this example.

The facet design approach does effectively specify a limited domain and the items that can be generated within that domain. However, this approach is limited to those content domains that can be structured into a mapping sentence. Therefore, the facet design approach is not widely applicable.

THE ITEM FORM/ITEM FRAME APPROACH. This approach is very similar to the facet design approach, because it focuses on the use of fixed and variable components to generate items within a domain. The item form approach is characterized by the following: (1) it uses a fixed syntactical structure (the item form shell) to generate items; (2) it contains one or several variable elements; and (3) it specifies replacement sets for each of the variable elements and thereby defines a class of item sentences (Osburn, 1968, p. 98).

A single example of this approach is the generation of items for a test of knowledge of cranial nerve function as presented below:

Item Form Shell: The function of cranial nerve (a) can be tested by (b).

Replacement Sets:	(a)	(b)
	I	Checking vision
	II	Checking strength of facial muscles
	III	Checking hearing
	IV	Having client swallow
	V	Having client shrug shoulders
	VI	Checking for gag reflex
	VII	Checking extraocular movements
	VIII	Having client protrude tongue
	IX	Checking client's ability to taste
	X	Checking the pupil's reaction to light
	XI	Using the Weber test
	XII	Having client clench teeth

In this example, the elements in column (a) or replacement set (a) are the numbers of the specific cranial nerves. The elements in column (b) or replacement set (b) are the specific behaviors that are required to test the function of various cranial nerves that are elements in set (a). By selecting one element from replacement set (a) and one from replacement set (b), the item form shell is completed and an item is generated which could be a true-false item. Using various combinations from the item sets, it is possible to generate 144 items with the same syntactical structure. These 144 items make up a content domain. The item form approach is very similar to the facet design approach, because it consists of using variable elements that can be selected and placed within a fixed frame similar to the mapping sentence. Martuza (1977) suggests that the item form approach may actually be a special case of the facet design strategy.

The item frame approach is a modification of the item form strategy that is capable of generating several parallel tests. Instead of using an item form shell, this approach employs an item frame, which is a statement in which one or more variable elements have been identified. Instead of specifying the replacement set for each variable element, generation rules are provided that guide the test constructor about how sets for the variable elements should be generated. For a more detailed presentation of this variation of the item form approach the reader is referred to the work of Price, Martuza, and Crouse (1974).

Item forms and item frames are quite specific in the manner in which they define the content domain and generate items. However, a major disadvantage of this approach, as with the facet design approach, is that it is suitable only for highly structured types of content.

THE LINGUISTIC TRANSFORMATION APPROACH. Linguistic transformation involves transforming part of a passage from a text or other written material by using a rule to directly generate test items. The segment from the text or written material along with the transformational rule specifies and defines the relevant item domain. Advantages of this approach are that it is relatively simple, and different item writers will generate the same items if they are given the same written material and the same transformational rule.

Bormuth (1970) and Anderson (1972) suggest several transformational rules that can be applied in the linguistic transformation approach. The rules for transforming original textual material into test items vary in complexity. Several examples—echo, tag, Yes/No, and noun deletion transformations—and the use of paraphrase are presented in Table 6-1. Echo consists of restating the original base sentence and adding a question mark. The tag is similar to echo in that it is a restatement of the original base sentence, but it includes a supplemental phrase which turns the original base sentence into a question. The Yes/No transformation is accomplished by varying the form of the original base sentence into a question that requires a Yes/No response. In the noun deletion transformation, the subject of the base sentence is deleted and the original base sentence is then re-

TABLE 6-1 Base sentence: Glucosuria is one symptom of hyperglycemia

Transformation Name	Item
1. Echo	Glucosuria is one symptom of hyperglycemia?
2. Tag	Glucosuria is one symptom of hyperglycemia, isn't it?
3. Yes/No	Is glucosuria one symptom of hyperglycemia?
4. Noun deletion	What is one symptom of hyperglycemia?
5. Paraphrase	Is the presence of glucose in the urine a sign of excessive glucose in the blood?

stated in a question form that would encourage the elicitation of the noun in the original base sentence as a response. Paraphrase occurs when two statements are equivalent in meaning but have no substantive nouns, verbs, or modifiers in common. The original base sentence and its paraphrase are related in respect to meaning but are unrelated in regard to their words and form.

Except for paraphrase, all of the examples cited and most other transformations test recall. Anderson (1972) suggested paraphrase as a transformational technique for testing comprehension. In fields such as nursing in which many technical and scientific terms have no synonyms, items that measure comprehension may be difficult to create using the paraphrase technique. Another problem with this approach is its tendency to assess trivia. For a fuller discussion of the rules for creating the transformations cited above and for other more complex rules, the reader is referred to Bormuth (1970) and Anderson (1972).

ITEM REVIEW AND SELECTION

A preliminary review of all test items (or tasks) should be done once the generation of items has been completed. Items are reviewed by content specialists and those that are not well formulated or congruent with objectives are identified, revised, or discarded. In some instances a fairly large number of items may be generated to test one content domain. When a large sample of items is developed to test one objective, a predetermined number may be selected for inclusion in the measure by random sampling. Similarly, if several unrelated objectives are being assessed and a large number of items have been developed for each objective, a sample of items of a predetermined number can be selected for each objective. Martuza (1977) asserts that the same approach can be used to sample objectives when the number of objectives is large. The random selection of the predetermined number of objectives would, of course, require that their accompanying items be the only ones included in the measure. The goal is to construct a measure representative of the content domain defined by the objective. Any sampling method that maintains the domain-referenced status of the test would be appropriate.

SETTING STANDARDS FOR INTERPRETING RESULTS

Once the domain of a measure has been defined and items to measure the domain have been generated and selected, the next step in the construction of a criterion-referenced measurement tool often is to establish standards or cut score(s). However, standards or cut scores are not a necessary feature of all criterion-referenced measures (Linn, 1982), for example, those that assess domain status by percentage scores only. A standard or cut score is a point along the scale of test scores that is used to classify a subject to reflect level of proficiency relative to a particular objective. Sometimes several cut scores may be established so that a subject may be assigned to one of several levels of proficiency.

If a test or measure consists of items that assess more than one objective, different standards will be set in relation to sets of items that measure the different objectives. In other words, items that measure different objectives are separated out and used like individual tests, and cut scores are established in order for criterion-referenced interpretations to be made of the results. This is done because one cannot subject results to criterion-referenced interpretations when performance on different objectives is reflected in one score. The use of one score to represent performance on a number of different objectives does not communicate what a subject can actually do, because the pooling of results will mask performance relative to each specific objective (Airasian and Madaus, 1972).

Whenever possible, the domain score is computed for each objective, since it represents knowledge, skills, or attitudes in relation to the specified content domain. The percentage score is the domain score. Whereas the percentile rank is used in norm-referenced measurement as an indicator of relative performance, the percentage score often is used in criterion-referenced measurement as a measure of absolute performance. The percentage score is the proportion of the maximum raw score points that have been earned by the subject and is calculated by the formula below.

Formula 6-1 To convert a raw score to a percentage score:

$$\text{Percentage score} = \frac{\text{subject's raw score on the measure}}{\text{the maximum possible raw score on the measure}} \times 100$$

That is, the percentage score is the subject's raw score on a measure divided by the maximum possible raw score on the measure times 100.

Example: A raw score of 10 on a 20-item test is equivalent to a percentage score of:

$$\text{Percentage score} = \frac{10}{20} \times 100$$

$$= 0.50 \times 100$$

$$= 50$$

The percentage score represents the proportion of a content domain that an individual has mastered or responded to appropriately. Hence, it indicates an individual's level of performance in relation to the possible minimum and maximum raw scores on a measure.

How are standards or cut scores determined? The answer to this question will depend on the nature of the measure and the content domain that is the focus of measurement. The key idea in criterion-referenced measurement is to determine critical behaviors that distinguish those objects that possess the attribute in question from those that do not. In some situations it is quite a simple matter to make these distinctions. However, in other situations these distinctions are not clear. It also is apparent that the standard level will vary from measure to measure depending upon the nature of the objective assessed and the critical behaviors or attributes that must be observed in order to make a criterion-referenced interpretation. For instance, it is easier to determine if a child possesses the psychomotor skills to jump double dutch than to determine if the child possesses the psychomotor skills appropriate for his age and stage of development. In the former case, 100 percent mastery of the domain would likely be required in order to make the judgment that the child could indeed jump double dutch. However, making a criterion-referenced judgment in the latter case is not so simple, nor is 100 percent mastery of the items that might be used to measure psychomotor development for a particular age and stage of development a likely expectation.

Because the determination of standards for making criterion-referenced interpretations is often not a simple matter, a number of approaches to standard setting have been suggested. Several researchers have reviewed or catalogued most of the available methods (Glass, 1978; Hambleton and Eignor, 1979; Hambleton, et al, 1978; Jaeger, 1976; Meskauskas, 1976; Millman, 1973; Shepard, 1976). Most standard-setting methods can either be categorized as judgmental, empirical, or combination. Judgmental methods subject the individual items on the measure to the inspection of judges who are asked to assess how a person who is minimally competent would perform on each item. When empirical methods are used, data are collected and cut scores are based on the results of data analysis. Some blend of both judgmental and empirical methods are used in combination methods for setting cut scores.

No matter what standard-setting method is used, judgment is involved, and the standard in that regard is arbitrary. If a standard is set too high the chances of making false-negative criterion-referenced interpretations and decisions are increased; that is, there will be increased chances of wrongly classifying persons or objects as not meeting the standard, when they in actuality do meet it. Similarly, false-positive classifications are made when persons or objects are categorized as having met the standard when in actuality they do not. When standards are set too low the chances of false-positive results are increased. Figure 6-6 illustrates groups that have been classified as masters and nonmasters of a content domain. The area designated masters incorrectly classified represents false-negatives, and the area specified nonmasters incorrectly classified indicates false-positive classifications. The optimal outcome in establishing a standard is to set cut scores in a manner whereby chances of false-positive and false-negative results are at a minimum. However, depending on the use that will be made of the results, standards may electively be set high by the user to reduce the chances of making false-positive interpretations at an increased expense of making more false-negative interpretations, and vice versa.

Several authors have suggested judgmental methods that provide a means for setting a standard or cut score. The judgmental methods offered by Martuza (1977), Nedelsky (1954), and Ebel (1979) will be presented here, because they are rather clear-cut approaches that are recognized and used by measurement specialists.

Martuza (1977, p. 270) suggests a rather simple three-step process to the establishment of cut scores. First, content specialists examine each item and carefully rate its importance relative to the objective on a 10-point scale ranging from of little importance to extremely important. The second step

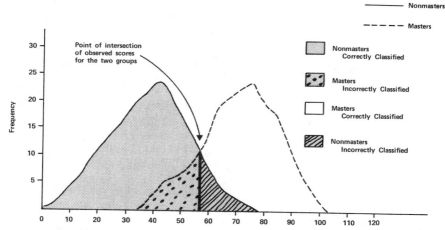

FIGURE 6-6. Frequency polygons of criterion-referenced test scores for masters and nonmasters.

involves averaging each judge's ratings across all items in the test. Finally, the averages are converted into a proportion. The proportion could then be used as a cut score for the test. If more than one judge independently rate the items, the mean of the averages from all judges would be used to calculate the proportion that would be used as a cut score. If the proportion that resulted was 85 percent, then this would be the standard. The cut score might be adjusted upward or downward based on the potential for guessing, sampling error, the relative cost of false-negative and false-positive results, or other factors that might influence the results or how they are used.

Ebel (1979) has proposed a judgmental approach to establishing cut scores which requires content specialists to rate each item within a measure along two dimensions: relevance and difficulty. Four levels of relevance (essential, important, acceptable, questionable) are used along with three levels of difficulty (easy, medium, and hard). These results are presented in a 3 × 4 grid with 12 cells. Judges examine each item and locate the items in the proper cell, based upon their level of difficulty and relevance. Once all test items have been located within cells, the judges assign a percentage to each cell which they agree is representative of the percentage of items in the cell to which the minimally qualified subject should be able to respond correctly. The percentage is then multiplied by the number of test items in each cell, and the sum of all the cells is divided by the total number of test items to obtain the standard (cut score). Figure 6-7 presents an example of Ebel's method.

Nedelsky (1954) has offered a method to establish cut scores for tests with multiple-choice items. Judges are asked to review each item and to identify distractors for each item that D-F students or students who are minimally competent should be able to eliminate as incorrect. The reciprocal of the remaining alternatives is the minimum passing level (MPL) on that item for the student who is minimally competent. It is the probability

		Relevance		
		Essential	Important	Acceptable	Questionable
	Easy	1,20,21 100%	4,15,27,28 100%	3,10 100%	6 100%
Difficulty	Medium	5,14,22,23 100%	2,7,19,16,30 60%	8,13,18 33.3%	17 0%
	Hard	9,26 100%	11,25,29 33.3%	12,24 50%	

$$\text{Standard (cut score)} = \frac{\Sigma \text{ No. of items in cell} \times \text{cell percentage}}{\text{Total no. of test items}}$$

$$\text{Standard (cut score)} = \frac{300 + 400 + 200 + 400 + 300 + 100 + 200 + 100 + 100 + 100}{30}$$

$$\text{Standard (cut score)} = \frac{2200}{30}$$

$$\text{Standard (cut score)} = 73.3\%$$

FIGURE 6-7. An example of Ebel's grid for standard-setting.

of a correct response as a function of remaining answer choices. For instance, if an item had five options from which the student could select an answer and the judges determined that the minimally competent student could eliminate one distractor as incorrect, this would leave four alternatives from which the student would really have to select. The minimum passing level for that item would be $1/4$ or 0.25. If 3,2, and 1 items remained, the minimum passing level for the items would be 0.33, 0.50, and 1.00, respectively. Once the minimum passing level for each item has been determined by the judges, the minimum passing levels are summed across the test items to obtain a standard. All of the judges' standards are then averaged to obtain a standard or cut score for the test.

Nedelsky recommends a method for adjusting cut scores in order to reduce the chances of false-negative or false-positive interpretations, depending on the user's needs. He assumes that if the standard deviation of the individual judges' standards is computed, a distribution synonymous with the hypothesized distribution of scores of borderline students will result. This standard deviation is then multiplied by a constant K, which is subtracted from or added to the standard. The constant is decided upon by the test user and would regulate the approximate number of borderline students who will pass or fail the test.

Two combination methods for setting standards on classroom tests suggested by Zieky and Livingston (1977) have applicability for other nursing situations as well. They are the Borderline-Group and the Contrasting-Group methods. In both methods, experts are used as judges and standards are based on subjects rather than items. For illustrative purposes, assume that a nursing supervisor is trying to establish a cut score for acceptable performance on a rating scale of staff nurse team leadership. In the

Contrasting-Group method, the supervisor identifies those staff nurses exhibiting definite acceptable and unacceptable team leadership behavior after defining minimally acceptable performance. The distributions of scores obtained by the two groups are then plotted. The point of intersection of the two groups is taken as the standard. (Refer to Figure 6-6 for an illustration of the point of intersection.)

In the Borderline-Group method, the evaluator defines the minimally acceptable performance on the content domain assessed, after which a list is made of a group of subjects who are borderline in performance; that is, their performance is so close to being both acceptable and unacceptable that they cannot be classified into either group. The median of the test scores from this borderline group is taken as the cut score.

As can be noted from the methods presented here, the rigor and applicability of the standard-setting methods vary. Different approaches are required from measure to measure, depending on the purpose, content domain, and intended use of the results. The decision-making context and the resources available to aid in the standard-setting process also need to be taken into consideration. Analysis of the decision-making context consists of viewing the short-term and long-term implications of decisions or conclusions that will be made using the measure. Possible psychological, social, financial, and educational consequences that may result and the number of people that might be affected must be given careful thought before making a final decision about the approach to establishing a standard for a measure.

The actual resources that will be needed to implement a standard-setting method also need consideration. The degree to which resources (e.g., personnel, time, effort, money, material, and expertise) are expended would best be determined by the decision context for which the measure will be used and the availability of such resources to carry out the task. The actual number of judges needed for the standard-setting process, when they are used, is usually the decision of the user. However, approximately three or four content specialists should be employed when a high degree of precision is needed in the estimation of the cut score. Hambleton (1980, p. 114) offers several suggestions and insights that are particularly pertinent for the standard-setting process.

Regardless of how technically sound or how content valid the test is, considerable care and attention must be given to the standard-setting process. The best test can be sabotaged by an inappropriate standard. Therefore, the test developer should:

a. Select a standard-setting method that can be efficiently and effectively handled by judges.
b. Ensure that all relevant groups have an opportunity to be involved in standard setting.
c. Train the judges so that they understand their tasks during the standard-setting process.
d. Ensure that the judges understand the purpose of the testing program, know the characteristics of the group of subjects to be tested or assessed, and have the same perspective or definition of a master and a nonmaster of test content.

e. Pilot test the measure. Decision-validity* information should be provided for several standards of test performance. Both test results from subjects and independently derived standards from judges can be used to set a revised standard.
f. Review standards occasionally.

CONSTRUCTION OF MEASURES WITH DESCRIPTIVE DOMAINS

In nursing many of the criterion-referenced measures that are used assess physical attributes or purely descriptive domains. Specificity and precision in the measurement of descriptive domains are needed in clinical nursing and in nursing research as a means to facilitate precise measurement of client conditions and states. Nominal- and ordinal-level measurements are often employed for descriptive purposes in these situations. A number of examples of such descriptive domains were cited earlier in this chapter, for example, the results of pregnancy tests, which are interpreted as either positive or negative; or the measurement of acetone in the urine, which is given as negative, trace, or 1+, 2+, or 3+. Although such measures appear rather simple and easy to construct and use, the reader is reminded that these criterion-referenced measures must adhere to the same measurement principles as are required in the measurement of behavioral domains. In addition, the same principles that undergird the construction of measures to test behavioral domains also apply for descriptive domains, although the approach varies somewhat.

As noted previously, the goal of criterion-referenced measurement is to assess a specified domain and to determine the domain status of some object in regard to the attribute of interest. The outcome or result of criterion-referenced measurement is that the object is classified or categorized according to the attribute that is the focus of measurement. When the attribute is a cognitive or psychomotor skill the person is classified on a pass/fail basis or is categorized in some other relevant manner in terms of the specified content domain. When an object is assessed in regard to a descriptive content domain, the major difference is that a number of items or tasks are not generated in order to determine the domain status of the object. A woman is either pregnant or not. The breath sounds of the lungs are described and categorized by level of intensity, pitch, and duration as vesicular, bronchovesicular, or bronchial, because no clinical measurement equipment exists that can measure this variable as a continuous variable at the interval level of measurement. There is no pool of items or tasks that can be generated to facilitate measurement of these descriptive domains. However, it is desirable that they be assessed in a way that provides an accurate classification of an object's status within the domain.

---

*Decision validity as used in this instance refers to the accuracy with which objects are classified into specific groups based on the set of standard(s) for categorization.

There are a number of important steps that must be followed in the development of measures with descriptive domains that are similar to those required in the construction of measures that test behavioral domains. When considering the steps, one will notice the marked similarity to those presented in Figure 6-2.

1. Formulate the purpose of the measure; domain definition.
2. Prepare specifications for the formulation of classes or categories.
3. Determine content validity of classes or categories with the assistance of content specialists.
4. Revise classes or categories, if indicated.
5. Administer the measure.
6. Assess the reliability and validity of the measure.

The initial step in the construction of a criterion-referenced measure with a descriptive content domain, as with any other type of measure, is to provide conceptual clarity about what is being measured. Therefore, a clear definition of the central concept or variable that is the focus of the measurement is obtained. The definition must provide conceptual clarity about the scope and limitations in conceptualization of the variable. The purpose of the measure is stated in terms of this definition and thereby defines the content domain of the measure.

The next step is to specify and define the nonoverlapping categories within which phenomena may be classified. The goal is to describe accurately and specifically the distinguishing attributes or dimensions of each category in order to provide a basis for the classification process. Figure 6-1 presents a sample measure for the classification of primary skin lesions. In this example, the descriptions of the categories are based on several dimensions: size, shape, color, and configuration of skin lesions. Descriptions must be precise and unambiguous so that no entity can be classified in more than one category.

The content validity of the classes or categories is judged by content specialists who review each category to determine if there are overlapping categories or one or more categories in which the same object might be classified. The judges also determine if the dimensions used in the categorization scheme are appropriately followed and if there are missing categories. A missing category would be indicated if the categories that had been identified and described did not provide for the categorization of an object or phenomenon that is included in the content domain according to the domain definition. Additional revisions of the classes are made, if indicated, prior to administering the measure. Reliability and validity data can then be investigated.

SUMMARY

After clarifying the definition of criterion-referenced measurement, the application of this measurement framework in nursing was reviewed. The approach to developing criterion-referenced measures was discussed and a presentation of various strategies for item generation and test construction was provided.

Criterion-referenced measures are used to determine an object's status in relation to a specified domain rather than for a comparison group, as is the case in norm-referenced measurement. Criterion-referenced measures have been heavily used and broadly applied in nursing education, research, and practice.

Although criterion-referenced measures should be domain-referenced, the two terms are not synonymous. Domain-referenced refers to the representativeness of the items within a measure for measuring a specified domain. Criterion-referenced refers to the frame of reference used to interpret results.

Three steps are of particular importance in the construction of criterion-referenced measures: (1) the domain to be tested must be clearly explicated; (2) the measure must include a relatively homogeneous collection of test items or tasks that assess the specified domain; and (3) a standard or cut score must be determined with as much accuracy as possible.

A number of approaches have been offered as a means to facilitate construction of criterion-referenced tests and to generate content-valid homogeneous items. Among the approaches discussed were test specifications, linguistic transformation, facet design, and item form/item frame. There is no one approach that is best in all situations. Each has strengths and limitations. These approaches should not be considered as entities to be used in isolation but perceived as complementary processes that may be used in combination with each other or alone, depending upon the nature of the content domain that is measured.

Several methods for establishing standards or cut scores for criterion-referenced measures also were explored. Different approaches to standard-setting are best for different measures depending upon the decision-making context in which they will be used and available resources that would be required for the standard-setting process.

The construction of the criterion-referenced tools for purely descriptive content domains was discussed and it was noted that the principles that are applicable for the construction of measures for behavioral domains are also applicable for this case. The major difference is that usually there is not a pool of items or tasks that can be generated to facilitate measurement of descriptive domains as in behavioral domains so that the domain status of objects or phenomena may be classified.

In Chapter 7, attention turns to the discussion of issues related to establishing the reliability and validity of criterion-referenced measures.

REFERENCES

ANASTASI, A: *Psychological Testing, 4th edition.* Macmillan Publishing Co., New York, 1976.

ANDERSON, RC: "How to construct achievement tests to assess comprehension." *Review of Educational Research* 42:145–170, 1972.

ARASIAN, PW AND MADAUS, GF: "Criterion-referenced testing in the classroom." *Measurement in Education* 3(4), 1972.

BERK, RH (ed.): *Criterion-referenced Measurement: The State of the Art.* Johns Hopkins University Press, Baltimore, 1980.

Block, JH and Burns, RB: "Mastery learning." In Shulman, LS (ed.): *Review of Research in Education, Vol. 4*, F.E. Peacock, Itasca, IL, 1976.

Bloom, BS: "Learning for mastery." *Evaluation Comment* 1(1), 1968.

Bloom, BS (ed): *Taxonomy of Educational Objectives, Handbook I. The Cognitive Domain.* David McKay, New York, 1956.

Bormuth, JR: *On the Theory of Achievement Test Items.* University of Chicago Press, Chicago, 1970.

Carroll, JB: "A model of school learning." *Teachers College Record* 64:723–733, 1963.

Carroll, JB: "Problems of measurement related to the concept of learning for mastery." *Educational Horizons* 48:71–80, 1970.

Ebel, RL: *Essentials of Educational Measurement.* Prentice-Hall, Englewood Cliffs, NJ, 1979.

Frankenburg, WK, Dodds, JB, and Fandal, AW: *Denver Developmental Screening Test Manual, Revised Edition.* University of Colorado Medical Center, Denver, 1970.

Gagne, R: *The Conditions of Learning.* Holt, Rinehart, and Winston, New York, 1965.

Glaser, R: "Instructional technology and the measurement of learning outcomes: Some questions." *American Psychologist* 18:519–521, 1963.

Glass, GV: "Standards and criteria." *Journal of Educational Measurement* 15:237–261, 1978.

Guttman, L: *Integration of Test Design and Analysis.* Proceedings of the 1969 Invitational Conference on Testing Problems. Educational Testing Service, Princeton, 1969.

Hambleton, RK: "Test score validity and standard-setting methods." In Berk, RA (ed): *Criterion-Referenced Measurement: The State of the Art.* Johns Hopkins University Press, Baltimore, 1980.

Hambleton, RK, and Eignor, DR: *A Practitioner's Guide to Criterion-referenced Test Development, Validation, and Test Score Usage.* Laboratory of Psychometric and Evaluative Research, Report n. 70. School of Education, University of Massachusetts, Amherst, MA, 1979a.

Hambleton, RK, and Eignor, DR: "Competency test development, validation, and standard-setting." In Jaeger, RM and Tittle, CI (eds): *Minimum Competency Achievement Testing.* McCutchan, Berkeley, CA, 1979b.

Hambleton, RK, Swaminathan, H, Algina, J, and Coulson, DB: "Criterion-referenced testing and measurement: A review of technical issues and developments. *Review of Educational Research* 48:1–47, 1978.

Jaeger, RM: "Measurement consequences of selected standard-setting models." *Florida Journal of Educational Research* 18:22–27, 1976.

Krathwohl, DR, Bloom, BS, and Masia, B: *Taxonomy of Educational Objectives. Handbook II. The Affective Domain.* David McKay, New York, 1964.

Linn, RL: "Two weak spots in the practice of criterion-referenced measurement." *Educational Measurement,* Spring 1982, 12–13.

Mager, RF: *Preparing Instructional Objectives.* Fearon Publishers, Belmont, CA, 1962.

Martuza, VR: *Applying Norm-referenced and Criterion-referenced Measurement in Education.* Allyn and Bacon, Boston, 1977.

Mayo, SI: Mastery learning and mastery testing. *Measurement in Education, National Council on Measurement in Education* 1(3):1–4, 1970.

Meskauska, JA: "Evaluation models for criterion-referenced testing. Views regarding mastery and standard-setting." *Review of Educational Measurement* 46:133–158, 1976.

Millman, J: "Criterion-referenced measurement." In Popham, WJ (ed): *Evaluation in Education: Current Applications.* McCutchan, Berkeley, CA, 1974.

Millman, J: "Passing scores and test lengths for domain-referenced measures." *Review of Educational Research* 43:205–216, 1973.

Nedelsky, L: "Absolute grading standards for objective tests." *Educational and Psychological Measurement* 14:3–19, 1954.

Nunnally, JC: "Vanishing individual differences—Just stick your head in the sand, and they will go away." *Journal of Instructional Psychology* 3:28–40, 1976.

OSBURN, HG: "Item sampling for achievement testing." *Educational and Psychological Measurement* 28:95–104, 1968.

POPHAM, WJ: *Criterion-referenced Measurement.* Prentice-Hall, Englewood Cliffs, NJ, 1978.

POPHAM, WJ: "Domain specification strategies." In BERK, RA (ed): *Criterion-Referenced Measurement: The State of the Art.* Johns Hopkins University Press, Baltimore, 1980.

POPHAM, WJ AND BAKER, EL: *Writing Tests Which Measure Objectives.* The Prentice-Hall Teacher Competency System, Prentice-Hall, Englewood Cliffs, NJ, 1973.

PRICE, JR, MARTUZA, VR, AND CROUSE, JH: "Construct validity of test items measuring acquisition of information from line graphs." *Journal of Educational Psychology* 66(1):152–156, 1974.

SHEPARD, LA: "Setting standards and living with them." *Florida Journal of Educational Research* 18:23–32, 1976.

ZIEKY, MJ AND LIVINGSTON, SA: *Manual for Setting Standards on the Basic Skills Assessment Tests.* Educational Testing Service, Princeton, NJ, 1977.

7

RELIABILITY AND VALIDITY OF CRITERION-REFERENCED MEASURES

In Chapter 6, the construction of criterion-referenced measures was discussed. Information was provided about the initial steps in the development of criterion-referenced measures, that is, domain definition, item generation, test specification strategies, and the establishment of criteria or standards. Although the production of a measure to assess a specified domain includes the major aspects involved in developing a measure, the process is not complete until there is information about how consistently and how well the measure functions. In other words, the development of a measure is not complete until there is evidence that it is a reliable and valid measure of the specified domain.

In this chapter, consideration is given to reliability and validity as they function in terms of criterion-referenced measurement. It will become apparent that many similarities exist between norm- and criterion-referenced reliability and validity concepts and procedures; however, there also are some major differences. Reliability of criterion-referenced measures will be addressed initially, followed by a discussion of validity.

RELIABILITY

Reliability refers to the consistency with which a measuring device assesses a content domain. As in the norm-referenced case, reliability in the criterion-referenced context deals with the extent to which measurements are free from measurement error and the degree to which observed scores reflect true scores. However, in the case of criterion-referenced results, the range of variability is often quite reduced, particularly when scores have been divided into two gross categories, for example, master and nonmaster. In the norm-referenced case, scores are usually highly variable and reliability is calculated on the basis of parametric correlational analyses. With criterion-referenced measurement the resulting scores are generally less variable than in the norm-referenced case, so reliability is often determined with nonparametric procedures. However, when domain status is estimated with percentage scores, some of the procedures used to estimate reliability in the norm-referenced case may be appropriate to assess the reliability of a criterion-referenced measure (Popham, 1978).

In some cases, a criterion-referenced measure may yield scores that are quite variable as far as the actual scores are concerned, but the interpretation of the range of scores would have reduced variability. For example, if a nursing instructor uses a test to determine if a student has mastered the requisite knowledge in maternity nursing, the potential score range might be 0 to 100. However, assume that the cut score for mastery is set at 80. If the student scores 75 on the test, then the student has not mastered the content. Based on the way in which the scores on the test are interpreted and used, the concern for testing reliability is on the consistency with which the measure classifies the subjects within the specified categories of the content domain. Even if a whole class of 20 students is tested by the measure, with the scores reflecting marked variability, the primary concern would be the consistency with which the measure classifies each student as master or nonmaster in terms of the stated criterion standard, the cut score. This brings to mind another very important point. In the case of the criterion-referenced measurement, unless the standard or cut score has high validity, the computation of a reliability index has little significance. A high reliability index in a situation in which the standard has been improperly set may mean only that the measure consistently classifies objects or phenomena incorrectly.

In the criterion-referenced framework, reliability is usually estimated by employing test-retest, parallel form, and intrarater and interrater agreement procedures.

TEST-RETEST PROCEDURE

As in norm-referenced measurement, the test-retest procedure is used in the criterion-referenced case to determine the stability of measurements over time. The focus of the test-retest procedure for criterion-referenced measures is on the stability of the classification of persons by a measure on two separate measurement occasions, that is, the ability of a measure to consistently classify objects or persons into the same categories on two separate occasions. The extent to which a criterion-referenced measure is able to reflect stability of results over time is an indication of the degree to which it is free from random measurement error.

To estimate the test-retest reliability for a given criterion-referenced measure, the nurse would follow the same general guidelines in administering the measure as described for the norm-referenced case in Chapter 5. However, the calculation of the reliability index would be different because of the difference in the way criterion-referenced test results are interpreted and used.

Two statistics have been identified that may be employed to assess the stability of criterion-referenced test results for the test-retest procedure, regardless of the number of categories established by the measure: P_o and Kappa (K). P_o is the proportion of objects or persons consistently classified in the same category on both measurement occasions. Thus, P_o is the proportion of observed agreements in classifications on both occasions. K, also referred to as Cohen's K, is the proportion of persons consistently classified in the same category on both occasions beyond that expected by chance. Hence, K is P_o corrected for chance agreements. P_o, also termed percent agreement, is computed by the following formula.

Formula 7-1 (Subkoviak, 1980):

$$P_o = \sum_{k=1}^{m} P_{kk}$$

where:

m = the number of classification categories

P_{kk} = the proportion of objects or persons consistently classified in the kth category

For illustrative purposes, assume that a criterion-referenced measure that is designed to assess a nurse's attitudes toward elderly clients is administered to 30 nurses at two-week intervals to determine test-retest reliability. Results are illustrated in Table 7-1. The P_o would be the proportion of student nurses consistently classified with positive/positive and negative/negative attitudes on both testing occasions. Thus, P_o would be the total proportion of the values in cells A and D. Hence:

$$P_o = \frac{15}{30} + \frac{12}{30}$$
$$= 0.50 + 0.40$$
$$= 0.90$$

Therefore, in this example 0.90 or 90 percent of the classifications made by the measure on both testing occasions were in agreement. However, some small portion of this estimate can be attributed to chance and 0.90 is, therefore, an overestimate of the stability of the test. The proportion of chance agreements (P_c) in Table 7-1 can be computed by the product of the corresponding row and column totals as indicated by Formula 7-2.

Formula 7-2 (Subkoviak, 1980):

$$P_c = \sum_{k=1}^{m} P_{k.}P_{.k}$$

TABLE 7-1 Hypothetical test results matrix for 30 nurses for computing P_o and K on a measure of nurse attitudes toward elderly clients

		First Administration		
		Positive	Negative	Totals
Second Administration	Positive	(A) 15	(B) 2	(A + B) 17
	Negative	(C) 1	(D) 12	(C + D) 13
	Totals	(A + C) 16	(B + D) 14	(A + B + C + D) 30

where:

  m   = the number of classification categories

  $P_k.P_k.$ = the proportion of objects or persons assigned to category k on each measurement occasion, respectively.

In this situation P_c would be computed by the proportions for (A + B) (A + C) + (C + D) (B + D). Thus,

$$P_c = \left(\frac{17}{30}\right)\left(\frac{16}{30}\right) + \left(\frac{13}{30}\right)\left(\frac{14}{30}\right)$$
$$= (0.57 \times 0.53) + (0.43 \times 0.47)$$
$$= 0.30 + 0.20$$
$$= 0.50$$

The proportion of nonchance agreements is provided by Kappa (K) (Cohen, 1960). P_o, observed agreements, and P_c, chance agreements, are used to calculate K as follows:

Formula 7-3 (Martuza, 1977; Subkoviak, 1980):

$$K = \frac{P_o - P_c}{1 - P_c}$$

In the present example, K is computed by:

$$K = \frac{0.90 - 0.50}{1 - 0.50}$$
$$= \frac{0.40}{0.50}$$
$$= 0.80$$

Several points should be kept in mind regarding the interpretation of P_o and K values. The value of P_o can range from 0 to 1.00. Total disagreement in observed test classifications is reflected by a P_o value of 0, while total agreement in observed results is reflected by a P_o value of 1.00. As indicated by the formula for K, the value of K is always less than or equal to P_o. The size of the difference between P_o and K is always a function of the size of P_c or chance agreements. The value of K always lies within an interval between -1.00 (which represents complete inconsistency of test results) and 1.00 (which reflects total consistency of results). The upper limit of 1.00 for K is fixed; however, the lower-bound value may fluctuate from one situation to another depending upon several influencing factors. Both P_o and K are affected by factors such as test length, number of response alternatives (e.g., when items are multiple choice), the value of the cut score used to classify subjects, and the homogeneity of the group of subjects. At this time, guidelines related to these factors (which would facilitate further interpretation of P_o and K values) have not been explicated. Whenever P_o and K are used to describe the reliability of a criterion-referenced test, these influencing factors should be clearly described because of their impact on the values of P_o and K (Martuza, 1977).

An upper-bound K value of 1.00 will result only when the marginal distributions for two administrations have the same proportions in them, for example, when the proportions in the right upper cell (A + B) and in the bottom left cell (A + C) of the table are the same. One can determine the maximum possible value of K for a specific situation by adjusting the values within the cells of the table to reflect the maximum number of consistent test classifications that are congruent with the observed marginal proportions (marginal proportions are not changed); and by calculating a revised version of K using the adjusted values. When this is done the resulting value is K_{max}, which represents the upper limit value that K could take on with a particular distribution of results. The K_{max} value provides information that can facilitate a better interpretation of a specific K value. When the K/K_{max} ratio is calculated, it provides a value that can be interpreted on a standard scale. The upper limit of this ratio is 1.00.

The computation of K_{max} for the information provided in Table 7-1 is conducted by first transforming all of the values in Table 7-1 to proportions as shown in Table 7-2. The proportions in the cells of Table 7-2 are then adjusted to reflect the maximum number of agreements that are congruent with the observed marginal proportions as shown in Table 7-3. At this point K_{max} can be calculated using the formula for K. Hence:

TABLE 7-2 Data from Table 7-1 expressed as proportions

		First Administration		
		Positive	Negative	Totals
Second Administration	Positive	(A) 0.50	(B) 0.07	(A + B) 0.57
	Negative	(C) 0.03	(D) 0.40	(C + D) 0.43
	Totals	(A + C) 0.53	(B + D) 0.47	(A + B + C + D) 1.00

TABLE 7-3 Adjustments required in Table 7-2 for the calculation of K_{max}

		First Administration		
		Positive	Negative	Totals
Second Administration	Positive	(A) 0.53	(B) 0.04	(A + B) 0.57
	Negative	(C) 0.00	(D) 0.43	(C + D) 0.43
	Totals	(A + C) 0.53	(B + D) 0.47	(A + B + C + D) 1.00

$$K_{max} = \frac{0.53 + 0.43 - (0.57)(0.53) + (0.43)(0.47)}{1 - (0.57)(0.53) + (0.43)(0.47)}$$

$$= \frac{0.96 - 0.50}{1 - 0.50}$$

$$= \frac{0.46}{0.50}$$

$$= 0.92$$

The K value for the present example is 0.80 and the K_{max} value is 0.92. Based on these findings it can be assumed that the measure classified the nursing students with a relatively high degree of consistency, since K/K_{max} is 0.87.

THE PARALLEL FORMS PROCEDURE

There are some situations when more than one form of a measure is desirable. For instance, in situations in which subjects are measured before and after a nursing intervention, it may be preferable to administer a parallel form on subsequent administrations. The test-retest procedure has a potential pitfall which makes that approach to the study of the reliability questionable, since significant events may occur during the between-testing interval that might interfere with results on the second administration. The use of parallel forms of a measure could help remedy such situations. However, a major concern in instances in which parallel forms of a measure are used is whether the two forms produce a substantial degree of agreement or consistency in the classification of subjects in a specified group.

Two criterion-referenced measures are considered parallel if they assess the same content domain, that is, if they were constructed with the same set of test specifications, and items are relatively homogeneous. Parallel forms of a criterion-referenced measure may be created through random item selection from a pool of items constructed with the same test specifications or the same item generation rules (Popham, 1978).

The approach to the estimation of the reliability of parallel forms involves administering the two alternate forms of the measure to one specific group on the same measurement occasion or on two separate occasions. The nurse would then calculate P_o and K in the same manner used in the test-retest case. Data from the two forms would be compiled and placed in a matrix as shown in Table 7-1. However, the labels First Administration should be changed to Form 1, and Second Administration to Form 2. If the two forms have high parallel form reliability there will be a high consistency in the classification of subjects into categories. In the parallel forms procedure, high P_o and K values reflect consistency between the alternate forms of a measure.

INTERRATER AND INTRARATER AGREEMENT PROCEDURES

As with the test-retest and the parallel forms procedures, P_o and K can be employed to estimate interrater agreement and intrarater agreement. The focus of interrater agreement in the criterion-referenced case is on the consistency of classifications of two (or more) different raters who classify a specified group of objects or persons using the same measurement tool on the same measurement occasion. For example, if a rating tool designed to measure the environmental safety of nursing units is used, two nurse raters could be employed to independently classify a group of nursing units as either safe or unsafe one at a time. Once results are obtained, P_o and K could be calculated to determine interrater agreement for the classification of the safety of the nursing units. The values of P_o and K are computed in the same manner as indicated previously and used as the index of interrater agreement. Prior to computing P_o and K the data would be set up in a matrix table similar to Table 7-1, but with the appropriate label changes, that is, changing First Administration to Rater 1, Second Administration to Rater 2, Positive to Safe, and Negative to Unsafe.

Intrarater agreement for criterion-referenced measurement situations is the consistency with which a single rater classifies a group of persons or objects, using a specified measuring tool after rating each person or object on two separate occasions. In instances when intrarater agreement is used, there is a danger that the first rating might affect the second rating. Steps would be taken to minimize this problem by using such techniques as obscuring the identification of the persons or objects being rated, altering the order in which ratings are done and reordering the pages of the rating tool if appropriate. Data are arrayed in a matrix in the manner discussed previously, with the proper labeling changes. P_o and K are then calculated to provide an index of intrarater agreement (Martuza, 1977).

VALIDITY

Once a measure has been constructed it is crucial to ascertain if it is valid; that is, if it measures what it purports to measure. Thus, once the initial construction of the measure has been completed, it is necessary to subject it to validity testing. When indicated, based on validity information, the measure is revised to enhance its validity. The process of tool development is therefore a cyclical process that involves testing, revision, and retesting the measure until there is sufficient evidence that it is valid.

The validity of a criterion-referenced measure can be analyzed at the item and test levels to ascertain if the measure functions in a manner consistent with its purposes. As Berk (1980b, p. 47) so aptly pointed out, the focus of item validity for criterion-referenced measures is "how well each item measures its respective objective (item-objective congruence)" and helps classify persons or objects into their appropriate category (item discrimination). Test validity focuses on the representativeness of a cluster of items in relation to the specified content domain (content validity), the significance of test results in relation to the initial conceptualization of the measure (construct validity), the decisions that result from the scores on the measure (decision validity), the extent to which future performance on a measure can be predicted from performance on a prior measure (predictive validity), and the extent to which an individual's performance on one measure can be used to estimate an individual's performance on a criterion measure (concurrent validity). For instance, in a test designed to measure whether or not a nurse understands the concept of homeostasis, item-objective congruence would relate to how well a specific item in the test matched or tested content related to the respective test objective. Item discrimination would depend on how well a specific item helped to screen nurses who understand homeostasis from those who do not. Content validity of the test would depend on how well the group of items in the test represented the range of potential items that would measure a nurse's knowledge of homeostasis. If one could predict a nurse's ability to apply the basic principles of homeostasis to the care of a patient with a potential for fluid and electrolyte imbalance, then the test could be said to have criterion-related validity. If the standard of test performance or cut score classified nurses who understand the principles of homeostasis as masters and classified those who do not understand homeostasis as nonmasters at a high level of probability, then the test would have a form of construct validity called decision validity. It is important to remember that item validity is a prerequisite to test validity. Hence, evidence of item validity is supportive of the establishment of the total validity of the measure and the validity of inferences based on the results.

Since criterion-referenced measures result in the classification of phenomena in relation to the domain of interest, the validity of standards or cut scores assumes special significance. In essence, validity in terms of criterion-referenced interpretations relates to the extent to which scores result in the accurate classification of objects in regard to their domain status. The measure also must be content valid, that is, its items or tasks must adequately represent the domain that is the focus of measurement. Since validity of the content of the measure is requisite to the validity of the total measure or test, attention is now given to a discussion of content validation of criterion-referenced measures.

CONTENT VALIDITY

As pointed out previously, content validity relates to how well the content of a test or measure matches the objective to be measured or domain specifications. Unless the items or tasks in a criterion-referenced measure assess the objective, any use of scores obtained will be questionable. As indicated previously, the major role of a criterion-referenced measure is to provide a clear description of an object's domain status. If a criterion-referenced measure does not fulfill this function, then it is fundamentally invalid. In order for a measure to provide a clear description of domain status, the content domain must be consistent with its domain specifications or objective. Thus, content validity of a criterion-referenced measure is the first type of validity that should be established and is prerequisite for all other types of validity.

Content is considered at the item and test levels. Item content validity is the extent to which each item is a measure of the content domain. At the total test level, content validity relates to the representativeness of the total collection of test items or tasks as a measure of the content domain. In Chapter 6, a discussion of test specifications and item generation strategies is provided. The major purpose of these approaches to the construction of the criterion-referenced measures is to facilitate the generation of content-valid test items. When highly structured rules are applied in the formulation of test items, such as with linguistic transformation and the facet design approach, then a logical connection between items and the content domain can be demonstrated which supports the validity of the measure. The use of highly structured item generation rules can be considered an a priori approach to content validity, because such rules assure the validity of items and the representativeness of the domain. In most instances it is not possible to use such structured rules to generate items, and the quality of items then must be assessed independently after they have been formulated. This is an a posteriori approach to the validation of test items.

Two approaches are useful for an a posteriori content validation. The most frequently used approach uses content specialists to assess the quality and representativeness of the items within the test for measuring the content domain. Content specialists examine the format and content of each item and assess whether it is an appropriate measure of some part of the content domain of interest as determined by test specifications. The second approach is an objective approach that uses empirical techniques in much the same manner in which empirical techniques are used to validate norm-referenced measures. Some empirical procedures used in the validation of norm-referenced measures can be used in criterion-referenced test validation. However, these statistics must be used and interpreted correctly in the context of the criterion-referenced framework. Rovinelli and Hambleton (1977) suggest that empirical methods used for item discrimination indices have limited usefulness, because they can only be used to identify aberrant items without any intention of eliminating items from the item pool. It is not appropriate to rely on item statistics to select the items for criterion-referenced measures, because this would theoretically alter the content domain and thereby weaken the interpretability of the domain score (Berk, 1980a; Hambleton, Swaminathan, Algin, and Coulson, 1978; Millman, 1974; Millman and Popham, 1974). Therefore, obtaining content specialists' ratings holds the most merit for assessing item validities for determining which items should be retained or discarded; empirical item discrimination indices should be used primarily to detect aberrant items in need of revision or correction (Hambleton, 1980). The procedures discussed below are designed to determine if items that have been developed for a measure are valid either singularly or as a group.

VALIDITY ASSESSMENT BY CONTENT SPECIALISTS. Several procedures have been developed that use the judgment of content specialists for the assessment of the validity of test items or the group of items within a measure. In such procedures the role of content specialists is to interpret a measure's descriptive scheme or content in terms of how well it satisfies the domain specifications or objective. Content specialists selected for such a task should be conversant with the domain treated in the measuring tool. Care is taken to select individuals with expertise in the area by identifying appropriate criteria to guide the selection process. In most instances, two or more content specialists are employed; however, the number depends on the type of procedure.

Of the content validity procedures discussed, item-objective congruence focuses on the content validity at the item level, while the other procedures primarily place emphasis on the content validity of the group of items within a measure. Remember that if more than one objective is used for a measure, the items that are measures of each objective should be treated as separate tests.

Item-Objective Congruence. A procedure for the determination of item-objective congruence was demonstrated by Rovinelli and Hambleton (1976; 1977), which provides an index of the validity of an item based on the ratings of two or more content specialists. In this method content specialists are directed to assign a value of $+1$, 0, or -1 for each item, depending upon the item's congruence with the measure's objective. Whenever an item is judged to be a definite measure of the objective, a value of $+1$ is assigned. A rating of 0 indicates that the judge is undecided about whether the item is a measure of the objective. The assignment of a -1 rating reflects a definite judgment that the item is not a measure of the objective. Hence, the task of the content specialists is to make a judgment about whether or not an item falls within the content domain as specified by the measure's objective. The data that result from the judge's ratings are then used to compute the *index of item-objective congruence*.

The index of item-objective congruence provides useful information about the agreement between content specialists' ratings as to whether each item in a test measures the intended objective. The limits of the index range from -1.00 to $+1.00$. An index of $+1.00$ will occur when perfect positive item-objective congruence exists, that is, when all content specialists assign a $+1$ to the item for its related objective and a -1 to the item for all other objectives that are measured by the test. An index of -1.00 represents the worst possible value of the index and occurs when all content specialists assign a -1 to the item for what was expected to be its related objective and a $+1$ to the item for all other objectives. An advantage of the index of item-objective congruence is that it does not depend on the number of content specialists used nor on the number of objectives measured by the test.

The index of item-objective congruence is provided by the following formula.

Formula 7-4 (Martuza, 1977)

$$I_{ik} = \frac{(M - 1)\, S_k - S'_k}{2N\,(M - 1)}$$

where:

I_{ik} is the index of the item-objective congruence for item i and objective k

M is the number of objectives

N is the number of content specialists

S_k is the sum of the ratings assigned to objective k.

S'_k is the sum of the ratings assigned to all objectives, except objective k.

Based on the information provided in Table 7-4, the index of item-objective congruence can be calculated in the following manner.

It should be noted that in this case:

$I_{ik} = I_{11}$

$M = 4$

$N = 3$

$S_1 = 2$

$S'_1 = (-3) + (-2) + (-3) = -8$

Hence:

$$
\begin{aligned}
I_{11} &= \frac{(4 - 1)\,(+2) - (-8)}{2(3)\,(4 - 1)} \\
&= \frac{6 + 8}{18} \\
&= \frac{14}{18} \\
&= 0.78
\end{aligned}
$$

When the index is used to determine which items should be retained during the measure's development process, an index cut-off score to separate valid from nonvalid items within the test should be set. The setting of this index cut-off score is usually derived by the test developer. Hambleton (1980) suggests that this should be done by creating the poorest set of con-

TABLE 7-4 Judges' ratings of item-objective congruence for a hypothetical item 1

Content Specialist	Objective			
	1	2	3	4
A	+ 1	− 1	− 1	− 1
B	+ 1	− 1	− 1	− 1
C	0	− 1	0	− 1
S_k	+ 2	− 3	− 2	− 3

tent specialists' ratings that the test developer is willing to accept as evidence that an item is within the content domain of interest. After computing the index for this set of minimally acceptable ratings, the resulting index serves as the index cut-off score for judging the validity of the items. It serves as the criterion against which each item within the measure is judged, based on its index of item-objective congruence, which resulted from content specialists' ratings. If, for instance, the index cut-off score is 0.75, then all items with an index of item-objective congruence below 0.75 are deemed nonvalid, while those with an index of 0.75 or above are considered valid. Those with an index below 0.75 are discarded from the measure or analyzed and revised to improve their validity.

Determination of Interrater Agreement. Rating scales frequently are used to assess validity of the group of items within a measure. Content specialists are provided with the domain specifications or the objective for the measure along with a set of items. The content specialists then independently rate the relevance of each item to the specified content domain.

One technique involves a four-point rating scale whereby two content specialists rate the relevance of each item to a domain as $1 =$ not relevant, $2 =$ somewhat relevant, $3 =$ quite relevant, or $4 =$ very relevant. If, for example, a 30-item measure is constructed to assess adjustment to parenthood by new parents, then two judges could be employed to rate the relevance of each item to the specified domain by using the four-point rating scale. The two content specialists' ratings are used to compute P_o and K as measures of *interrater agreement*. A content validity index (CVI) also can be obtained. Suppose the ratings obtained from the judges are as shown in Table 7-5. P_o then is the proportion of items given a rating of not/somewhat relevant (1 or 2) and quite/very relevant (3 or 4) by both content specialists. Hence, in the case of content validity determination, P_o is representative of the consistency of judges' ratings of the relevance of the group of items within the test to the specified content domain. As noted previously, K is P_o corrected for chance agreements. P_o and K are calculated as described in Formulas 7-1 and 7-3.

Once obtained, what do the values of P_o and K mean? An acceptable level of interrater agreement varies from situation to situation. However, safe guidelines for acceptable levels are P_o values greater than or equal to 0.80, or K greater than or equal to 0.25. If P_o and K or either of these values is too low, one or a combination of two problems could be operating. First, this could be an indication that the test items lack homogeneity and that the domain is ambiguous or is not well defined. Second, the problem could be due to the raters who might have interpreted the rating scale labels differently or used the rating scale differently (Martuza, 1977). Refinement of the domain specifications is required if the former is the case. If the latter is the problem, the raters are given more explicit directions and guidelines in the use of the scale to reduce the chances of differential use.

The index of content validity (CVI), as discussed in Chapter 5, can be calculated from the content specialists' ratings and is the proportion of items rated as quite/very relevant (3 or 4) by both judges. In the present case the CVI is 24/30 = 0.80.

TABLE 7-5 Hypothetical content specialists' ratings of the relevance of 30 items for assessing adjustment to parenthood

		Judge 1		
		not/somewhat relevant (1 or 2)	quite/very relevant (3 or 4)	Totals
Judge 2	not/somewhat relevant (1 or 2)	(A) 3	(B) 2	(A + B) 5
	quite/very relevant (3 or 4)	(C) 1	(D) 24	(C + D) 25
	Totals	(A + C) 4	(B + D) 26	(A + B + C + D) 30

$$(1) \quad P_o = \frac{3 + 24}{30} = 0.90$$

$$(2) \quad P_c = \left(\frac{5}{30}\right)\left(\frac{4}{30}\right) + \left(\frac{25}{30}\right)\left(\frac{26}{30}\right)$$
$$= 0.022 + 0.722$$
$$= 0.74$$

$$(3) \quad K = \frac{P_o - P_c}{1 - P_c}$$
$$= \frac{0.90 - 0.74}{1 - 0.74}$$
$$= 0.62 \text{ (rounded)}$$

As indicated earlier, low values of P_o and K may be due to lack of homogeneity of items because of an inadequate domain definition. As noted in Chapter 6, a clear and precise domain definition and domain specifications function to communicate what the results of measurements mean to those people who must interpret them, and what types of items and content should be included in the measure to those people who must construct the items. Content specialists' ratings can be used to help check the descriptive clarity of the domain definition of a measure when indicated (Popham, 1978). Suppose that three content specialists are used to judge the congruence of the items in a measure of the specified domain, and that items were developed by 10 item writers who contributed 3 items each. The *proportion of homogeneous items*, as determined by each rater, will be useful in assessing the adequacy of the domain definition. For each judge the number of items rated as congruent divided by the total number of items in the measure yields the proportion of homogeneous items. For example, if a judge rated 20 of the items in a 30-item measure as congruent, the proportion of homogeneous items would be 20/30 = 0.67. Suppose the proportion of homogeneous items for the three content specialists are 0.67 (20 out of 30), 0.50 (15 out of 30), and 0.60 (18 out of 30). If, upon inspection of the item-by-item ratings of the judges, the majority of the item writers had at least one item that was judged not/somewhat relevant (1 or 2) by the three content specialists, then this would be support for lack of clarity in the domain definition.

Assume that the proportion of homogeneous items for the three content specialists are 0.90 (27 out of 30), 0.93 (28 out of 30), and 0.93 (28 out of 30). After scrutinizing the items, it becomes apparent that each of the items judged to be unlike the rest had been prepared by one item writer. In this case the flaw is not likely to be in the domain definition as specified, but in the interpretations of the one item writer.

Average Congruency Percentage. The content validity of a test also can be estimated by an *average congruency percentage* (Popham, 1978). Suppose four content specialists are identified and asked to read the domain specifications for a measure and then judge the congruence of each item on a 20-item measure with the specifications. The proportion of items rated congruent by each judge is calculated and converted to a percentage. Then the mean percentage for all four judges is calculated to obtain the average congruency percentage. For example, if the percentages of congruent items for the judges are 95, 90, 100, and 100 percent, the average congruency percentage would be 96.25 percent. An average congruency percentage of 90 percent or higher can be safely considered acceptable.

When using content specialists, accuracy of each can be checked by including a specified number of irrelevant or incongruent items in the item pool. The effectiveness of content specialists can be determined by the number of such aberrant items detected. Ratings of any content specialist who does not meet a set minimum level of performance in detecting these bad items are discarded from the analysis.

CONSTRUCT VALIDITY

Measurements obtained through the use of criterion-referenced measures are used to describe and to make decisions based on an object's domain status. It is therefore imperative that a criterion-referenced measure function in the manner consistent with the purpose for which it is designed and used. Even though content validation of a measure is an important initial step in this direction, content validity evidence alone does not insure a measure's construct validity. For example, a criterion-referenced measure that is designed to measure a diabetic patient's understanding of self care may actually only measure the patient's ability to recall factual information without truly measuring understanding. However, on the basis of content validation evidence, it may appear to measure understanding. Hence, evidence of the content representativeness of a measure does not guarantee that the measure is useful for the intended purpose. Although "we may say that a test's results are accurately descriptive of the domain of behaviors it is supposed to measure, it is quite another thing to say that the function to which you wish to put a descriptively valid test is appropriate" (Popham, 1978, p. 159). Thus, the major focus of construct validation for criterion-referenced measures is to establish support for the measure's ability to function in accordance with the purpose for which it is being used. Approaches used to assess construct validity for criterion-referenced measures are presented below.

EXPERIMENTAL METHODS AND CONTRASTED-GROUPS APPROACH. Experimental manipulation and the contrasted-groups approach can be used to generate support for the construct validity of criterion-referenced measures. The basic principles and procedures for these two approaches are the same for criterion-referenced measures as for norm-referenced measures (see Chapter 5). Since criterion-referenced measures yield nominal or ordinal data, nonparametric statistical procedures may be required when comparative statistical analysis is conducted. Experimental methods or the contrasted-groups approach may be used to assess the decision validity of a measure.

DECISION VALIDITY. The measurements obtained from criterion-referenced measures often are used to make decisions. For example: (1) a nursing student may be allowed to progress to the next unit of instruction if test results indicate that the preceeding unit has been mastered; (2) a woman in early labor may be allowed to ambulate if the nurse assesses, on pelvic examination, that the fetal head is engaged (as opposed to unengaged) in the pelvis; or (3) a diabetic patient may be allowed to go home if the necessary skills for self care have been mastered. These are just a few of the many examples of how criterion-referenced results can be used for decision making. The decision validity of criterion-referenced measures that are used for such decisions takes on special significance. The decision validity of a measure is supported when the set standard(s) or criterion classifies subjects or objects with a high level of confidence.

In most instances, two criterion groups are used to test the decision validity of a measure: one group known to be low in the attribute of interest and the other high. For example, suppose a measure is designed to test mastery of skills of application of aseptic technique. Also, suppose that students in a fundamentals of nursing course, who have no prior exposure to aspetic technique, are randomly assigned to one of two groups: one receiving instruction on aseptic technique, and the other receiving no instruction in the area. If the test has decision validity, a much higher percentage of students in the group receiving instruction should be classified as masters after instruction than nonmasters, and a higher percentage of those receiving no instruction should be classified as nonmasters by the test than as masters. The decision validity of the test would be calculated "by summing the percentage of instructed students who exceed the performance standard and the percentage of uninstructed students who did not" (Hambleton, 1980, p. 98). It is assumed that these are the groups who are correctly classified by the testing procedure. Thus, decision validity can range from 0 to 100 percent, with high percentages reflecting high decision validity.

Criterion groups for testing the decision validity of a measure also can be created if individuals can be classified prior to testing according to whether they are known by independent means to be low or high on the attribute tested. The congruence between the classifications resulting from the measure and the known classifications is used to calculate the decision validity of the measure. For example, assume that the validity of a nurse's assessments of the position of the fetal presenting part on pelvic examination during labor is considered. Suppose the fetal positions are also determined via sonography. The congruence between the nurse's assessments and the results from sonography is used to determine the decision validity of the nurse's assessments.

Decision validity is influenced not only by the quality of the measure, but also by the appropriateness of the criterion groups, the characteristics of the subjects, and the level of performance required or cut score. Of course, decision validity is necessary only in instances in which scores or results are used to make decisions (Hambleton, 1980).

CRITERION-RELATED VALIDITY

The functional usefulness of criterion-referenced measures is supported by criterion-related validity evidence. Criterion-related validity, particularly predictive validity evidence, establishes support that a measure functions as it should (Popham, 1978). Criterion-related validity studies of criterion-referenced measures are conducted in the same manner as for norm-referenced measures. The reader is referred to Chapter 5 for a thorough discussion of criterion-related validity approaches.

EMPIRICAL ITEM ANALYSIS PROCEDURES

Item analysis is useful in criterion-referenced as well as in norm-referenced measurement. However, as indicated earlier, in the criterion-referenced case, empirical item analysis procedures are used primarily to evaluate each item separately in order to help identify aberrant items that need revision. Criterion-referenced item analysis procedures determine the effectiveness of a specific test item to discriminate subjects who have acquired the target behavior and those who have not. It is important that the content of the measure be kept as representative of the specified content domain as possible. Therefore, caution should be exercised before items are discarded from a criterion-referenced measure based on empirical item analysis procedures. The nature of the subjects, the treatment, or intervention may result in an item discrimination index that may imply that the item does not function well, when it is actually content valid. However, if there is sufficient evidence that an item is not functioning as it should and also is not content valid, it is recommended that it be discarded from the measure.

In criterion-referenced item analysis procedures, empirical data are obtained from respondents in order to evaluate the effectiveness of the items of the measuring tool. The major goal is to evaluate if items function in the intended manner. The most commonly used item analysis procedures employ either pretest-post-test measurements with one group, or two independent measurements with two different groups. The selection of the groups to use depends upon the purpose of the measure. Groups chosen for item analysis of criterion-referenced measures are often referred to as criterion groups. Two approaches are used for identifying criterion groups: (1) the *criterion-groups technique,* which also may be referred to as the *uninstructed-instructed groups approach,* when the focus of measurement is knowledge; and (2) *pretreatment-post-treatment measures approach,* which in appropriate instances may be called *preinstruction-postinstruction measurements approach.*

The criterion-groups technique involves the testing of two separate groups at the same point in time—one group that is known by independent means to possess more of the specified trait or attribute, and a second group known to possess less. For example, if the purpose of a criterion-referenced measure is to identify parents who have and who have not adjusted to parenthood after the birth of a first child, two groups of parents would be of interest—those who have adjusted to parenthood and those who have not had a previous opportunity to adjust to parenthood. A group of parents who have previously experienced parenthood might then be contrasted with a group of inexperienced parents who have just had their first child. The subjects chosen for each of the groups should be as similar as possible on relevant characteristics, for example, social class, culture, and age. In addition, the proportional distribution of relevant characteristics between groups should be equivalent. The only real difference between the groups should be in terms of exposure to the specified treatment or experience.

The criterion-groups technique has a major advantage in that it is highly practical. Item analysis can be conducted at one point in time if a group that is known to possess more of the specified trait or attribute is available at the same time as a group that is low or lacking in the trait or attribute of interest. However, one disadvantage is the difficulty of defining criteria for identifying groups. Another is the requirement of equivalence of groups. It is often difficult to randomly assign persons to groups, such as when using instructed and uninstructed groups. Differences in group performance might be attributable to such characteristics as socioeconomic background, age, sex, or levels of ability, if groups are not proportionately balanced on relevant characteristics.

The pretreatment-post-treatment measurements approach involves testing one group of subjects twice—once before exposure to some specified treatment (pretreatment), and again after exposure to the treatment (post-treatment). Subjects are usually tested with the same set of items on both occasions, or a parallel or equivalent set of items can be administered on the second testing. In the case in which instruction is the treatment, testing would occur before instruction (preinstruction) and after instruction (post-instruction).

This approach has the advantage of allowing analysis of individual as well as group gains. However, a major limitation is the impracticality of administering the post-test. Item analysis cannot be done until after the treatment or instruction has been completed. A second limitation is the amount of time that may be required between the pretest and post-test. When the period between testings is short, there is a potential problem for *testing effect,* which could influence performance on the post-test. The use of parallel or equivalent items helps to obviate testing effect. If this is not possible because of practical constraints or the nature of the content domain, the period between administrations might be extended to reduce the carry-over effect of memory from the initial testing. The period between the pre- and post-test should not extend beyond four months to reduce the chances of a history or a maturation effect. Intervening events or simply growing older can influence individual performance or results on the post-test. Improvement in performance due to history or maturation or both can become inextricably mixed with the treatment or effects of instruction. Item analysis is designed to focus only on the change in responses to items because of treatment or instruction (Berk, 1980a).

Computation of the item statistics for the criterion-groups approach and the pretreatment-post-treatment measurements approach can be expedited by displaying item scores in a respondent X item matrix (Berk, 1980a). Table 7-6 illustrates item scores (0,1) on a hypothetical measure of parental adjustment for 12 experienced parents and another group of 12 inexperienced parents. A similar presentation is provided in Table 7-7 for a group of 10 students who were administered 8 items before and after instruction. An item is assigned a score of 0 for an incorrect response or no response, and a score of 1 is assigned if the item is answered correctly. Item difficulty level (also called item p level) and item discrimination indices can be easily calculated from item scores displayed in this manner.

ITEM DIFFICULTY. Because of the purpose of criterion-referenced measures, it is appropriate to examine the difficulty level of items and compare them between criterion groups. Separate item p levels should be calculated for each item in the measure for each of the criterion groups. As noted in Chapter 5, an item p value can range from 0 to 1.00 and is the proportion of persons in a group of respondents who answer the item correctly or appropriately. The higher the item p level, the easier the item. The item p levels for each item are compared between groups to help determine if respondents would have performed similarly on an item, regardless of which group they are in. The item p level should be higher for the group that is

TABLE 7-6 Item scores for a group of experienced parents and a group of inexperienced parents on a hypothetical measure of parental adjustment (Criterion-groups technique)

	Inexperienced Parents						Experienced Parents				
			Item						Item		
Parent	1	2	3	4	5	Parent	1	2	3	4	5
A	0	0	0	1	0	A	1	1	0	1	1
B	1	0	0	0	0	B	1	1	1	1	1
C	0	0	0	0	1	C	1	0	1	1	1
D	0	0	0	0	0	D	0	1	1	0	1
E	1	0	1	0	0	E	1	1	1	1	1
F	0	0	0	1	0	F	1	1	1	1	1
G	1	0	1	0	0	G	1	0	1	1	1
H	0	0	0	0	0	H	1	1	1	1	0
I	1	1	0	0	0	I	1	0	0	0	1
J	0	0	0	0	1	J	0	1	1	1	1
K	0	0	0	0	0	K	1	1	1	1	0
L	0	1	0	0	0	L	1	1	1	1	1

TABLE 7-7 Item scores for preinstruction-postinstruction measurements for a group of students (Pretreatment-post-treatment measurements approach)

| | Preinstruction | | | | | | | | | Postinstruction | | | | | | | |
| | Item | | | | | | | | | Item | | | | | | | |
Student	1	2	3	4	5	6	7	8	Student	1	2	3	4	5	6	7	8
A	0	0	0	1	0	0	0	0	A	1	1	1	1	1	0	1	1
B	0	0	1	0	1	1	0	0	B	0	1	0	1	1	1	1	1
C	1	0	0	0	0	0	0	1	C	1	1	1	1	1	1	1	0
D	0	1	0	0	0	1	0	0	D	1	1	1	0	1	1	1	1
E	0	0	0	1	0	0	0	0	E	1	1	1	1	1	1	1	1
F	0	1	0	0	0	0	0	0	F	1	0	1	1	1	1	1	1
G	0	0	0	0	0	0	0	1	G	1	1	1	1	1	1	1	1
H	0	0	0	0	1	0	0	0	H	0	0	1	0	0	1	0	1
I	0	0	1	0	0	0	0	0	I	1	0	1	1	1	1	0	0
J	1	0	0	0	0	1	0	0	J	0	1	0	1	0	1	1	1

known to possess more of a specified trait or attribute than for the group known to possess less. Hence, the item p level should be substantially higher on a measure of parental adjustment for a group of experienced parents, who have had an opportunity to adjust to parenthood previously, than for a group of inexperienced parents. If this were the case, this would be positive evidence of item validity. Likewise, the item p levels of a group should be higher on a post-test after a relevant treatment has been provided than on the pretest. For example, if the instructional treatment relevant to the objectives of the measure is known to be reasonably effective, then a substantial increase in the item p level from pretest to post-test would be support for the validity of the item.

ITEM DISCRIMINATION. The focus of item discrimination indices for criterion-referenced measures is on the measurement of performance changes (e.g., pretest-post-test) or differences (e.g., experienced parents-inexperienced parents) between the criterion groups. Criterion-referenced item discrimination (generally referred to as D') is directly related to the property of decision validity, since it is reflected in the accuracy with which persons are classified on the domain of interest. Items with high positive discrimination indices improve the decision validity of a test. Although a vast array of item discrimination indices for criterion-referenced measures has been described in the literature, those discussed here are considered practical in terms of their ease of calculation and meaningfulness for the test development process (Berk, 1980a).

A rather simple item discrimination index, which can be used with data obtained via the criterion-groups technique, is the criterion groups difference index (CGDI) (also known as the uninstructed-instructed group difference index). The CGDI is the proportion of respondents in the group known to have less of the trait or attribute of interest who answered the item appropriately or correctly subtracted from the proportion of respondents in the group known to possess more of the trait or attribute of interest who answered it correctly.

Formula 7-5

$$CGDI = \begin{bmatrix} \text{the item p level for} \\ \text{group known to possess} \\ \text{more of the attribute} \end{bmatrix} - \begin{bmatrix} \text{the item p level for} \\ \text{group known to have less} \\ \text{of the attribute} \end{bmatrix}$$

Three item discrimination indices that can be employed when the pretreatment-post-treatment measurements approach is used are: (1) pretest-post-test difference, (2) individual gain, and (3) net gain. The *pretest-post-test difference index* (PPDI) is the proportion of respondents who answered the item correctly on the post-test minus the proportion who responded to the item correctly on the pretest.

Formula 7-6

$$PPDI = \begin{bmatrix} \text{the item p level} \\ \text{on the post-test} \end{bmatrix} - \begin{bmatrix} \text{the item p level} \\ \text{on the pretest.} \end{bmatrix}$$

The *individual gain index* (IGI) is the proportion of respondents who answered the item incorrectly on the pretest and correctly on the post-test. For example, in Table 7-8, which shows the response data on an item by 50 respondents, IGI would be the value in cell C divided by the total number of respondents as given below in Formula 7-7.

Formula 7-7

$$IGI = \frac{C}{A + B + C + D}$$
$$= \frac{35}{50}$$
$$= 0.70$$

The *net gain index* (NGI) is the proportion of respondents who answered the item incorrectly on both occasions subtracted from the IGI. Thus, NGI is an extension of IGI which considers the performance of all respondents who answered the item incorrectly on the pretest. Given the information in Table 7-8, the NGI could be calculated in the following manner:

Formula 7-8

$$NGI = IGI - \frac{D}{A + B + C + D}$$
$$= \frac{0.70 - 7}{50}$$
$$= 0.56$$

The selection of an item discrimination index is determined by the criterion groups providing the data for analysis. CGDI is the only index dis-

TABLE 7-8 Hypothetical response data on an item by 50 respondents

		Post-test		
		Correct	**Incorrect**	**Total**
Pretest	**Correct**	(A) 5	(B) 3	(A + B) 8
	Incorrect	(C) 35	(D) 7	(C + D) 42
	Total	(A + C) 40	(B + D) 10	(A + B + C + D) 50

cussed for the criterion-groups technique. Of the three indices appropriate for pretreatment-post-treatment groups, NGI provides the most conservative estimate of item discrimination and uses more information. NGI also provides a greater range of possible values than IGI (Berk, 1980a).

The range of values for each of the indices discussed above is -1.00 to $+1.00$, except for IGI which has a range of 0 to $+1.00$. A high positive index for each of these item discrimination indices is desirable, since this would reflect the item's ability to discriminate between criterion groups. The nature of the content domain and the measure's objective, along with the method used to compute discrimination, would influence the level at which the item discrimination index would be deemed acceptable. At the very least, an item discrimination index should be positive. A summary of criterion-referenced item discrimination indices discussed above is presented in Table 7-9.

A useful adjunct item discrimination index is provided through the use of P_o or K to measure the effectiveness of an item in relation to the total test in classifying subjects into categories (Martuza, 1977). For example, groups of masters and nonmasters can be created after the fact as determined by the relevant cut score for a test. The proportion of subjects who are classified as masters and nonmasters by the test are checked against the proportion of masters and nonmasters on the item. If, for example, the data (expressed as proportions) in Table 7-10 reflect classifications by a specific item and the test for a group of subjects, agreement between these two classifications could be considered an index of item discrimination. Thus, in this case there is 38 percent agreement between the item and the test as determined by the value of K.

At this point, the value of K_{max} can be calculated to determine the maximum possible agreements consistent with the observed marginal proportions in Table 7-6. The tabular adjustments required are presented in Table 7-11. The value of K_{max} in this instance is 0.69. When K is considered in terms of the value of K_{max}, there is evidence that the item discriminates between masters and nonmasters, since K/K_{max} is 0.55.

When item p levels and discrimination indices do not support the validity of the item, the problem could be explained in terms of the item itself, the objective, or the nature of the treatment. When an item p level is much

TABLE 7-9 Summary of selected criterion-referenced item discrimination indices

Index	Range of Values	Definition	Comments
Criterion groups difference index (CGDI)	−1.00 to +1.00	The proportion of respondents in the group known to possess more of the attribute of interest who answered the item correctly minus the proportion of respondents in the group known to possess less of the attribute who answered it correctly.	Commonly referred to as the uninstructed-instructed group difference index when used in instructional context. Index is only sensitive to group differences. Does not focus on individual performance differences.
Pretest-Post-test difference index (PPDI)	−1.00 to +1.00	The proportion of respondents who answered the item correctly on the post-test minus the proportion who responded to the item correctly on the pretest.	Index is only sensitive to group changes in performance and not to individual performance gain or loss.
Individual gain index (IGI)	0 to +1.00	The proportion of respondents who answered the item incorrectly on the pretest and correctly on the post-test.	Reflects change in performance in group based on performance changes by the individuals within the group who shifted from incorrect to correct response from pretest to post-test.
Net gain index (NGI)	−1.00 to +1.00	The proportion of respondents who answered item incorrectly on both the pretest and post-test subtracted from IGI.	Considers performance of all respondents who answered item incorrectly on the pretest. Yields values that are more conservative than preceding indices.

Adapted from: Berk, R.A. Item analysis. In R.A. Berk (ed.): *Criterion Referenced Measurement: The State of the Art.* Johns Hopkins University Press, Baltimore, 1980, p. 49–79.

TABLE 7-10 Joint mastery classifications of examinees by one item and the total test score expressed as proportions

		Test Classifications		
		Master	**Nonmaster**	**Totals**
Item	**Master**	(A) 0.70	(B) 0.05	(A + B) 0.75
Classifications	**Nonmaster**	(C) 0.15	(D) 0.10	(C + D) 0.25
	Totals	(A + C) 0.85	(B + D) 0.15	(A + B + C + D) 1.00

$$P_o = 0.70 + 0.10 = 0.80$$

$$P_c = (0.75)(0.85) + (0.25)(0.15) = 0.68$$

$$K = \frac{P_o - P_c}{1 - P_c}$$

$$= \frac{0.80 - 0.68}{1 - 0.68}$$

$$= \frac{0.12}{0.32}$$

$$= 0.38$$

higher than expected on the pretest or in a group with less of the specified attribute, it is possible that there has been previous exposure to the content domain. If the p level is much lower than expected on a post-test, the objective may be too difficult or the treatment may have been ineffective. A much lower than expected item discrimination index could be due to one or a combination of the problems cited above (Berk, 1980a).

When the item itself is suspected of being faulty, then it must be carefully scrutinized. Usually a negative discrimination index is due to a faulty item. Examination of the structure of the item and each response alternative is in order. Ambiguity, ineffective distractors, and more than one correct answer on a multiple-choice test should be considered. It is a good idea to get item reviews from respondents at the time the tool is administered, when the purpose of the administration is to obtain data for item analysis. Respondents can be asked to identify confusing items, items with no correct answer or more than one correct answer, and other problems encountered while progressing through the test. Such information can be used when identifying and revising poor items.

TABLE 7-11 Tabular adjustments required in Table 7-10 for computation of K_{max}

		Test Classifications		
		Master	**Nonmaster**	**Totals**
Item	**Master**	(A) 0.75	(B) 0.00	(A + B) 0.75
Classifications	**Nonmaster**	(C) 0.10	(D) 0.15	(C + D) 0.25
	Totals	(A + C) 0.85	(B + D) 0.15	(A + B + C + D) 1.00

$$K_{max} = \frac{1 - [\,(0.75)\,(0.85) + (0.25)\,(.15)\,]}{1 - [\,(0.75)\,(0.85) + (0.25)\,(.15)\,]}$$

$$= \frac{0.90 - 0.68}{1 - 0.68}$$

$$= \frac{0.22}{0.32}$$

$$= 0.69$$

SUMMARY

In this chapter attention has been focused on the reliability and validity of criterion-referenced measures. Although several similarities were noted between norm- and criterion-referenced reliability and validity conceptions, a number of substantial differences also were noted. As in the norm-referenced case, criterion-referenced measurements always involve some error that can be reduced with sound measurement approaches.

When measurements are subjected to criterion-referenced interpretations, the estimation of the correct domain classification is the primary concern. The focus of reliability estimates within the criterion-referenced framework is the consistency with which measures classify phenomena. Several reliability estimation approaches were discussed, including test-retest, parallel forms, and intrarater and interrater agreement procedures. The concern of criterion-referenced validity is not only with whether a measure assesses what it is purported to measure, but also whether it functions in accordance with the purpose for which it is designed and used. Content validity and the assessment of construct validity and criterion-related and decision validity are important for criterion-referenced measures. As with norm-referenced measures, the validity of criterion-referenced tools may be assessed at the test or item levels. Item validity is a prerequisite to test validity and may be estimated by the determination of item-objective congruence with the use of content specialists or estimated via empirical means. Item validity estimates provide important information that can be used to revise and improve criterion-referenced measures, thereby improving test validity. However, the validity of standards or cut scores takes on special significance and has a direct impact on the validity of the measure, because criterion standards or cut scores are used to classify phenomena in relation to a specified content domain.

REFERENCES

BERK, RA: "Item analysis." In BERK, RA (ed): *Criterion-Referenced Measurement: The State of the Art.* Johns Hopkins University Press, Baltimore, 1980a, p. 49–79.

BERK, RA: "Item and test validity." In BERK, RA (ed): *Criterion-Referenced Measurement: The State of the Art.* Johns Hopkins University Press, Baltimore, 1980b, p. 47–48.

COHEN, J: "A coefficient of agreement for nominal scales." *Educational and Psychological Measurement* 20:37–46, 1960.

HAMBLETON, RK: "Test score validity and standard-setting methods." In BERK, RA (ed): *Criterion-Referenced Measurement: The State of the Art.* Johns Hopkins University Press, Baltimore, 1980, p. 80–123.

HAMBLETON, RK SWAMINTHAN, H, ALGINA, J, AND COULSON, DB: "Criterion-referenced testing and measurement: A review of technical issues and developments." *Review of Educational Research* 48:1–47, 1978.

MARTUZA, VR: *Applying Norm-referenced and Criterion-referenced Measurement in Education.* Allyn and Bacon, Boston, 1977.

MILLMAN, J: "Criterion-referenced measurement." In POPHAM, WJ (ed): *Evaluation in Education: Current Applications.* McCutchan, Berkeley, CA, 1974, p. 311–397.

POPHAM, WJ: *Criterion-referenced Measurement.* Prentice-Hall, Englewood Cliffs, NJ, 1978.

ROVINELLI, RJ AND HAMBLETON, RK: "On the use of content specialists in the assessment of criterion-referenced test item validity." *Dutch Journal of Educational Research* 2:49–60, 1977. Also in *Laboratory of Psychometrics and Evaluative Research, Report No. 24.* The University of Massachusetts, Amherst, MA, 1976.

SUBKOVIAK, MJ: "Decision-consistency approaches." In BERK, RA (ed): *Criterion-Referenced Measurement: The State of the Art.* Johns Hopkins University Press, Baltimore, 1980, p. 129–185.

8

STANDARDIZED APPROACHES TO MEASUREMENT

It has long been recognized in the physical sciences that measurement must be carried out in a rigorous and consistent manner; thus, considerable effort has been devoted to standardizing the measurement process in laboratory settings. For example, measurement devices such as balances, thermometers, and spectrophotometers are carefully constructed according to rigorous specifications, and their accuracy is checked regularly by comparison with recognized standards. Also, procedures for using the devices are prescribed in detail and in many instances are automated in order to maintain consistency. Defined rules or procedures are applied in assigning a value to a given result, and results are often interpreted using published tables showing the normal distribution of possible values. These activities and procedures represent attempts to *control* the measurement process in order to reduce error. Analogous standardized approaches to measurement are currently being advocated and used in the behavioral sciences and in nursing in order to approximate the rigor of a laboratory setting.

DEFINITION

Broadly defined, a standardized measure is a controlled measure. It is one that is constructed, administered, scored, and interpreted in a prescribed, precise, and consistent manner in order to reduce external influences that compromise reliability (Risley, et al, 1978; McGaghie, et al, 1978).

In order to be considered standardized, a measure must be carefully developed, rigorously tested before general use, consistently administered

213

and scored, and interpreted on the basis of established norms. Thus, standardized measures are considered a subset or special case of norm-referenced measures, distinguished by the explicit and conscious exercise of control in all aspects of their development, use, and interpretation.

At present there is no uniform set of criteria for defining standardized measures. As used in this text, the term standardized is applied to measures that have four essential characteristics:

1. A development process that involves testing, analysis, and revision in order to assure high technical quality;
2. A fixed set of items or operations designed to measure a clearly defined concept, attribute, or behavior;
3. Explicit rules and procedures for administration and scoring; and
4. Provision of norms to assist in interpreting a given score.

In the light of these criteria a variety of instruments and procedures may be considered standardized measures. Examples include published paper-and-pencil tests designed to measure cognitive achievement; tests designed to measure complex abilities, such as verbal and quantitative skill, problem-solving, abstract reasoning, spatial perception, or manual dexterity; tests to measure personality characteristics, emotional adjustment, attitudes, and interests; tests to assess the developmental level of infants and children; and tests designed to measure anatomical and physiological characteristics. A standardized approach can be applied in measuring a wide range of attributes and behaviors of interest in nursing. The defining characteristics of a standardized measure refer to the properties of the measure itself rather than to the nature of the entity being measured.

STANDARDIZED VERSUS NONSTANDARDIZED MEASURES

Standardized measures are similar in many respects to informal or nonstandardized measures that have been carefully constructed. Some informal measures may not meet all of the defining characteristics of a standardized measure, even though elements of control are included in many aspects of their construction. In this sense, standardization may be considered a matter of degree. It is possible to compare informal measures in terms of the degree to which they approximate the model for standardized measures. Some differences between standardized and informal measures are described below.

CONSTRUCTION

Standardized measures are constructed by following a number of sequential steps, many of which are also used for nonstandardized measures. Although there is some variation, the following procedure is generally used (Gronlund, 1976; Tinkelman, 1971; McGaghie, et al, 1978):

1. Objectives, specifications, and a blueprint are developed;
2. Items are written or operations identified;
3. The items are pretested and analyzed using item statistics;

4. Acceptable items are assembled into a preliminary form (or preliminary equivalent forms) of the measure;
5. The preliminary form of the measure is experimentally administered to criterion groups of examinees to determine or verify the adequacy of time limits and instructions, difficulty level, discriminating power, reliability, and validity;
6. Revisions are made to eliminate items or operations that are unnecessary or do not contribute to the measure's reliability and validity;
7. A final form of the measure is assembled;
8. Uniform mechanisms for administration and explicit instructions for scoring are established;
9. The final form of the measure is administered to carefully selected referent groups in order to develop norms; and
10. The final version of the measure, a manual, and supplementary materials are made available for use.

This process is time consuming and complex, often taking several years. Because of the effort and time involved, standardized measures are usually developed for widespread use. Ideally their development incorporates the joint efforts of content and measurement experts throughout. The considerable effort expended is directed toward producing a measurement instrument or device that is of high technical quality and that can be used with consistency in a variety of settings.

Nonstandardized measures, even those that are carefully developed, generally do not involve as rigorous a construction procedure. Unique features of the construction of standardized measures include:

1. Development by experts;
2. Extensive pretesting and revision;
3. The development of prescribed procedures for administration and scoring; and
4. Most importantly, the administration of the final form of the instrument to specified groups for the purpose of establishing norms as a basis for interpretation.

CONTENT

Because they are designed for widespread and consistent use, standardized tests are characterized by content that is (1) sufficiently generic to be applicable in a variety of settings; (2) not time-bound or rapidly outmoded; and (3) fixed or predefined. In contrast, the content of nonstandardized measures is typically specific, geared to use in a given setting, and has potential to be flexible; thus, content may be updated frequently and adapted to accommodate minor changes.

Selection of content for any norm-referenced measure is based on a statement of purpose and a blueprint that specifies the elements or dimensions of the domain of behavior or cognition that is to be sampled and the relative emphasis that is to be given to each element. The purposes of a standardized measure are generally stated in terms that are not situation-specific, for they must be acceptable to a variety of potential users. Similarly, the blueprint reflects a definition of the domain to be measured that is potentially acceptable across settings and defensible on the basis of published research or expert opinion. Such a blueprint would eliminate content that is relevant only in a particular setting or situation or that is specific to a particular theory.

Consider, for example, the difference between the content of an informal classroom test to be administered in one school of nursing to measure achievement in a medical-surgical nursing course and that of a standardized achievement test designed to be administered across the nation to all students studying medical-surgical nursing. The former would reflect a theoretical perspective and content that had been defined by an individual faculty member or small group as important or that had been included in a required text. It could include reference to a given theory or to specific information taught only in that setting. The standardized test, however, would have to reflect content that is taught in schools nationally in order to be useful. The blueprint for the standardized test would therefore be based not on one person's definition but on systematic analysis of a variety of medical-surgical texts and course syllabi, the input of experienced medical-surgical nursing practitioners and educators, and relevant literature in the field. One example in which generic content that is not bound to a particular theoretical perspective has been identified for a standardized measure is the California Q-Sort, discussed in Chapter 9. Careful screening of content using the above approaches helps to eliminate conflicting or controversial ideas and new information that has not yet gained widespread acceptance. Neither would be appropriate for a standardized measure.

Because standardized measures are very time consuming to develop, they are generally used for several years without modification. Hence, content that can become rapidly outdated is generally precluded. Cognitive or affective behaviors that assume or indicate a knowledge of current events or very recent advances in the field are more appropriately included in informal than in standardized measures.

By definition, the content of a standardized measure is *pre-established*. Items or operations are carefully selected and tested. They cannot be changed or deleted by the user of the measure without modifying its known properties (reliability and validity), thus negating the essence of standardization. Nonstandardized measures are not content constrained. Thus, an important difference between the two types of measures is that the content of a standardized test is fixed well in advance of its general use, whereas the content of informal measures is generally defined by the developer-user. Importantly, when an informal measure that has been tested and used previously is modified for subsequent use, it in effect becomes a different measure, and former estimates of reliability and validity no longer apply.

ADMINISTRATION AND SCORING

In order to assure consistency, standardized measures are characterized by prescribed administration and scoring procedures. The method for administering the measure is determined in advance by the developer and is pretested. Once it is final, explicit instructions are provided for users in a test manual. Specific administration procedures obviously vary from measure to measure. They specify such elements as time limits, directions that are to be given the individual being measured, environmental conditions under which the measure is to be administered, and (for laboratory devices) the way in which the instrument is to be used. For some laboratory tests a standard administration may be assured by means of automation. Some standardized measures can be administered only by an individual who has been specifically trained and certified. Examples are the Brazelton (1973) Neonatal Assessment Scale and the Nursing Child Assessment Tools (Barnard and Earles, 1979).

Rules for scoring a standardized measure are explicit. For paper-and-pencil tests scoring keys will be provided if the instrument is to be hand scored. In some instances completed instruments are mailed to a central scoring facility for computer-assisted scoring. Standardized measures that involve observation include detailed rules for scoring to assure that any given behavior will be assigned the same numerical value by different raters and that identical behaviors will receive the same score. Advances in computer technology have resulted in highly automated scoring procedures for many physiological laboratory measures; in effect, scoring rules have been incorporated in designing the machinery and are applied automatically in processing the entity to be measured.

Informal or nonstandardized measures may incorporate uniform procedures for administration and scoring; however, they are usually more flexible, less detailed, and less explicit than procedures for standardized measures. The developer-user generally is free to define the procedures; however, the same cautions noted above apply in terms of redefining a procedure that has been previously established for use as an informal measure. If the administration and scoring procedures differ from one application to another or from the procedure designed by the developer, results are not truly comparable.

INTERPRETATION

Standardized measures are those for which norms have been established by administering the measure to groups that are representative of the population for which the measure is designed. Scores derived from standardized measures are assigned meaning on the basis of comparison with established norms; that is, interpretation of a given score involves comparing the score of an individual being measured with scores of larger samples of similar individuals. Frequently the norm (comparison) group is composed of individuals from widely distributed geographic areas, so that an individual's score is interpreted in comparison with a national distribution. Further, since norms are provided in published form (usually in the accompanying manual) and since procedures for interpretation may be clearly specified or automated, the meaning assigned to a given score is likely to be consistent across different settings and over time. Norms, norming procedures, and interpretation will be discussed in greater detail in later sections of this chapter. The crucial point is that for a standardized measure interpretation is comparative and carried out with reference to a well-defined, external group whose distribution of scores is known. Informal or nonstandardized measures generally do not have established norms to aid in interpretation. Score comparisons and interpretations, therefore, are limited to a given situation.

COMPARATIVE ADVANTAGES

The comparative advantages and disadvantages of standardized and nonstandardized measures are summarized in Table 8-1. Review of this table suggests that standardized measures are desirable for some purposes but not for others; hence, a standardized measure is not always better by definition than an informal one. For example, if a nurse researcher wished to assess the developmental level of abused children in relation to national norms, a standardized measure of child development would be appropriate. On the other hand, if the purpose were to compare the developmental level of children before and after a short hospitalization, a standardized measure would be of little value.

Because standardized and informal measures can provide different types of information that is useful for decision-making, evaluating, or understanding a particular phenomenon, the two types of measures are often used complimentarily. For example, schools of nursing often use both informal teacher-made tests and standardized National League for Nursing tests to measure student achievement in a given subfield of nursing. Schools may require as a basis for admission decisions both standardized aptitude tests (such as the Scholastic Aptitude Test) and informal aptitude tests developed by the school in relation to specific abilities deemed relevant to its particular curriculum. A clinician or researcher wanting to measure preoperative anxiety might combine a standardized laboratory procedure (e.g., measurement of catecholamines in the urine), a standardized measure of anxiety (e.g., the State-Trait Anxiety Inventory, Spielberger, et al, 1970), and an informal measure specific to the preoperative situation or a particular type of surgical procedure. Decisions about the use of standardized or nonstandardized measures must be based on the purposes for which the information will be used and the types of questions that must be answered.

NORMS

As used in reference to standardized measures, norms refer to statistical information that describes the scores earned by members of a defined population or defined reference group (or generated from a defined set of observations) with which the score earned by a particular individual (or generated from a given observation) can be compared. Some terminological confusion frequently is encountered in discussions of norms and standards. A standard is an ideal—an object or state defined by authority or consensus as the basis for comparison. It represents what ought to be, whereas a norm represents what is. For many aspects of physical and chemical measurement (e.g., weight, length, temperature) standards have been established and serve as the basis for scoring a given result. For example, in the measurement of length, a standard has been developed by the National Bureau of Standards that serves as the basis for constructing measurement devices (e.g., rulers), determining their accuracy, and scoring results. Norms or distributions of scores describing the lengths or heights of representative samples of objects (including people) also have been generated to depict what is. Standards are used to answer the question, "How does this score compare with the ideal score?" Norms are used to answer the question, "How does this score compare with those generated from a representative sample of identical observations?"

TYPES OF NORMS

Norms can be classified on the basis of the scope of the population from which they were generated or the units in which they are expressed. *National* norms are those describing scores earned by a national sample of subjects. They have been established for many of the standardized tests used in nursing and are useful for comparison with individuals from a wide variety of locales and backgrounds. National samples are characterized by their heterogeneity; that is, they contain individuals who vary in sociodemographic characteristics such as age, sex, race, urban-rural residence, social status, and educational background. As a result, national norms may be too general to permit specific interpretation and action. In order to supply information that will be useful, national norms may be provided in terms that display the distribution of the sample as a whole *(total group norms)* as well as the distributions of subgroups selected according to relevant characteristics *(differentiated norms)*. Examples of differentiated norms are sex-specific norms, age-specific norms, and occupation-specific norms. National norms may be based on a representative sample of the nation's population or on a nationwide sample of a select, but relevant, group of individuals. Norms for the NLN achievement tests are not based on a sample of the U.S. population but on a sample of students from nursing education programs across the country.

Regional and *local* norms are those established on the basis of more geographically circumscribed samples. Although the developer of a nationally standardized measure may supply norms specific to given multistate regions of the country, local norms are generally established by users themselves: teachers, counselors, administrators, and practitioners. Local norms are established on the basis of samples of subjects in a given school, agency, or district. Because these samples are generally more homogeneous than regional or national samples, local norms are valuable as a basis for decision making in specific settings. For example, schools of nursing may find local norms for a standardized aptitude test derived from a sample of current students more useful than national norms in admission decisions, because the former constitute a more relevant basis for comparison.

Norms may also be classified by the statistical units in which they are expressed. Examples are percentile norms and standard score norms. The strengths and weaknesses associated with expressing norms in terms of these units were addressed in Chapter 4.

TABLE 8-1 Comparative advantages and disadvantages of standardized and non-standardized measures

Standardized Measure	Nonstandardized Measure
Construction	
Advantages: Involves input of experts; method of construction is designed to enhance technical quality, reliability, and validity; procedure used in construction and testing is usually described.	Advantages: May be carried out in situations in which time and resources are limited; short span of time is required between planning and use of the measure.
Disadvantages: Costly, time consuming; requires adequate resources.	Disadvantages: Construction procedure is variable and does not necessarily assure high quality; procedure generally is not described in detail; amount of expert input is variable and may be unknown.
Content	
Advantages: Measures attributes or behaviors that are common to a variety of settings and situations; is applicable to many settings; reflects widespread consensus rather than localized emphasis; is applicable across time and locale; is well defined and fixed, allowing consistent comparison; parameters are usually specified.	Advantages: Well adapted to specialized needs and emphasis; flexibility allows adaptation to changes in materials or procedures; allows inclusion of controversial or timely information.
Disadvantages: Inflexible; cannot be adapted to local or specialized situations; may reflect consensus views that are incongruent with specialized needs and purposes; precludes innovative, controversial, or time-bound material.	Disadvantages: May reflect unique views or biases that are not deemed relevant by recognized authorities. Time- and situation-specificity precludes widespread use.
Technical Properties	
Advantages: Reliability (internal consistency and test-retest) is high, hence yields stable results; procedures to establish reliability and validity are reported, hence known to the user; items and operations have high discriminating power.	Advantages: Technical properties to be optimized are determined in light of the purposes of the measure.
Disadvantages: Stability of scores results in insensitivity to minor fluctuations that may be desirable to measure.	Disadvantages: Technical properties are frequently unknown and may be highly variable, depending on the construction procedures used.

ESTABLISHING NORMS

The process used to establish norms involves several steps.

1. A sample group (or groups) of individuals who are representative of those for whom the measure is designed is selected.

2. The final form of the measure is administered to these individuals according to the set procedure or protocol that has been developed and

TABLE 8-1 Continued

Standardized Measure	Nonstandardized Measure
Administration and Scoring	
Advantages: Established procedures provide consistency, hence comparable results; effects of different testing conditions and environments are minimized; centralized or automated scoring is cost efficient for large-scale efforts.	Advantages: Procedures can be developed in the light of specific needs and resources; flexible procedures permit last-minute alterations; local and/or hand scoring is cost efficient for small samples; time lag between administration and scoring is determined by the user.
Disadvantages: Inflexibility precludes altering to fit individual circumstances and resources; may be costly and time consuming; scheduling of administration and return of scored results may be controlled externally.	Disadvantages: Consistency between different administrations of the same measure is variable; different rules may be applied in scoring, thus yielding incomparable results.
Interpretation of Scores	
Advantages: Scores can be uniformly compared with norm groups, often at the national level; interpretation is likely to be consistent across applications; explicit instructions may be provided to facilitate interpretation.	Advantages: Comparisons and interpretations can be geared to specific needs and unique circumstances; amenable to situations for which comparison to a defined group is not an appropriate way to assign meaning to a score.
Disadvantages: National norms may be inappropriate for unique purposes; utility for decision making in specific settings is variable; inappropriate for purposes that do not require comparison with the status quo.	Disadvantages: No established basis for interpretation exists; consistency and accuracy of interpretation is variable, depending on the procedure used and the statistical skill of the interpreter.

under conditions that are identical to those recommended for administration.

3. Raw scores of the sample individuals are plotted in a frequency distribution, and descriptive statistics are computed.

4. A decision is made regarding the statistical units that will be used to express the norms and these statistics are computed.

5. Tables or graphs displaying the norms are prepared.

6. Norms are updated as necessary by reapplying steps 1 through 5. Since the norming procedures used are critical determinants of the accuracy and usefulness of the norms generated, each of these steps will be addressed in detail.

SELECTING THE STANDARDIZATION SAMPLE. The scores of individuals selected for the standardization or referent group serve as the basis for comparing all subsequent scores on the measure; thus, it is mandatory that these individuals accurately represent the larger population of individuals for whom the measure was designed. Using the purposes of the measure and the blueprint, the population of intended subjects must be clearly specified. Because most measures are designed for a specific purpose and are not universally applicable across all ages, cultures, educational levels, and situations, the relevant population is limited to some extent by the test purposes and blueprint. Many cognitive measures, for example, are designed to be age-specific, that is, they are applicable only to persons from the general population who fall within a specific age range. Other measures are designed only for persons in specific settings or circumstances or who have had certain experiences. For example, some nursing measures may be designed only for hospitalized patients or only for students who have completed an undergraduate nursing curriculum.

The relevant population is also determined by the scope of the norms to be developed. Examples of populations appropriate for establishing national norms would be all students enrolled as seniors in baccalaureate nursing programs, all adult patients hospitalized in public psychiatric institutions, or all three-week-old infants who have no known birth defects. Populations for local norms might include, for example, all students enrolled in a given school of nursing, all adult patients who had been hospitalized in a given institution, or all persons living in a defined geographical area. The important point is that the relevant population must be specified to include all individuals to whom the measure can appropriately be applied.

In specifying the population for establishing norms for any standardized measure it is important to consider that a variety of personal characteristics of potential subjects may be correlated with scores on that measure. For example, scores on an aptitude test to measure problem-solving potential may be related to the subject's educational level and background, age, or sex, as well as to the region or type of residential community. Scores on a measure of job satisfaction may be related to age, stage in career, sex, salary level, type of occupation, and so forth. The specific characteristics that are likely to be correlated with the concept, attribute, or behavior being measured should be identified on the basis of related literature. As noted above, some of these characteristics will have been taken into account in the test purposes and blueprint, and their impact on possible scores will have been controlled or held constant by limiting the relevant population to particular categories of individuals. Other characteristics assumed to be correlated with scores on the measure are not held constant by virtue of the population definition. Rather, they are acknowledged to be variables that potentially will influence the scores obtained from the population. It is important that these variables be specified in advance and that the relevant population include individuals who differ with respect to their status on these characteristics. Let us assume, for example, that it is known that an adult's educational level influences response to paper-and-pencil measures of anxiety. It would be important to specify that the relevant population for such a measure includes adults with a variety of educational levels, if, in fact, the measure is to be used across all segments of society. Including those with a range of educational backgrounds would potentially allow a wider range of possible scores to be obtained than limiting the population only to those with high school education or above. Remembering that norms make up the basis for comparing scores on the measure and therefore should reflect a wide range of possible scores, it is critical that the nature of the population that will ultimately be measured be specified as clearly as possible and that attempts be made to assure diversity with respect to characteristics that may have an impact on the scores obtained.

Once the relevant population for the measure has been identified, it is necessary to select a sample that is representative of the population to make up the referent group, that is, the group that will be used as the basis for establishing norms. The selection of a referent group that is truly representative of the individuals for whom the measure is intended is the most important and most difficult task in the standardization process. The norms for the measure are established on the basis of scores from the members of this sample (referent group) and serve as the basis for comparing scores from subsequent administrations of the measure. Thus, if a referent sample is atypical of the population that will ultimately be measured, there will not be an accurate basis for interpreting scores. If there is bias in the norms (i.e., if they do not represent the true distribution of the scores in the population), this bias will be transmitted in all subsequent interpretations of a given score.

Certain sampling procedures are more likely than others to yield a referent group that is representative of the test population. *Probability sampling* refers to a class of sampling procedures in which the process of selecting an individual for the sample is prescribed, such that each individual in the population has a known probability of being selected into the sample. Probability samples are selected at random; that is, the basis for the selection of a given individual is chance rather than conscious choice. Thus, it is possible to assume that by drawing a random sample any differences between the sample and the population will be randomly (or normally) distributed. The primary advantages of probability sampling for selecting a referent group for establishing norms are that bias is minimized and sampling error can be estimated. Several types of probability samples that can be used for selecting referent groups are described in Table 8-2.

Those probability sampling procedures that require enumerating each individual in the population (simple random sampling, systematic sampling, or stratified random sampling) are usually impractical for selecting referent groups for most standardized tests because of the large numbers of individuals included. *Cluster samples*, which involve identifying groups or clusters of individuals as the primary sampling units, are more efficient when the population is large. Such groups or clusters might include communities, census tracts, schools, hospitals, classrooms, or patient units. Once the clusters in the population are listed, a random sample of clusters is drawn and individuals within the randomly selected clusters make up the referent group. In establishing national and regional norms that involve a very large population, *multistage clustering sampling* is usually employed. This is a procedure that involves dividing the initially selected clusters into subunits or secondary sampling units, which are, in turn, randomly selected. The procedure can be continued through several stages involving successively smaller clusters until individuals can be enumerated and randomly sampled. An example of a multistage cluster sampling procedure is included in Figure 8-1. Cluster samples are more convenient and efficient than those that require enumerating the entire population; however, considerably larger sample sizes are required to achieve the same

TABLE 8-2 Probability samples used to select referent groups

Type of Sample	Procedure	Comments
Simple Random	1. List and number all individuals in the population. 2. Randomly select the sample using a random number table or other device.	1. Complete listing is often difficult to construct. 2. The procedure is costly and time consuming.
Stratified Random	1. Subdivide the population into two or more groups (strata) that are homogeneous with respect to a given characteristic. 2. From each group (stratum) randomly select a sample. 3. Numbers of subjects may be selected in proportion to the size of each stratum in the population (proportionate stratified random sample), or sampling fractions may differ from stratum to stratum (disproportionate stratified random sample).	1. Some characteristics of the population must be known in advance. 2. Can be used to assure representativeness on the selected characteristic(s) used for stratification. 3. Can be used to assure inclusion of sufficient numbers of subjects within selected subgroups. 4. The procedure is costly and time consuming.
Systematic	1. List all individuals in the population. 2. Determine the width of the selection interval (K) to be used by dividing the total number in the population by the number of sample cases desired. 3. Select a starting point at random (termed the random start) within the first selection interval using a random number table. 4. After the random start, select every K^{th} case.	1. Can be applied to stratified or unstratified listings. 2. Generally is more efficient and convenient than simple random sampling. 3. Is subject to bias if there is periodic or rhythmic tendency inherent in the list (e.g., if every K^{th} element has more or less of a given characteristic than the others). 4. Is subject to bias if there is a linear trend in the list. 5. Effects of periodicity and linearity can be minimized by shifting random starts part-way through the list.
Cluster	1. List the largest (most inclusive) unit in which population elements are found (termed the primary sampling units). 2. Randomly select a sample of these units. 3. Subdivide the sampled units into smaller units (secondary sampling units). 4. Randomly select a sample of these units. 5. Repeat the procedure in steps 3–4 as many times as necessary until the final stage is reached.	1. In all but the final stage, clusters or groups are sampled rather than individuals. 2. Stratification can be used for any part of the multistage process. 3. Is cost and time efficient, particularly for large, dispersed populations. 4. Sampling errors are greater with cluster samples than with other samples of the same size. 5. Special statistical procedures should be employed for data analysis.

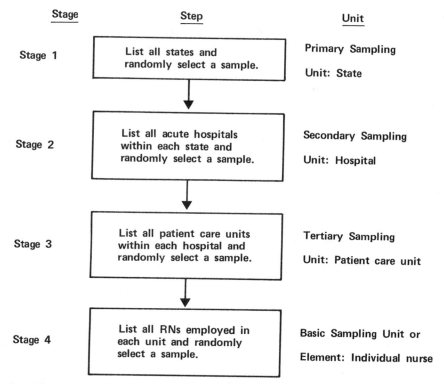

Stage	Step	Unit
Stage 1	List all states and randomly select a sample.	Primary Sampling Unit: State
Stage 2	List all acute hospitals within each state and randomly select a sample.	Secondary Sampling Unit: Hospital
Stage 3	List all patient care units within each hospital and randomly select a sample.	Tertiary Sampling Unit: Patient care unit
Stage 4	List all RNs employed in each unit and randomly select a sample.	Basic Sampling Unit or Element: Individual nurse

FIGURE 8-1. Steps in selecting a cluster sample.

reliability of norms than would be achieved by simple random sampling (Angoff, 1971).

When some characteristics of the population related to the measure are known, it is possible to stratify within each cluster for any stage of the sampling process. This procedure, called *multistage stratified cluster sampling*, involves dividing the sampling units into homogeneous strata or subunits on the basis of one or more characteristics which are related to the measure (i.e., the score), then sampling at random within strata. In the example shown in Figure 8-1, let us assume that the size of the hospital in which a nurse works is a variable believed to be related to job satisfaction. In order to introduce more precision into the sampling procedures and to assure that the referent group includes nurses from large and small hospitals, stratification can be employed at Stage 2. Once all hospitals are listed, two strata can be formed, provided bed capacity is known. Stratum 1 would consist of all hospitals within the selected state that have 500 or more beds and Stratum 2 would consist of all hospitals with less than 500 beds. Hospitals would be randomly selected from within each stratum. The primary advantage of stratified sampling is that it increases the precision of the norms generated. However, this holds only if the variables selected as the basis for stratification are those that are related to the measure for which norms are being developed. Stratification is frequently impossible because the characteristics of the population are not sufficiently well known to permit subdivision into homogeneous groupings.

If the desire is to represent as closely as possible in the sample the proportions of nurses working in large and small hospitals, it is desirable to select into a sample the number of hospitals in each stratum that corresponds to its percentage of the total number of hospitals in the state. Assuming that small hospitals make up 25 percent of the 160 hospitals in State A and 50 percent of the 200 hospitals in State B, and that a 10 percent sample of hospitals is to be drawn, then in State A 4 small and 12 large hospitals would be chosen and in State B, 10 small and 10 large hospitals would be selected. A sampling procedure that involves sampling from each stratum at a rate proportionate to its distribution in the population is called *proportionate* sampling. It is employed to assure representativeness with respect to variables that are believed to be correlated with the measure being standardized. Disproportionate sampling, wherein strata are sampled at rates that are not proportionate to their distribution in the population (e.g., if equal numbers of large and small hospitals had been selected irrespective of their proportions), may be employed to assure sufficient variety in the reference group or to assure inclusion of members of a stratum that may include a small number of individuals (or units) who may be theoretically very important. For detailed information about probability sampling procedures the reader is referred to Angoff (1971), Kish (1964), Connell (1960), and Lazerwitz (1968).

Probability sampling is critical to increasing the likelihood that the referent group will be representative of the population for which the measure is intended. However, because it is time consuming and involves the development of a detailed sampling frame, test developers may employ other sampling methods that are easier but that allow the introduction of bias and do not permit the accurate estimation of error. Examples include (1) convenience samples, selected on the basis of availability; (2) samples in which respondents can volunteer or select themselves into the sample; (3) purposeful samples, selected because they are thought to be typical; (4) samples that experts say represent an appropriate target population; and (5) samples that are drawn from listings that may incorporate an inherent bias (e.g., telephone directories, voluntary organization rosters, listings of individuals who have contacted a given health agency). Such procedures are likely to result in an atypical or nonrepresentative referent group. Also problematic because of potential bias are probability samples derived from outdated or incomplete population lists and samples that include a high percentage of nonresponse or nonparticipation (Angoff, 1971).

In addition to the sampling method used to select the referent group, it is necessary to consider the size of the sample to be used. As a general principle, all else being equal, the larger the sample, the more likely it is to be representative of the population. The size of the sample needed is based on mathematical calculation of sampling error which would result from using a given sample size and a given sampling procedure. In addition, consideration must be given to the degree of precision required in the norms, in light of the purposes for which they will be used and the decisions that will be made. The greater the precision required (the smaller the sampling error that can be tolerated), the larger the sample size must be. Sample size is, in part, determined by practical considerations such as the time and cost involved. In selecting the referent group for establishing norms, the most fundamental considerations (more crucial than sample size) are that the population be clearly specified in advance and that the sample be selected randomly from that population.

THE NORMING ADMINISTRATION. Rigid control over the conditions of administration to assure uniformity is critical to the concept of standardization. Norms can be a meaningful reference for comparison only if they have been derived from administration of the measure under established and completely identical procedures. Detailed instructions for administration and instructions for the subjects must be final before the norming administration and followed precisely. The term norming administration refers to administration of the measure to the representative referent group. In actuality, for most standardized measures a series of norming administrations is required in order to encompass the entire referent sample, which may be geographically dispersed. In each instance the measure is administered according to the same specifications and under conditions identical to those that will be used in subsequent administrations. For example, if the measure is designed for administration to nurses in a group setting and within a specific time limit, these conditions must prevail during each norming administration in order to assure comparability of results. At the time of the norming administration supplementary data about characteristics of the referent sample members are often collected. These data are later used to prepare differentiated norms specific to particular subunits of the referent group.

STATISTICAL ANALYSIS. After the measure has been administered to the referent group, it is scored in a prescribed and accurate manner. Raw scores earned by the entire referent sample are then represented in a frequency distribution, as described in Chapter 4. If the measure has several component parts (subscales), a separate frequency distribution is developed for each part. If personal characteristics are believed to be related to the score on the measure, it is desirable to categorize the referent sample on the basis of one or more of these characteristics and develop separate frequency distributions for each category. For example, if sex is a characteristic assumed to be highly related to the score, separate frequency distributions would be developed for males and females. Subgroups based on age, occupation, educational level, field of study, and residence are frequently identified, because they are likely to represent distinct subpopulations that differ with respect to the scores earned. There is no set number of variables that should be used to identify subgroups. The principles are that data should be available about as many subpopulations as will be useful for comparison purposes and that the characteristics selected are those that influence the score.

For each frequency distribution summary statistics are calculated as described in Chapter 3. In addition to measures of central tendency (mean, mode, median), statistics that describe the spread of scores (range, variance, standard distribution) and the shape of the distribution (skewness and kurtosis) are computed. The latter statistics allow one to evaluate how closely the obtained distribution of scores approximates the theoretical normal curve. The measures of central tendency and dispersion calculated for the referent group (and subgroups) serve as the basis for assigning meaning to any given raw score.

Developers of standardized tests must make decisions about the most meaningful way to communicate to others the nature of the data derived from the standardization administration so that these data can be effectively used for subsequent comparisons and interpretation. The decisions are based on the nature of the measure and its intended use, as well as on statistical considerations. The objective is to describe the data in a manner that is clear and definite and has direct meaning. As noted in Chapter 4, raw scores lack meaning and must be converted into some type of derived score in order to be interpreted.

The types of derived scores most commonly used to convey information about referent groups for standardized measures relevant to nursing are *percentile scores* and *standard scores*. These scores describe the standing of a given score in relation to the distribution of scores obtained from the referent group. The computation of percentile and standard scores was described in Chapter 4. Percentile scores, which indicate the percentage of scores that fall below the given score, have the advantage of being easily interpretable. However, one limitation is that percentile units are not equal at all points on the scale of raw scores, because a large number of individuals obtain scores near the middle of the distribution. Thus, a percentile difference of eight points near the middle of the scale (e.g., 48th versus 56th percentile) represents a much smaller difference between raw scores than does a percentage difference of equal magnitude at either end of the distribution (e.g., 5th versus 13th percentile).

Standard scores express the raw score in terms of standard deviation units above or below the mean. They have the advantage of providing equal units, such that a given difference between two standard scores represents the same difference between raw scores anywhere along the distribution. Their interpretation is conceptually less apparent than percentile scores, however, and must be based on the assumption of a normal distribution. This assumption is generally appropriate for referent samples, since numbers of subjects are sufficiently large. However, standard scores are not advantageous when a nonnormal distribution of scores in the referent group reflects actual peculiarities in the distribution of the attribute or behavior measured. Several types of standard scores can be measured as the basis for describing norms. The Z-score, described in Chapter 4 using Formula 4-1, ranges between -4.0 (a score four standard deviation units below the mean) and $+4.0$ (a score four standard deviation units above the mean). Because of the potential risk of error when minus signs are used, Z-scores are frequently transformed to another standard score that uses only positive numbers. Examples of standard scores that use positive numbers are T-scores and stanines. The T-score is obtained by multiplying the Z-score by 10 and adding the product to 50, which is the mean of the T-score distribution (see Formula 4-2). *Stanines* present norms on a 9-point scale of equal units, each the width of one half of a standard deviation unit. Stanine scores have a mean of 5 and a standard deviation of 2.

Standard scores have the advantage that, regardless of the value of the mean and standard deviation of a distribution, the interpretation of a given standard score is consistent. This feature facilitates comparison across several measures. Standard scores can also be interpreted in terms of percentile rank, assuming a normal distribution. As described in Chapter 4, each standard deviation unit in a normal distribution contains a fixed percentage of the cases. Thus, a raw score one standard deviation above the mean can be expressed as a Z-score of $+1.0$, a T-score of 60, a stanine score of 7, or a percentile score of 84.

For some measures of early cognitive and physical development the performance of the referent group may be expressed in terms of *age equivalents*. These norms are based on the average scores obtained by individuals of different ages. For example, if children in the referent group who are two years and three months of age have an average score of 30 on the measure, this score is assigned an age equivalent of 2-3. Age equivalents are expressed in terms of two sets of numbers, the first representing the year and the second the month of age. They represent average or typical performance for a given age group. Because patterns of growth vary at different ages, age equivalents do not have uniform meaning across all age groups and are easily misinterpreted. They are declining in popularity, being replaced by age-specific norms (i.e., norms differentiated on the basis of age), which are calculated using the frequency distributions for specific age groups and presented as percentile or standard scores.

Once the decision has been made about which types of derived scores are to be used to represent the data from the referent group, necessary calculations are carried out, generally by computer. For every possible raw score, corresponding derived scores are calculated, thereby assuring that any score earned subsequently will be assigned the same meaning. The exact procedure that was used for transforming raw scores as well as all relevant summary statistics is made available to subsequent users of the measure.

TABULAR AND GRAPHIC DISPLAY. After derived scores have been calculated, tables and graphs are prepared to summarize the referent group data, that is, to display the norms. Since the purpose of these tables is to communicate to others the exact nature of the referent group and to provide a basis for interpreting specific scores, accuracy, clarity, and precision are required. Specific instructions for use of the table or graph should be provided.

UPDATING NORMS. The establishment of norms for a standardized measure cannot be viewed as a one-time occurrence, despite the time and cost involved in generating them. Norms become outmoded due to societal changes. Changes in nutrition, sanitation, life style, and health care have made decade-old physiological norms obsolete. Increases in the average level of schooling and changes in educational curricula and in media programming tend to affect the scores earned on tests of general mental ability, thus rendering norms established for such measures even five years ago inaccurate as a basis for current comparison. Such changes necessitate repeating at periodic intervals the procedure described previously for developing norms. The frequency with which the norming procedure must be repeated and new norms established depends on the likelihood that the attribute or behavior being measured has been influenced by recent changes. In addition to monitoring the occurrence of external or societal events or patterns that might be correlated to the measure, it is desirable to make systematic and ongoing comparisons between distributions of current scores and those of the referent group. Such comparisons are easily made when a measure is centrally scored and all data from subsequent administrations of the measure are available to the test developer and publisher. Current research using the measure is another source of comparative information.

ADEQUACY OF NORMS. The process for establishing norms has been described in detail, because it provides the basis for judging the adequacy of any set of norms generated. The adequacy of norms is, in turn, a prime consideration when selecting a standardized measure for use and when interpreting results. Criteria for determining the adequacy of norms include the following:

1. The norms were established on the basis of a representative sample from a clearly specified population.

2. The norms were established using a referent group with known (accurately described) characteristics.

3. The norms were established under conditions of uniform administration and scoring.

4. The date of the norming administration is known.

5. The statistical procedures used in deriving the norms were appropriate and accurately described.

6. The norms are clearly presented, with instructions for interpretation provided.

7. Differentiated norms are available to reflect relevant differences among subgroups with specific characteristics.

8. The norms are up-to-date.

Standardized measures vary in the degree to which information is provided to assess the adequacy of the established norms. Ideally information about the method of sampling, the size and characteristics of the norm sample, the conditions of administration, and the date of testing is included with the norm values and tables in an accompanying manual, which must be carefully studied. When such information is not automatically supplied by the publisher, manufacturer, or developer, it is advisable to request it directly and to review published literature related to the measure.

EMPLOYING AND INTERPRETING STANDARDIZED MEASURES

In many instances nurses engaged in clinical practice, education, administration, and research do not have sufficient resources (time, money, expertise) to develop standardized measures themselves, yet seek the technical quality, consistent information, and precise comparative interpretation that a standardized measure can provide. In this section of the chapter, procedures and considerations to be taken into account in selecting, using, and interpreting standardized measures are discussed.

SELECTING THE MEASURE

Selection of any measure must be based on careful consideration of the nature of the concept, attribute, or behavior about which information is being sought and the purposes to be achieved by acquiring the information. The initial step in selecting a measure is to clearly define the kind of information required. This in itself is a time-consuming procedure, which often involves the combined efforts of a variety of people. However, its importance cannot be overemphasized.

Each standardized measure is unique in its assumptions and specific content and in the aspects of behavior, cognition, affect, or skill that it measures. Similarly nurses have, within the context of a given situation, unique needs for particular kinds of information. It is critical to remember that only those who require information for particular purposes are in a position to define the exact nature of the information needed and that they must do so before seeking a measure. The defined needs provide the primary criterion for selecting measures to meet them.

Many nursing decisions made on the basis of information gained from measurement have considerable impact on the decision-makers and others. Examples are admissions decisions, promotion decisions in educational and clinical settings, and clinical decisions regarding the use of particular nursing interventions. Given the potential impact of nursing decisions, it is important that the process of defining the need for information be carried out thoughtfully, with attention given to goals to be achieved and the consequences of the decisions. During this process it is necessary to identify not only local requirements and conditions, but also the values that underlie the specification of goals. Desired outcomes (goals), of necessity, reflect values whether or not they are recognized and acknowledged. Decision-makers who identify and rank in importance the values that they wish to maximize are able to set priorities for their information needs accordingly. Measures can then be selected and their relative importance determined on this basis, heightening the probability that they will yield the information needed for a sound decision (McGaghie, et al, 1978).

It should be noted that the process of acknowledging and setting priorities for values and determining information needs frequently involves prolonged discussion in order to achieve agreement. Individuals who are in a position to evaluate the potential consequences of the decisions to be made are vital participants. To cite an example, faculty members with intimate knowledge of a given nursing curriculum, its objectives, and the capabilities required of students to complete it successfully are in an optimal position to determine the values that are to underlie admissions decisions and the relative importance of those values. Their priorities supply the model for identifying the specific attributes that are to be measured and the importance that each is to be assigned. Let us assume that a faculty decision-making group determines that the value to be given highest priority is academic potential, with verbal aptitude more highly valued than quantitative aptitude, but decides that creativity is relatively unimportant. The implication is that information will be sought about applicants' academic potential via measures such as aptitude tests and previous grade point average, whereas information about applicants' creativity will not be solicited. A further implication is that verbal aptitude will be given greater importance in the admission decision than quantitative aptitude, and hence, should be measured more extensively and weighted more heavily in the final decision. Ideally, the outcome of the first step in the measurement selection process will be a rank-ordered and weighted list of the values to be maximized and a correspondingly weighted list of the information required.

Once information needs are defined and priorities are set, it is necessary to consider which ones can best be fulfilled by standardized versus non-standardized measures. As noted in an earlier section of this chapter, standardized measures are inappropriate for situations in which flexibility, adaptability to specific circumstances, and sensitivity to minor fluctuations are required and in which interpretation by way of comparison to a defined and relatively heterogeneous reference group is not desirable. Given the comprehensive listing of information needs it is necessary to differentiate those that can best be met by standardized measures from those for which other measures are preferable. Having determined the specific needs to be met by standardized measures, the next step is to identify those measures that have potential to provide the information desired. A number of resources are available to aid in the search. Particularly helpful are the well-known publications by Buros, *Tests in Print* (1970) and *Mental Measurement Yearbooks* (e.g., Buros, 1978). The former includes a description of all known standardized tests including title, author, publisher, age levels covered, publication dates, special comments, number and type of scores provided, and references to test reviews and publications using the test. The latter include evaluative information about the tests as well as additional descriptive information. Other sources of information are books that describe standardized instruments (e.g., Anastasi, 1976; Mehrens and Lehmanon, 1975), test publishers' and instrument manufacturers' catalogs, and articles in professional journals. These publications are described in more detail in the Appendix.

Sample sets of those measures deemed potentially useful and accompanying test manuals can be ordered for review and evaluation. These should be examined carefully for evidence of high technical quality and characteristics that are desired for the particular use intended. According to Gronlund (1976, p. 365), the review of test materials must be done critically and with a certain degree of skepticism. He notes that statements about technical features or the adequacy of norms should be disregarded, unless they are supported by detailed descriptions and statistical evidence.

The following is a list of questions that can serve as the basis for evaluating standardized measures.

1. Purpose: Are the stated purpose and recommended uses for the measure congruent with the purpose for which it will be employed? Will the measure yield the desired information?

2. Conceptual basis: Is the theoretical model that guided development of the measure identical to (or at the very least compatible with) the model being employed? What are the assumptions and potential biases underlying the measure? Are the values inherent in the development of the mea-

sure congruent with those that are to be maximized in the current situation?

3. Content: Is the content of the measure appropriate (without modification) for the use intended? Is it up-to-date? Is the content appropriate for the ages, reading abilities, and frames of reference of potential subjects?

4. Technical quality: What type of reliability and validity have been established? What is the nature of evidence supporting the reliability and validity of the measure? How was the measure developed and tested? What were the qualifications of the individuals involved?

5. Norms: How were norms established? How was the referent group selected and what are its characteristics? Are the norms appropriate and sufficiently detailed for use as a basis of comparison? Are the norms clear and easily interpretable? Are they up-to-date?

6. Administration: Are clear and explicit instructions provided for administration? What resources are required for administration? How easy, costly, and time consuming is the administration?

7. Scoring: Is the measure hand or machine scored? What costs or special equipment are required? How likely are errors to occur in scoring? What is the time required for scoring?

8. Interpretation: Can scores be easily and consistently interpreted? Are materials provided to aid in interpretation?

9. Cost: What is the cost for employing the measure, including purchase, administration, and scoring costs? What is the cost (if any) to subjects? Are the costs proportional to the relative importance of the information that will be obtained?

10. Critical Reviews: What are the evaluations provided by others who have used the measure? What problems, strengths, and weaknesses have been identified?

Each measure being considered should be evaluated in the light of these considerations and its advantages and disadvantages identified. Those features deemed most important should be given highest priority in the evaluation. In addition to the general considerations listed above, criteria specific to the particular situation in which the measure is to be used should be identified in order to facilitate the selection process. For example, a faculty group planning an applicant selection process for the graduate program in a school of nursing may determine in advance that it wishes to consider only those standardized aptitude measures that are administered abroad as well as in the United States and that provide norms specific to individuals with an undergraduate major in nursing. A nurse researcher contemplating a survey of large numbers of adults may decide to consider only measures that are machine-scored by a centralized facility, whereas a group of clinicians choosing a standardized measure to be used in patient assessment may desire a measure that can be hand scored within a matter of minutes. The final selection is based on comparative evaluation within the context of priorities established by the user.

ADMINISTERING AND SCORING THE MEASURE

It is known that blood pressure readings cannot be meaningfully compared unless certain procedures are carried out consistently across all measurements. For example, the cuff and stethoscope must be positioned identically, the same extremity must be used, and patient position must be consistent. Similarly, if the values resulting from the use of a standardized measure are to have the desired meaning in comparison to established norms, the measure must be administered under standard, consistent conditions. The most important requirement for administering a standardized measure is that the procedure prescribed by the developer must be followed exactly. Even minor alterations yield incomparable results and render the measure nonstandardized.

The requirement for standard administration procedures and conditions places responsibility on the measure's developer to provide explicit instructions that leave little latitude for error. As noted above, in the case of complex administration procedures, special training and certification may be required to assure consistency. This requirement also places considerable responsibility on the user to become thoroughly familiar with the procedures in advance and to anticipate and try to eliminate potential threats to consistency. Assembling all necessary materials in advance and selecting a quiet location for administering the measure are examples of steps that might be taken to prevent delays and distractions during administration.

Any unanticipated alteration of the prescribed protocol should be noted carefully so that it can be taken into account in interpreting results. Such alterations might include (1) distractions that would affect an entire group of subjects (e.g., a fire alarm); (2) systematic errors in executing the procedure itself (e.g., inaccurate time keeping); and (3) influences unique to an individual score (e.g., a subject is called away from the administration momentarily or receives additional instructions). In addition, it may be important to note special circumstances external to the test administration that might alter the performance of an individual or group. For example, if a nurse researcher was measuring staff nurses' perceptions of the leadership style of the supervisors in a public health agency, an event such as the recent dismissal of a staff nurse colleague would be likely to influence results and should be noted. Although not all distractions or idiosyncratic circumstances can be eliminated, the user of the standardized measure must: (1) try to prevent altering the established procedures to the greatest extent possible; (2) record any unanticipated alterations that do occur; and (3) evaluate the potential impact of any alterations in order to determine whether the results are usable. Many manuals for standardized measures now include instructions about how to handle unexpected problems that may occur during administration.

As with administration, the procedure for scoring standardized measures is predetermined by the developer. A fixed and explicit set of rules is applied so that the same numerical value (score) will be assigned consistently to a given performance on the measure; that is, any number of raters scoring an individual's performance on the measure should arrive at the same result. The primary considerations in scoring are consistency in following the scoring rules and accuracy in computation. Machine scoring by optical scanners and computers is being used increasingly with standardized measures, because it is, in general, more accurate and cost efficient than hand scoring. Whether hand or machine scoring methods are used, random periodic checks of accuracy are advisable. For machine scoring, this generally entails rescoring a random sample of measures by hand or machine and comparing the results with the original computation. For hand scoring, a random sample of measures is selected and rescored by a different individual. The two sets of scores are then compared by computing interrater reliability as described in Chapter 5.

INTERPRETING SCORES

In order to discuss the interpretation of scores on standardized measures it is necessary to differentiate the meaning of a given piece of information (in this case the score itself) and the use of that information. Ultimately, interpretation takes into account both the generic meaning of the score as it derives from the process of standardization itself and the purposes and context within which the information ultimately will be used. Given the way in which any standardized measure is developed, the meaning of a given score is determined with reference to established norms. The meaning derives from comparison of an individual score with the scores earned by others (the defined referent group) on the same measure. Importantly, the comparison is with performance that is *typical* of the referent group and should not be construed as comparison with an ideal or standard to be achieved. The generic meaning of any score on a standardized measure, therefore, is always normative, that is, defined in terms of interindividual comparison with the typical performance of a referent group.

The scores on standardized measures are most frequently used for the purposes of making interindividual or intergroup comparisons. Examples of interindividual comparisons would include ranking a group of applicants prior to selecting the one most qualified for a position or evaluating the anxiety level of a given patient as high or low in comparison with that of the typical adult. An intergroup comparison would be exemplified by the determination that the average job performance ratings of staff nurses in Hospital A are higher than those in Hospital B or are higher than the national average. In some instances, however, the score on a standardized measure may be used to make intraindividual (also termed ipsative) comparisons, such as comparing an individual's performance at two points in time, or comparing scores earned on a number of separate measures or on subscales measuring different dimensions of behavior or cognition. In some cases a standardized measure score may be used to compare an individual's performance with a standard that has been established on the basis of previously gathered data regarding the relationship between typical performance on the measure and other salient variables. For example, after gathering data about the relationship between the Scholastic Aptitude Test scores of entering students and their grade point averages throughout an undergraduate nursing curriculum, a school may determine that a particular percentile score on the SAT is necessary for successful completion of the program. Subsequently that score can be used as a standard for comparing the scores of applicants. Similar procedures are used in businesses to select candidates for leadership positions, using data from standardized personality measures. In the realm of clinical practice a given score on a standardized measure could be used to identify individuals who are at high risk relative to a particular condition. In each case, the standard that is used for evaluating performance on the measure is established on the basis of normative data and only after systematic study of the ability of the measure to predict outcomes on another variable.

The generic meaning assigned to a score on a standardized measure involves a complex set of considerations related to the procedures used to develop the measure and to establish the norms, the nature of the comparison (referent) group, the type of norms established, and the meaning of the statistics used. A score that is compared with national norms that have been differentiated on the basis of age and converted to percentile ranks would have a different meaning from one that is compared with local norms expressed as age equivalents. Developers and publishers or manufacturers of standardized instruments generally supply aids to help assign meaning to raw scores. These include tables, guidelines, examples, and in some instances even computerized printed explanations that provide the appropriate meaning for a given score. However, it is ultimately the responsibility of the user to make an informed judgment about the meaning of a score. The following guidelines should be kept in mind:

1. The conceptual meaning of whatever derived score is used should be clear to the user.

2. The score has meaning only in relation to the specific measure from which it was derived; thus, the meaning that can be inferred is limited by the purpose, scope, and content of the measure itself.

3. The score has meaning only in relation to the referent group used to establish norms; thus, the characteristics of the referent group must be studied carefully.

4. Measurement error must be taken into account; that is, the subject's true score is recognized to fall not exactly on the point of the obtained score but within a range of scores, the limits of which are one standard error of measurement above and below the obtained score.

5. To the extent that they are provided and address relevant characteristics of the subject(s), differentiated norms should be used as the basis for comparison, because they allow for more precise meaning to be inferred.

6. Relevant characteristics of the subject(s) should be taken into account. These include not only demographic characteristics, which help to identify subgroups for whom a given measure or set of norms may be inappropriate, but also abnormal circumstances, which may have influenced performance on the measure.

It was noted above that standardized measures are sometimes used to make intraindividual or ipsative comparisons, that is, comparisons involving two or more scores earned by a single individual. Such comparisons are often used to identify an individual's strengths and weaknesses. In order to assist with interpreting intraindividual comparisons, a profile chart is often developed. This is a graphic representation of the individual's scores on various measures (or subscales of a more inclusive measure), which are plotted on comparable score scales. The median scores (scores that fall at the 50th percentile) of a group on several measures may also be plotted on a profile. An example of a profile for one individual depicting scores on three measures is shown in Figure 8-2. Scores can be displayed either as bands that extend one standard error of measure above and below the obtained score (as in Figure 8-2) or as specific points on the scale (as in Figure 8-3). The former style is preferable, because it allows the interpreter to take into account the inaccuracy of the scores in determining whether a difference actually exists between the scores on different measures. In Figure 8-2 the subject's scores can be interpreted as essentially identical on Tests A and B and higher on Test C.

In order to construct a profile based on comparable score scales, it is necessary that the norms be comparable across all measures; that is, they must be converted to the same system of numbers (derived scores) and must have the same shape distribution. Ideally, all measures included in the profile should be normed on the same referent sample and should be independent of one another. The interpretation of a profile is both normative and ipsative, in that it involves a comparison of the individual's scores with one another as well as with those of the referent group.

An individual's profile is sometimes compared with the profile of a particular group, with the group profile defined as the median (50th percentile) score for the group on each measure. While this procedure allows eval-

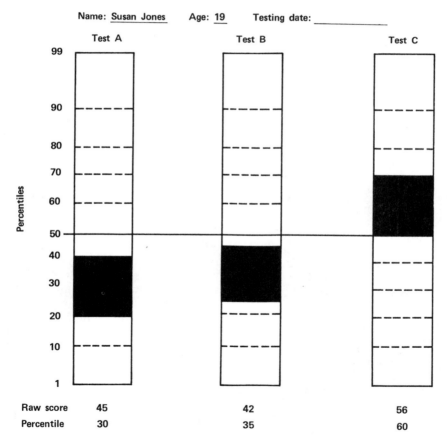

FIGURE 8-2. Example of a profile chart.

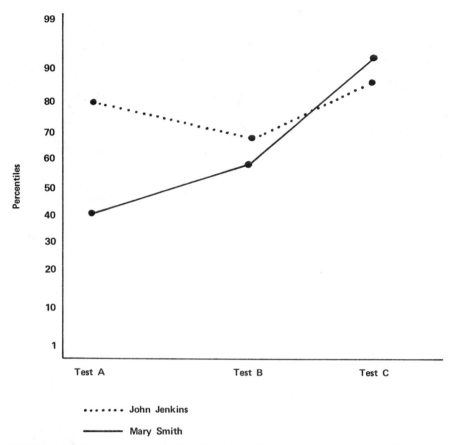

FIGURE 8-3. Example of a profile chart depicting the scores of two individuals.

uation of whether the individual's scores are different from the central tendency of the group (as defined by the median), it does not permit an accurate assessment of the difference, since the entire array of referent group scores is not represented. Profile charts may be used to depict the comparison of one individual's or group's scores with those of another or to compare one individual's score at different points in time. A profile comparing two individuals is shown in Figure 8-3. Profile charts are useful because of their flexibility, and because they provide a visual display, which is helpful in interpretation. Caution should be employed to assure that they are used appropriately (see Angoff, 1971, pp. 547–548).

The ultimate interpretation of any score on a standardized measure requires taking into account the purposes for which the information will be used. For example, given the generic meaning of a score (say, that a staff nurse scores in the 90th percentile, and hence ranks very high on a standardized measure of quantitative aptitude), that score would be interpreted differently, depending upon whether one was selecting applicants for advanced training in budget preparation or conducting research to determine the degree of improvement in medication accuracy resulting from a special training program for nurses with low quantitative ability. The intended use, therefore, provides the context in which a given score is interpreted.

Since the information derived from a standardized measure is often used alone or in conjunction with other measures for decision making, the development of a model defining and setting priorities for the values to be maximized and the information requirements was advocated as a necessary initial step in selecting appropriate measures. It is important to note that such a model also serves as a guide to interpreting scores in the light of the decision to be made. A model developed to set priorities for values and informational needs for admission decisions would provide guidelines, for example, to determine whether subscale scores on a measure should be interpreted individually or whether the total (overall) score should be interpreted. The model would also provide the basis for deciding whether the subscale scores should be given equal weight in the decision or differentially weighted in terms of their importance. The model would also specify the ways in which information from multiple standardized and nonstandardized measures should be combined to yield the basis for the decision. As an important cautionary note, all standardized measure scores are subject to an indeterminate degree of error because of unmet assumptions and uncontrolled conditions (Gronlund, 1976, p. 422). The best way to avoid making erroneous decisions is to base them on multiple indicators rather than on a single score. Thus, the final interpretation of a given score should be made only after assessing the extent to which it is congruent with other available information.

SUMMARY

Standardized measures are norm-referenced measures that are constructed, administered, and scored in a prescribed and consistent manner and that are interpreted with reference to established norms. Because they are carefully constructed, are of high technical quality, and are designed for widespread use, they have potential utility for measuring some types of nursing phenomena. They are useful for situations in which a normative interpretation is required (i.e., when scores are to be interpreted by means of comparison to a defined population) and in which the attributes or behaviors being measured are relatively stable and are common to a variety of situations and settings. They are not designed to be specific to a particular setting nor to discern minor fluctuations. Neither the content nor the administration of a standardized measure can be altered to meet local needs.

One of the key advantages of a standardized measure is that norms are provided to aid in interpreting results. Norms are statistics that describe the scores earned by a defined referent group with known characteristics, which is representative of the population of individuals for whom the measure is designed. They are established by administering the measure under controlled conditions. The scores of the referent group serve as the basis for comparing scores earned on all subsequent administrations of the measure, and hence, facilitate consistent interpretation.

The selection of a standardized measure for use in nursing is based on the defined needs for information, the stated purpose, assumptions and content domain of the measure, its technical quality, the adequacy of the norms, and the costs and procedures required for administration and scoring. Administration and scoring of the selected measure must be carried out with consistent adherence to prescribed procedures. Interpretation of the results occurs within the context of the defined needs. It is guided by the established norms but also takes into account the characteristics of the referent group and examinee(s) and technical features of the measure. Information gleaned from standardized measures should be interpreted in the light of information gathered from other sources as well.

REFERENCES

ANASTASI, A: Psychological Testing, ed. 4. Macmillan, New York, 1976.

ANGOFF, WH: "Scales, norms and equivalent scores." In THORNDIKE, RL (ed): Educational Measurement. American Council on Education, Washington, DC, 1971, pp. 508–600.

BARNARD, KE AND EARLES, SJ (ed): Child Health Assessment Part 2: The First Year of Life. USDHEW Pub. No. (HRA) 79–25, Washington, DC, 1979.

BRAZELTON, TB: A Neonatal Behavioral Assessment Scale. J.B. Lippincott, Philadelphia, 1973.

BUROS, OK: The Eighth Mental Measurements Yearbook. Gryphon Press, Highland Park, NJ, 1978.

BUROS, OK: Tests in Print II. Gryphon Press, Highland Park, NJ, 1970.

CONNELL, FG: "Sampling methods." In HARRIS, CW (ed): Encyclopedia of Educational Research, ed. 3. Macmillan, New York, 1960, pp. 1181–1183.

CRONLUND, E: Measurement and Evaluation in Teaching, ed. 3. Macmillan, New York, 1976.

KISH, L: Survey Sampling. Wiley, New York, 1964.

LAZERWITZ, B: "Sampling theory and procedures." In BLALOCK, HM AND BLALOCK, AB (eds): Methodology in Social Research. McGraw-Hill, New York, 1968, pp. 278–328.

MCGAGHIE, WC, ENGEL, JD, AND RISLEY, ME: "Standardized testing in health professions education: Problems and prospects." Evaluation and the Health Professions 1(2):10–24, 1978.

MEHRENS, WA AND LEHMANON, IJ: Standardized Tests in Education, ed. 2. Holt, Rinehart and Winston, New York, 1975.

RISLEY, ME, MCGAGHIE, WC AND ENGEL, JD: "Toward definition of a standardized test." Unpublished manuscript, Center for Educational Development, University of Illinois Medical Center, Chicago, 1978.

SPIELBERGER, CD, GORSUCH, RL AND LUSHENE, R: STAI Manual for the State-Trait Anxiety Inventory. Consulting Psychologist Press, Palo Alto, 1970.

TINKELMAN, SN: "Planning the objective test." In THORNDIKE, RL (ed): Educational Measurement. American Council on Education, Washington, DC, 1981, pp. 46–80.

9

STRATEGIES AND TECHNIQUES FOR DESIGNING NURSING TOOLS AND PROCEDURES

This chapter presents specific strategies and techniques for the design of selected tools and procedures with particular utility for the measurement of nursing variables. Tools and procedures were selected for inclusion in this chapter on the basis of their frequent use or misuse in nursing or on the basis of their realized or potential utility for employment in the measurement of nursing variables. More specifically, the following tools and procedures are addressed: (1) physiologic; (2) observational; (3) content analysis; (4) interviews; (5) questionnaires; (6) Delphi technique; (7) projective techniques; and (8) Q–sort methodology.

In each case, attention is given to the utility of the tool or procedure for measurement in nursing; step–by–step procedures for designing the measure are outlined; specific methods for investigating reliability and validity are detailed; and advantages and disadvantages of the approach are discussed. Although the focus of this chapter is on the design and testing of tools and procedures, in each case, care is taken to focus as well on the essential considerations to be made in selecting such measures in instances in which existing tools and procedures are to be employed.

PHYSIOLOGIC MEASUREMENT

This section provides an introduction to the principles of physiologic measurement or biometrics. *Biometrics* is the "branch of science that includes the measurement of physiological variables and parameters" (Cromwell, Weibell, and Pfeiffer, 1980, p. 6). A number of approaches used in biometrics are quite complicated and involved; therefore, no attempt will be made here to provide detailed information on the processes and procedures involved in the measurement of the numerous physiologic variables of interest to nurses. Rather, the discussion will focus upon the major types of physiologic measurement and common measurement concerns related to each. The reader is referred to basic laboratory manuals, such as the ones by Bauer, Ackerman, and Toro (1974); Cromwell, Weibell, and Pfeiffer, (1980); Weiss (1973); and Widmann (1979), for detailed information on specific laboratory procedures and the use and interpretation of laboratory values.

The focus of this discussion is on human biometry and will include measurements that may be conducted by nurses and those that may not be conducted by nurses but that are useful to nurses in providing care to clients and in conducting research. Physiologic measurements that are acquired through the use of various observational techniques and require the use of sensory organs (e.g., assessment of cyanosis, edema, or respiratory distress) will not be discussed, since they are measured via observational methods.

As nurses have become more involved in using physiologic indicators in making decisions about patient care, and as nurse researchers have become more attuned to the need for studying outcomes of care, physiologic measurement has taken on greater significance. Practicing nurses use the results of physiologic measurements to monitor the health status of clients, to alter the treatment regimen, and to make decisions about the counseling and learning needs of clients. For example, a test of the amount of glucose in the urine may indicate to a nurse who is caring for a patient with a sliding-scale insulin order whether to increase or decrease the dosage from that previously given. A cardiac monitor used in the care of a neonate will inform the nurse of episodes of bradycardia in the patient and could serve as the basis for the decision to provide immediate stimulation. A low hemoglobin level in a client may cue the nurse to obtain information about the person's dietary habits and fluid intake and to provide dietary couseling.

Nurse researchers use physiologic variables to document the effectiveness of nursing interventions. For example, a group of investigators (Kagawa-Busby, et al, 1980) evaluated the effects of three different temperatures of nasogastric tube feedings on gastric motility, total gastrointestinal transit time and diarrhea, and adverse subjective sensations and symptoms. A pressure transducer was used to measure changes in intragastric pressure as an indicator of gastric motility, and a thermistor probe was used to measure intragastric temperatures. (Other variables were measured by report of subjects.) Temperature of feedings was not related to gastric motility, although cold feedings were associated with gastrointestinal symptoms in some subjects. Nurse researchers use physiologic measures to operationalize independent and dependent variables, as done in this example.

TYPES OF PHYSIOLOGIC MEASURES

Three major categories of physiologic measures are (1) physical measurements; (2) chemical or biochemical measurements; and (3) microbiologic/microscopic measurements.

PHYSICAL MEASUREMENTS. Physical indicators are used as measures of the physical properties of the organism. Weight, height, temperature, volume, and pressure are some of the more common attributes measured. Other attributes include the electrical activity of organs, the density of organs, or the strength and speed of some event, such as nerve impulses.

In most instances, bioinstrumentation is required for measures to be obtained. Bioinstruments are tools that are used to measure biologic phenomena. Examples are phonocardiography, radiography, sonography, and various electronic devices. Information is gathered from the subject through such devices, and different physiologic events are measured. The electrocardiogram, electroencephalogram, electromyogram, galvanic skin response, and basal skin resistance are just a few of the records of measurement that can be obtained via electrical devices.

In most instances, some type of external stimulus is applied to the subject in order for measurements to be obtained through bioinstrumentation. Visual (e.g., a flash of light), tactile (e.g., a blow to the Achilles tendon), auditory (e.g., a tone), or direct electrical stimulation (e.g., evoked potential) of some part of the nervous system is required (Cromwell, et al, 1980).

Most electronic instruments use sensing equipment for measurement of variables. Sensing equipment consists of transducers that measure physical phenomena by converting the variable measured in the organism into an electrical signal. The electrical signal is an analog of the attribute being measured. Transducers may be used in the measurement of temperature, volume, flow, pressure, or other physiologic variables. The output from transducers is always an electrical signal which is representative of the phenomenon measured. Transducers also are used to convert bioelectric impulses into electronic potentials. Bioelectric impulses produced by the heart and brain are measured by transducers that have electrodes in them.

Once the transducer emits the electrical signal of the phenomenon being measured, signal-conditioning equipment prepares it for display or for recording. The signal from the transducer must be amplified or modified in most instances. For example, if information is received from more than one transducer, the signal-conditioning equipment combines or relates the outputs from the two or more transducers. Undesirable interference signals also are screened out. Hence, "the purpose of the signal-conditioning equipment is to process the signals from the transducers in order to satisfy the functions of the system and to prepare signals suitable for operating the display or recording equipment that follows" (Cromwell, et al, 1980, p. 15).

Display equipment transforms the signal, which has been modified or amplified by the signal-conditioning equipment, into a form amenable to detection by the human senses, that is, into visual or auditory output. For example, an oscilloscope allows for visualization of the wave form of a signal by displaying measures of the time, phase, voltage, or frequency of a physiologic input signal.

Recording, data processing, and transmission equipment often is incorporated into a bioinstrument and provides a permanent record of physiologic measurements for scrutiny and analysis. Data may be stored on a strip of paper or on a magnetic tape. Figure 9-1 illustrates the relationship between the subject and the instrument system.

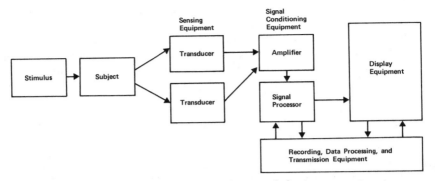

FIGURE 9-1. Relationship between the subject and the instrument system.

There are several problems which may be encountered in using bioinstrumentation for the measurement of physical variables. They are as follows (Cromwell, et al, 1980):

1. Certain variables are inaccessible to measurement. In some cases a medical operation would be required to place a suitable transducer in a position to make measurements, for example, in the measurement of dynamic neurochemical activity in the brain. This makes the measurement impractical for use with humans.

2. Many of the data obtained are highly variable due to variability in the body systems. Measurements taken at one point in time may be quite different from measurements taken under the same conditions at another point in time even within the same subject. Better understanding of physiologic relationships is required in order to make the best use of such measurements.

3. The presence of the transducer which has been placed to obtain a measurement may change the reading significantly. For example, a flow transducer placed within the bloodstream can cause a reduction of the blood flow by partially blocking the vessel and, thereby, reduce the accuracy of readings. In addition, the presence of the transducer in one system of the body can incite responses in other systems.

4. Artifacts, that is, extraneous components of a signal, can affect the readings. A major source of artifacts is movement by the subject, which causes movement of the transducer and variations in the output signal. Problems in calibration of the instrument also can affect measurements.

5. For many biomedical instruments a certain amount of energy must be applied to the body to obtain a measurement, for example, with x-rays or with the use of bioelectrical instruments. When dealing with living subjects, care must be taken not to inflict damage on cells or to affect measurements by energy concentrations used in instrumentation.

BIOCHEMICAL MEASUREMENTS. Biochemical measurement involves the use of chemical laboratory procedures for the identification or quantification of physiologic variables. Examples of biochemical variables are hormone, electrolyte (e.g., potassium and sodium), glucose, and urea levels.

The process of measuring biochemical variables consists of a number of steps and involves procedural details which vary according to the phenomenon measured. However, several general steps common to all procedures can be identified. The first step in the process is the collection of the specimen that will be subjected to measurement. Depending upon the attribute to be measured and the purpose of measurement, the specimen might be blood, urine, gastric juices, amniotic fluid, sputum, synovial fluid, cerebrospinal fluid, or some other physiologic medium in which the attribute of interest might be found. Care must be taken that the proper procedure for collection be followed. Contamination of the specimen is often a concern at collection and throughout the remainder of the measurement procedure. Contamination could alter the results of measurement. The person collecting the specimen should ensure that the proper amount of the specimen is obtained and placed in the correct receptacle. Some measurement procedures require only a small amount of the specimen, while others require much greater volumes. For some procedures, the type and size of the receptacle in which the specimen is placed are important to the measurement process.

Once the specimen has been collected, the next major step in the process of measuring biochemical variables often is the preservation and storage of the specimen. A number of specimens must be maintained at a certain temperature to prevent changes in the specimen and the biochemical components within it. For example, urine and blood must be refrigerated if there is an extended lag time between collection of the specimen and performance of the actual measurements. In some instances, chemical preservatives may be used. When this is the case, the preservatives must not alter the attribute of interest in a manner that would interfere with accurate measurement. Some specimens require storage in containers that protect them from light, since light rays may initiate chemical reactions that could alter the attribute of interest.

When measurement is conducted within the laboratory, various types of equipment, described in laboratory guides and manuals (Bauer, et al, 1974; Ferris, 1980), are employed. The individual conducting the biochemical measurements must be careful to follow established procedures to ensure accuracy of results. Equipment must be maintained in proper working order, and tests of equipment are required at regular intervals. Utensils and other supplies employed in the conduct of measurement must be properly prepared and cleansed. For many chemical measurements reagents are required. Reagents are substances employed to produce a chemical reaction within the specimen that is necessary to facilitate measurement. The type of reagent used depends upon the specimen and the variable under study. Therefore, the proper reagent must be used and the reagent should not be outdated.

The final step in the process involves the reading and recording of the results. Miscalculations in determining the results and transcription errors affect the validity of results. In some instances, the equipment produces digital or computer readings of values.

The accuracy of biochemical measurements can be assessed in the laboratory by comparing results obtained on specimens of known concentrations that have been analyzed previously. Results are rechecked with internal and external controls and standards. A standard is a substance for which the composition is known and the value of which has been determined by an analytic procedure different from that used in the clinical laboratory (Bauer, et al, 1974, p. 2). If the clinical laboratory procedure duplicates the value of the standard, then the procedure is considered accurate. The *accuracy* of a laboratory measurement is the closeness of the test results to the true value. It is important that standards be as pure as possible. The National Bureau of Standards (NBS) provides very pure substances for standards.

Controls are laboratory specimens that contain various substances of known concentration and that resemble the unknown specimen, for example, serum or urine controls. The control substances are assayed daily along with the substances with unknown quantities. The results of these assays form the basis for determining the precision of measurements. *Precision* is the "closeness of test results to each other and implies freedom from variation" (Bauer, et al, 1974, p. 2). Precision also may be determined by doing repeated analyses on the same specimen samples to ascertain the degree to which they duplicate each other. Standards are usually quite constant in their composition, while control specimens may vary in their composition over extended periods of time and if proper refrigeration is not maintained.

It should be noted that accuracy is analogous to validity, and precision is analogous to reliability. Hence, the use of controls and standards provides evidence of the reliability and validity of laboratory measurements.

MICROBIOLOGIC/MICROSCOPIC MEASUREMENT. Microbiologic/ microscopic measurement consists of identification or quantification of microorganisms within physiologic specimens (including bacteria, molds, and pathogenic protozoa), and the identification or quantification of structure and components of bodily tissues (including bacterial counts, identification of pathogens, and cell histology). The processes of collecting, preserving, analyzing, and recording the results of microbiologic/microscopic specimens are quite similar to those in biochemical measurement. Specific and proper procedures for the collecting and preserving of specimens must be followed. Representative and adequate specimens should be obtained from a suitable source, using proper techniques and under conditions that prevent contamination. Specimens need to be collected in sterile, labeled, covered containers. Instruments used for analysis must be properly calibrated. When microscopic examination of stained smears is done, there should be appropriate chemical reactivity of the staining agent.

For many microbiologic tests, cultures are grown in the laboratory. Care must be taken that the appropriate medium is employed for cultures. Since microscopic examination is required for a number of the microbiologic/ microscopic tests, technicians must be highly trained in the recognition and quantification of pathogens in specimens and in the identification and quantification of cell structures for histologic tests. Controls and standards also are used for the detection of errors in microbiologic/microscopic measurement.

RELIABILITY AND VALIDITY OF PHYSIOLOGIC MEASUREMENTS

Several potential sources of error in the measurement of physiologic variables have been presented in the discussion of the types of physiologic measurements. Major threats to the reliability and validity of measurements obtained via bioinstrumentation include improper procedure for use of the instrument, errors in measurement due to equipment problems, physiologic reactivity within the subject when in vivo measurements are done (i.e., when measurements are performed directly within the living organism), and the potential for instrumentation itself to alter the phenomenon measured. All of these problems can affect the results of measurement. The degree to which they come into play depends upon the type of procedure employed, the subject, and the instrument. The point is that there are a number of sources for error in the use of bioinstruments for measurement of physiologic phenomena. Although most of the instruments have demonstrated reliability and validity, the nurse should not be overconfident of the results from such measurement approaches.

Most of the measurement error that occurs in biochemical and microbiologic/microscopic measurements results from human error or equipment failure. The common sources of error for these types of measurements are listed below:

1. Failure to adhere to established rules and procedures for collection, preservation, and analysis of laboratory specimens.
2. Use of laboratory procedures that have been poorly tested or that may be adequate in normal ranges but inadequate in pathologic ranges.
3. An incorrect, inadequate, or contaminated specimen.
4. Improper use and calibration of laboratory equipment.
5. Use of improper reagents or reagents that have been stored in the wrong type of container or at the wrong temperature.
6. Inaccurate mathematical calculations by technicians in the quantification of results.
7. Transfer errors in the laboratory reporting system or entering results on the wrong person's record.

ADVANTAGES AND DISADVANTAGES

Although physiologic measurements are subject to measurement error as are other approaches to measurement, physiologic data obtained through bioinstrumentation and laboratory procedures generally have a high degree of accuracy. Most of these measurement procedures are highly sensitive and are generally confident measures of the variables of interest. They have the added advantage of being objective measures for the most part. It also is difficult for the subject to intentionally alter or distort measurements of physiologic functioning.

The high cost of physiologic measurement procedures because of the expense of instruments and supplies is a major disadvantage. However, most nurses have access to laboratories in hospitals which could decrease cost for researchers employing physiologic measurements. Generally, the expenses incurred as part of the accepted clinical care of patients are passed on to the client.

Breaks or interferences in the procedure for conducting physiologic measurements may have an impact on the results. It is often difficult for nurses and others who receive results from laboratories to determine if any such problems occurred during the processing of specimens.

When bioinstrumentation is employed with subjects, the measuring process itself can alter the variable of interest, and artifacts, such as random noise, can interfere with results. Some responses in subjects who are monitored by certain bioinstruments are quite unpredictable and poorly understood, and the measurement devices may stimulate one system and cause reactions in other systems (Polit and Hungler, 1978, p. 294). Bioinstrumentation is rarely unobtrusive and often requires application of energy to the body. Therefore, there is a potential for damage to the cells if high energy concentrations are employed in conducting measurements.

OBSERVATIONAL METHODS

The events and objects in a person's life are observed daily, and these observations are used to help form opinions, attitudes, and beliefs, and to make decisions. However, in the scientific sense observation is not a casual matter. Observation is a process whereby data are gathered through the senses in a systematic manner. It involves identifying and recording units of behavior or characteristics occurring in a concrete situation that is consistent with empirical aims of the observer. Behaviors may be observed in naturalistic settings or observations may be made of experimentally induced behaviors.

In nursing, observations are made of specific events or the behaviors of individuals. Most observations are concerned with collecting data about behavior. Behaviors observed include the interactions, communications, activities, and performance of living organisms in various situations. Although behavior is frequently the central focus of observation, environmental surroundings as well as the conditions and characteristics of the individual or event may be observed. Observations are made by nurses in clinical settings and by nurse educators and researchers on a daily basis. The nurse may want to observe clients' physical conditions via observations of breath sounds, skin turgor, visual acuity, or other observable signs. Such physiologic characteristics of clients are either directly observed through the senses or aided by equipment such as stethoscopes, x-rays, and other devices. The nurse educator uses observations to ascertain the skill attainment of students in the clinical setting, often aided by rating scales or checklists for recording observations. Observational methods can be employed by the nurse researcher to collect data for the measurement of variables under study. For example, the joint behaviors of mothers and infants were observed by Anderson (1981) to measure the reciprocity between mother-infant interactions after various nursing interventions. Hurley (1981) studied the communication patterns in marital dyads by observing couples' interactions. Observations of mothers' behavioral responses to the attachment behaviors of their chronically ill infants were conducted by Holaday (1981).

Observations can be conducted either directly via an observer who perceives and records the phenomenon of interest, or indirectly through observing the products of behavior and by collecting reports of behavior with interviews or questionnaires. Products of behavior include archival data and physical traces. Examples of archival data sources are records of births, deaths, and morbidity, and hospital records and other documents. Physical traces refer to deposits or erosion of environmental materials which reflect behavior (Kazdin, 1979), such as the number of cigarette butts left in a patient's ash tray as a measure of smoking behavior, and the number of pieces of incoming mail as a measure of the extent to which a psychiatric patient had contact with the community. This discussion is concerned only with direct observation as an approach to data collection.

OBSERVER ROLES

There are two observer roles which may be assumed: nonparticipant observer and participant observer. The nonparticipant observer attempts to adopt a completely passive role while observing phenomena of interest. The goal of the nonparticipant observer is to become an "unobtrusive bystander who observes and records information with a minimum of intervention" (Polit and Hungler, 1978, p. 303). Hence, the nonparticipant observer simply observes the situation without intentionally influencing the activities and behaviors under study.

Nonparticipant observers may either conceal their role or make no attempt to make observations covertly. Concealment of the observer role may be done to reduce the impact of the observer's presence on the behaviors of interest, because individuals may alter their behavior when they are aware of being monitored. A concern associated with concealment of the observer role is the ethics of observing and recording the behavior of individuals without their knowledge.

Participant observers try to become acceptable actors within the activity structure of the group under study. The observer becomes an intimate participant in the experiences of those being studied. An attempt is made to view the world of the subjects from their perspective by taking a flexible and relativistic stance. This demands that the participant observer respect and be sensitive to the subjects' style of dress and modes of gesturing and learn their language (Denzin, 1978a).

In order to immerse themselves in the experiences of their subjects, participant observers use several approaches to reveal all of the relevant aspects of the phenomenon studied. Direct participation in the activities of the subjects is attempted, introspection regarding experiences is used, interviews are conducted, documents are collected and analyzed when available, and direct observation is employed. The participant observer's role may be concealed or revealed to subjects; however, in most cases no attempt is made to conceal the observer's role. Identification of the observer has the advantage of allowing for probing and the elicitation of data that would not be readily available to the concealed observer.

The problem of behavioral alteration due to presence of an observer is called reactivity. Subject reactivity is perhaps the greatest overall limitation when either the nonparticipant or participant observer approach is used. Responses of subjects have been shown to differ markedly, even in naturalistic situations, when persons are aware that assessments are being made of their behaviors (Mercatoris and Craighead, 1974; Surratt, Ullrich, and Hawkins, 1969; White, 1977). The presence of observers may not necessarily influence the behavior of subjects directly but may provide cues to others in the setting who can influence the subjects' behaviors. For example, Johnson and Lobitz (1974) found that parents can influence observational data that are obtained on their children.

Some investigators use recording devices, such as tape recorders, audiotapes, and still and motion photography to aid observations. Subjects also are reactive to these devices and have been found to respond differently, depending upon whether they knew that recordings were being made or not (Robers and Renzaglia, 1965; Johnson, Christensen, and Bellamy, 1976).

In order to reduce subject reactivity, observations should be made as unobtrusively as possible. Several techniques may be employed to reduce reactivity. Whenever possible, continuous direct observation should not be employed. Observations of many phenomena can be made intermittently without negatively affecting the integrity of the data obtained. Observers can be instructed to restrict their observations to a prescribed number of seconds, for example, 10 seconds, and then to look away from the subject. The interval between observations also would be specified. Looking at and then looking away from the subject reduces reactivity, since the persons observed do not feel that all of their activities are being constantly monitored. This approach will not be useful in situations in which continuous observations are required, such as in the study of some behavioral interactions.

Subjects usually will habituate to an observer's presence after about 10 minutes. Therefore, observers should be in the setting for at least 10 minutes before actual data collection begins. During the preliminary period, observer behaviors should be consistent with those that will be displayed during the observational period. A change in the observer's behavior at any point during the observational period increases reactivity. Hence, the observer should remain constant in appearance, activity, and smell. Physical movement should be minimized as much as possible and no perfume or jewelry should be worn. Whenever the observer is required to leave and reenter an observational setting (e.g., when observations are made over several days or weeks), no major changes in clothing or hairstyle should be made. Clothing should be plain and, whenever possible, the same clothes should be worn during each observational period.

OBSERVING AND RECORDING

The selection of phenomena to be observed depends upon the problem that is the focus of investigation. Even after the problem has been specified, there often is a need to further delineate and select the behaviors to be observed. For example, Holaday (1981) studied mothers' behavioral response to the attachment behavior of crying in their chronically ill infants. Observations of mothers' behavioral responses were further specified as effective maternal intervention, nonroutine maternal behavior, and routine maternal behavior. Other behaviors also might have been selected as observational measures of mothers' behavioral response, for example, withdrawal or seeking assistance.

When selecting phenomena to be observed, decisions must be made concerning what constitutes a unit. Units of observation range from small and specific behaviors (molecular approach) to large units of behavior (molar approach). The molecular approach might, for example, require recordings of each movement, gesture, phrase, or action and each of these may be broken down into smaller units. In the molar approach a large unit of behavior, such as seeking help, may consist of a variety of verbal and nonverbal actions that together are construed as signaling the behavior of interest. The molecular approach has the potential disadvantage of causing the investigator to lose sight of behaviors that are central to the study at hand. The molar approach has the potential problem of allowing for distortions and errors by the observer because of the likelihood of ambiguity in the definition of units (Polit and Hungler, 1978). The approach to selecting units of observation largely depends on the investigator and the purpose for which observations are to be made.

SELECTING SAMPLES

When observational methods are employed, the approach to sampling and data collection will depend upon the problem that is studied, how variables are defined and operationalized, and the setting in which observations are to be made. Decisions about sampling and data collection will directly influence the reliability and validity of results as well as their general application.

Sampling involves "following a set of rules which place the observer in a situation to record or elicit a set of behaviors which are presumed to have some degree of relevance for a specific concept, hypothesis, proposition, or theory" (Denzin, 1978b, p. 79). These rules delineate a procedure that must be followed so that the general application and theoretical relevance of the behaviors to be observed or elicited are increased (Glaser and Strauss, 1976). The observer may observe one situation or a series of situations. The investigator draws the sample from a large population of behaviors, social situations, or events, or a small number for intensive observation. Before beginning to sample, the investigator must be able to enumerate the specific units that make up the larger population. This implies that the investigator has a clear definition of the population to which findings are to be generalized. If, for example, one is studying the role and functions of nurses who work in acute care settings, then a workable operational definition of acute care settings must be formulated. Depending upon the theoretical intentions of the investigation, an acute care work setting may be operationalized to include all types of units traditionally found in general hospitals, or it may be limited to medical and surgical units. An operational definition of nurse also is required.

After the operational definition of the population under study has been specified, the investigator then develops a complete list of all the elements that make up the population. In the example cited previously, this listing would be all of the acute care work settings in the geographical area that is to be sampled. Once the population has been defined and specified, then the investigator *randomly* selects units from that population to be included in the sample for observation. *Random sampling* gives each unit in the population the same chance of inclusion in the final set of observations. Several approaches to random sampling might be employed. Other approaches to sampling may be used, such as cluster sampling and stratified random sampling, which are described in Chapter 8.

It should be noted that the sampling process employed in observational approaches most often is multistage. The sampling procedure frequently is constrained by time and place, that is, by a specific point in time and by a specific geographical locality (Denzin, 1978a).

TIME SAMPLING

For some investigations, there may be a need to observe a behavior or activity that occurs continuously over several days, weeks, or months. When this is the case, it is not likely that an observer will be able to monitor the phenomenon of interest continuously. Time sampling can be used to select from the population of times those segments during which observations will be made. The time segments are selected randomly and may be parts of an hour, a day, or a shift, for example. Time segments selected will largely be determined by the focus of the investigation. If mother-infant interactions during feedings are to be studied, then it is possible that the times chosen for observations might be for one minute every five minutes. If a play therapy hour for a young child is to be observed, then the time segments selected might be the first ten, the middle ten, and the last ten minutes of the hour session.

The observer should consider rhythmicity of phenomena whenever time sampling is used. Certain activities or phenomena may occur on a specific time schedule, or phenomena may be quite different depending upon the time at which observations are made, such as with the administration of medications or treatments. Depending upon the purpose of the observations, the rhythmicity of phenomena may have a significant impact on the data. For example, data collected about the frequency of nurse-patient interaction on an acute care unit could be quite different from the usual if observations were made only during weekends, when the nurse-to-patient ratio might be lower than usual, or confined to times when medications or treatments were administered and nurse-patient interaction might be higher than usual. With such observations, random time sampling becomes particularly important.

EVENT SAMPLING

An alternative approach to time sampling, event sampling may be employed in situations in which events of interest occur relatively infrequently and are at risk of being missed if a strict time sampling procedure is used. In event sampling, integral events or behaviors are specified for observation. The observer must be in a position to take advantage of specific events; therefore, an awareness of the occurrence of the relevant events or behaviors is needed. For example, if an observer is recording the roles and functions of nurses in acute care settings, several events may be selected for observation, for example, change of shift, nursing rounds, care of a dying patient, or nurse-physician interactions. Observation of such events would be likely to provide the observer with data that would not be obtained if a time-sampling procedure were used.

Time sampling and event sampling are the most commonly used approaches for selecting observations; however, other approaches have been developed and used. Alternative approaches have been described by Altmann (1973) and Denzin (1978b).

OBSERVATIONAL APPROACHES

There are two basic approaches to the collection of data through observation: the structured approach and the unstructured approach. The structured approach is more amenable to use by the nonparticipant observer, while the unstructured approach is used more frequently by the participant observer.

Structured observational approaches specify behaviors or events for observation in a rather detailed manner, and a protocol for observing and record keeping is delineated in advance. Since structured observations are highly dependent upon the protocol and observational aids developed prior to observations, the kinds of phenomena observed are likely to be restrained.

Checklists and rating scales are the most frequently used observational aids employed. Checklists facilitate the classification or categorization of behaviors or characteristics observed. Each categorical system is designed to guide the observer in assigning qualitative phenomena into either a quantitative or qualitative system. Well-developed categorical systems facilitate accurate notation of phenomena within a common frame of reference. In most instances, checklists are devised to prompt the observer to record the absence or presence of a behavior or event; however, the frequency of occurrence may be recorded. The categorical systems of checklists used in observation should be nonoverlapping, mutually exclusive, and exhaustive.

Rating scales require the observer to classify behaviors or events in terms of points along a descriptive continuum. Observers may use rating scales during direct observations, or the observer may use rating scales to summarize an interaction or event after observation is completed (Polit and Hungler, 1978, p. 313). Rating scales are employed to record quantitative aspects of the phenomenon of interest, such as its intensity or magnitude, and thereby extend category systems beyond those generally found in checklists. Although rating scales are designed to generate more information about the behavior or event observed, immense demands are placed on the observer when the activity level of objects observed is high.

Unstructured observational approaches involve the collection of large amounts of qualitative information which describes the object, event, or group that is the focus of observation. There is no specific protocol for observations, nor are specific approaches to observing phenomena delineated. Hence, there are few restrictions on the types of methods used and on the types of data obtained. Interviews, life histories, visits, attendance at social events, and record review may be employed, as well as other appropriate strategies for data collection.

Logs and field notes are the most common methods of record keeping employed with unstructured observations. However, observational aids such as tape recordings, maps, and photographs also may be used. A *log* is a record of observations of events, objects, or conversations, which is usually kept on a regular basis during the time that the observer is in the observational setting. *Field notes* are more inclusive than logs and tend to extend observations by analysis and interpretation of relevant occurrences. Use of field notes is a method that combines data collection and data analysis.

Unstructured observation is very useful in exploratory investigations in which the identification and conceptualization of important variables are desired. This approach is flexible and allows the observer to obtain a more complete understanding of the complexities of the situation at hand. Proponents of unstructured observation point out that this approach allows for a better conceptualization of a problem. However, this approach to observation is more highly dependent upon the interpersonal and observational skills of the observer than structured observations. Two major concerns associated with employment of unstructured observation are observer bias and observer influence on the phenomenon that is observed.

RELIABILITY AND VALIDITY OF OBSERVATIONS

When structured observational approaches are used, the reliability and validity of observations depend upon the reliability and validity inherent in the observational aids and in the ability of the observer to identify and record the specified behaviors or events. Thus, the use of well-constructed and well-developed observational instruments and well-trained observers takes on special significance. Care should be taken to select reliable and valid observational aids, and observers should be trained prior to the initiation of data collection.

Observer training sessions should be held to familiarize observers with instruments, the nature of behaviors or events observed, the sampling procedure, and the purpose of the project. Trial experience in the use of instruments should be provided until observers have sufficiently mastered the art of observing and recording the phenomenon of interest. If more than one observer is employed, training should continue until there is sufficient interrater reliability.

Reliability and validity of unstructured approaches can be facilitated and assessed through the process of triangulation. Triangulation involves combining "multiple data sources, research methods, theoretical perspectives, and observers in the collection, inspection, and analysis" of observational specimens (Denzin, 1978b, p. 101). The reliability and validity of findings are evaluated by ascertaining the frequency of an observation by examining data obtained via multiple methods and multiple data sources. The more frequently an observed behavior occurs across time and space, the more likely it is to be valid. The lack of multiple instances of observation detracts from the validity of an indicator. Frequency of occurrence of a phenomenon should be observed across subjects or over and over again within the same individual. Validity of indicators also can be assessed by comparing records from different data sources, for example, interviews, diaries, or other documents. An indicator that results from an unstructured observation also can be assessed by the observability of behaviors or activities on which it is based. Less credence can be placed on those indicators that result from the observer's imputation of motives, attitudes, or intentions to others.

ADVANTAGES AND DISADVANTAGES OF OBSERVATIONAL METHODS

Several advantages and disadvantages of observation have been addressed during the discussion. This section will serve to highlight some of the major benefits and problems associated with observational approaches.

Observation provides a variety and depth of information that is difficult to obtain with other data collection methods. The approach can be quite flexible and allow an observer to get inside a situation in a manner that can reveal information that cannot be readily obtained via other methods. Hence, observational approaches can effectively facilitate and enhance conceptualization and understanding of phenomena. This approach is of particular benefit, because there are many problems that cannot be studied sufficiently by other means.

The major disadvantage of observational approaches is that data obtained through observation are readily amenable to bias and distortion. Perceptual errors by observers and insufficient skill in observing threaten the quality of data. This is less of a problem when the structured approach to observation is used rather than the unstructured. When the observer's presence is known, reactivity to the observer by subjects may distort behavior. However, concealment of the observer's presence or identity presents ethical concerns regarding subject's consent to be observed. Concealment of observer identity also can limit the depth and amount of data obtained.

The structured approach provides for better control of reliability and validity of measurements than the unstructured approach; however, it limits the kinds of phenomena that will be monitored and recorded. The unstructured approach provides for a large variety of data sources and data collection methods, but reliability and validity of measures are difficult to assess and control.

The problems and difficulties associated with observational methods need not be prohibitive. A clear conceptualization of the problem to be studied, operationalization of key variables, and a logical protocol for observing, recording, and interpreting data can help alleviate or decrease a number of concerns.

CONTENT ANALYSIS

Because recorded words and sentences are human artifacts, they provide rich and varied sources of data about the personalities, thoughts, attitudes, and preferences of the writers (or speakers), as well as about the interpersonal, social, political, and cultural contexts in which they are or were involved. In order to render these potential data sources usable for drawing reliable and valid scientific conclusions or clinical judgments, it is necessary to use procedures that are more objective and systematic than the intuitive judgments generally employed in everyday reading or listening. The term *content analysis* refers to a systematic, objective procedure for examining the content of recorded information. It is used for identifying, measuring, describing, and making inferences about specified characteristics within or reflected by written or verbal text.

Content analysis involves the systematic and objective reduction or simplification of recorded language to a set of categories or statistically manipulable symbols that represent the presence, frequency, intensity, or nature of selected characteristics (Markoff, et al, 1977, p. 5). Two key interrelated processes are involved: specifying characteristics of the content that are to be measured, and applying explicit rules for identifying and recording the characteristics (Stone, et al, 1966, p. 7).

Content analysis has several distinctive features which make it a useful measurement technique for nursing research, education, and practice. First, it is applied to *recorded* information, that is, information that has been written as text or recorded in a way that allows exact replay of the original communication. Either pre-existing materials that have been written or recorded for another purpose or materials produced for a particular investigation can be used. Examples of materials that can be used in content analysis include books, plays, newspaper articles and editorials, films, letters, notes, diaries, speeches, documents such as laws or minutes of meetings, written or tape recorded responses of subjects to questions, and audiotaped or videotaped recordings of communication. Through the use of content analysis, materials originally produced for a variety of different purposes can be used as data sources to answer questions relevant to nursing.

Second, emphasis is on the *content* of the written or verbal communication rather than its process or paralingual aspects (e.g., pitch, volume, rate, accompanying gestures). This is not to negate the importance of process or paralingual elements but to suggest that the procedures of content analysis are best suited to a content focus. Paralingual cues cannot be adequately analyzed unless they are consistently noted in textual form (Stone, et al, 1966, p. 13). Process analysis represents a different focus which is best handled using other tools and techniques designed specifically for that purpose, for example, Bales' Interaction Process Analysis (1951). However, inferences about processes (e.g., historical trends, information flow) can be made by comparing content expressed at different points in time or by different communicators. The analysis of materials can be directed toward either the manifest (overtly expressed) content of the communication or its latent content (unintentionally or unconsciously expressed). The analysis of latent content involves making inferences about what was intended or meant from that which was actually stated and is analogous to "reading between the lines."

Third, the procedure of content analysis is designed to achieve *objectivity* by incorporating explicit rules. Detailed rules for the examination of recorded information help to remove the effects of idiosyncratic characteristics of particular analysts or coders. Fourth, the procedure is *systematic*, in that specified criteria are consistently applied in selecting and processing the content to be analyzed. Selection and analysis procedures are therefore not arbitrary but predetermined and explicit and are applied consistently to all information being examined. These two defining characteristics of content analysis—that it is objective and systematic—make it appropriate for use in drawing scientific conclusions.

Finally, content analysis involves deliberate simplification that results in the loss of some of the individuality and richness of meaning in the original material in the interest of discerning regularities and patterns. The degree to which the material is simplified and the nature of the regularities discerned are determined by the purpose for the analysis and are not inherent in the procedure itself. Thus, content analysis has a wide variety of potential qualitative as well as quantitative applications in nursing.

Content analysis has been used by many disciplines as a research tool. The earliest applications were in the fields of journalism and political science in studies of the mass media and propaganda. More recent applications have ranged widely from studies of personality and psychological states of individuals to communication patterns within small groups, comparative cross-cultural studies, and studies of historical trends and social change (Stone et al, 1966; Gottschalk and Gelser, 1969; Gottschalk, 1979; Budd, et al, 1967; Carney, 1972).

Because content analysis can be successfully applied to many types of recorded information, its potential applications in nursing are many. The most frequently cited examples are research-oriented and include historical studies regarding trends in the profession and studies of interpersonal communication patterns; characteristics, opinions, and expressed values of individuals and groups; the impact of policy on health care; and current issues and trends. Content analysis can also be used as a means for validating other measures of the same concept or characteristic. Content analysis is potentially useful not only in the research arena but in practice contexts as well. For example, content analyses of the verbal responses of patients recorded preoperatively could be used to assess their level of anxiety, and content analyses of nursing notes or care plans could be used to evaluate the quality of care or the impact of an inservice education program.

EXAMPLE

A classic example of the application of content analysis techniques in nursing is a study of the content of public health nurses' home visits conducted by Johnson and Hardin (1962; Johnson, 1969). In this study 956 home visits were tape-recorded, and a sample of 287 home visits were ultimately analyzed. The home visits were also observed and nonverbal behavior and environmental dynamics were described in writing by the observer. A plan was devised for abstracting the sound symbols from each recording; these abstracts were then coded.

Each visit was subdivided into subject-matter sequences according to the dominant topics that arose, and each sequence was classified into one of the following major categories: (1) bodily states, processes, and symptoms; (2) treatment and control measures; (3) measures relating to the implementation of treatment/control procedures; (4) other aspects of the physical health status of individuals; (5) selected current individual and household activities having implications for health; (6) all other subject matter; (7) instrumental and irrelevant subject matter; (8) silences; and (9) unknown.

The time spent on each sequence and the number of occurrences of each topic were recorded.

In order to code data regarding the dynamic aspects of the visit, the frequency and length of other responses of nurses and patients were recorded. The three dimensions coded were communicative mechanisms, expressions of feeling states toward the subjects of discussion, and expressions of feeling states of participants toward each other. In order to assess such variables as the visit's dominance-passivity dimension, the degree of focus to the visit, the relative importance of the teaching dimension, and the affective quality of the visit, a variety of time-and-space measures were used. These included total verbal output, relative verbal output of the nurse, relative initiation of ideas by the nurse, relative time spent on questioning by the nurse, relative time spent on household responses to questions, relative time spent on advice-giving by the nurse, and number of episodes of laughter per unit of time. These measures were used to contrast cases that differed in such features as relative involvement of both nurse and household members in the visit and degree of focus on a particular topic such as physical health status.

The final data collection and analysis followed a 13-month pilot study during which time methods of data collection were tested. Observers and coders were trained in practice sessions. An estimate of interrater reliability was calculated using a subsample of 24 cases from the main sample and percentage of agreement ranged from 63 to 100 on the 16 dimensions so analyzed.

PROCEDURE

Content analysis involves a multistep procedure which is guided in all of its aspects by the purpose for the investigation, the questions to be answered, and hypotheses to be tested. For purposes of this discussion it is assumed that the purposes for the investigation have been identified, that the data source of relevant recorded information has been located, and that the investigator is ready to proceed with the content analysis.

STEP 1. DEFINE THE UNIVERSE OF CONTENT TO BE EXAMINED. The universe of content refers to the totality of recorded information about which characteristics will be described or inferences drawn. Examples would include all presidential addresses at the American Nurses Association conventions, all psychiatric nursing texts published in the United States between 1948 and 1965, all tape recorded responses to a telephone interview, or all nursing care plans generated by the staff of a community health nursing agency during one month. When a given universe of content is proposed, its appropriateness to the investigation must be assessed carefully. This entails consideration of the nature of the information included, its relevance to the purposes of the investigation, its completeness and ease of access, and the conditions under which the materials were produced. In many instances permission must be secured in advance to use the materials for the proposed investigation.

STEP 2. IDENTIFY THE CHARACTERISTICS OR CONCEPTS TO BE MEASURED. These vary widely from one investigation to another and are determined by the conceptual or theoretical background, research questions, or hypotheses. This step in the analysis consists essentially of answering the question, "What do I want to know about or learn from the content of the recorded information?" It is the initial phase of partitioning or subdividing the content into categories. There is no limit to the number of characteristics that can be examined; however, the selection should be dictated by the purpose for the investigation. For example, a nurse studying the relationship of nurses' educational preparation to their interviewing styles during history-taking interviews with patients might choose to examine such characteristics of interviewing style as orientation to self versus other; positivism versus negativism; or degree of activity versus passivity.

STEP 3. SELECT THE UNIT OF ANALYSIS TO BE EMPLOYED. Given the universe of content available and the variables to be measured, a decision must be made about which elements or subunits of the content will be analyzed. The selection is based on the type of unit that can be used most reliably as evidence for the presence, frequency, or intensity of the characteristics to be studied. Possible units of analysis range in complexity from letters or syllables—used primarily in linguistic research—to entire speeches or texts. The units most potentially useful in nursing are words, themes, items, and space-and-time measures (Berelson, 1954). Words are commonly chosen units for analysis, because they are easy to work with and are amenable to computer analysis. A frequently used procedure is to identify words or word combinations that are synonyms for or indicators of a more abstract concept or characteristic. Themes are sentences or propositions about something (Kerlinger, 1973, p. 528). Because they are more complex than words, they are more difficult to use reliably; however, they may impart more meaning than words taken alone. The term item refers to an entire production (e.g., story, book, interview, response to an open-ended question) that is analyzed as a whole in terms of a given characteristic. Time-and-space measures are physical measurements of content, for example, number of words or pages, or number of minutes of discussion. Generally speaking, the more complex the unit, the more difficult the attainment of high levels of reliability in measurement.

Depending on the number and complexity of the characteristics being measured, more than one unit of content analysis can be used to measure a given characteristic. In some instances a given unit may be appropriate for measuring one characteristic of the content but not another, and several units may be used within the investigation, each for a separate subanalysis. In the example cited above, the nurse might choose the following units of analysis:

Characteristic Dimension	Unit of Analysis
Self-other orientation	Word
Positivism-Negativism	Theme
Activity-Passivity	Theme and Time-and-space Measure

259

STEP 4. DEVELOP A SAMPLING PLAN. Once the unit of analysis has been identified, it is necessary to determine how the universe of content will be sampled. In some instances the entire universe will be examined; in others, only selected portions will be analyzed. A specific plan must be designed with explicit instructions provided as the basis for selecting the content to be analyzed. Random sampling of elements of the universe of content is preferable to nonrandom procedures. A frequent procedure is to use systematic random sampling wherein, after a randomly determined starting point, every n^{th} unit (word, phrase, paragraph, etc.) is sampled. Multistage sampling may be employed. For example, a random sample of textbooks might be selected from those available; then a random sample of three chapters selected from each book; then every third paragraph within those chapters content analyzed using the themes within each sampled paragraph as the unit of analysis. In the previous sample the nurse might select a five-minute segment from each recorded interview. A decision would have to be made whether to begin the segment at the same point in all interviews (e.g., the first five minutes) or whether to randomly select the starting point for the segment (e.g., determine the starting point by a random process such as using a table of random numbers to select a tape-counter reading at which to initiate the analysis).

STEP 5. DEVELOP A SCHEME FOR CATEGORIZING THE CONTENT. This is the most difficult and most important step in content analysis. As Berelson (1954) has noted: "Since the categories contain the substance of the investigation, a content analysis can be no better than its system of categories" (p. 147). Development of the categorical scheme can proceed deductively (deriving categories from the theory guiding the investigation) or inductively (deriving categories from the data themselves); or a combination of the two strategies can be used. An essential point to be remembered is that the categorical scheme links the theoretical or conceptual background of the investigation with the data and provides the basis for making inferences and drawing conclusions.

Having identified the characteristics to be measured (Step 2), the categorical system provides the basis for measuring the existence, frequency, intensity, or nature of each characteristic. Two or more categories are specified to classify the content with respect to each characteristic being measured. The categories are constructed so that each unit of the content can be assigned unequivocably to one category; that is, the categories for a given characteristic must be exhaustive and mutually exclusive, and criteria for assigning the content to a category must be clear and explicit. It is generally recommended that the categories in content analysis be semantically as close as possible to the wording in the original text, so the meaning is distorted as little as possible.

In many categorical schemes for content analysis the category consists of a list of language signs, such as words or phrases, which represent a given characteristic (variable) or level of that variable. The basic procedure is to determine which words or statements with similar meanings cluster together to form a category that is different from the others, identify these language signs when they occur in the text, and score them as instances of the category. In the example cited above, in order to develop a categorical scheme for measuring self-other orientation of the interviewer, the nurse researcher might generate a list of words indicative of self-orientation (I, me, mine, etc.) to form the self category and a list of words to form the other category (you, yours, their, etc). When these words are encountered they would be scored as instances of one of the two categories, and other words would be assigned to a neither category or disregarded as noninstances of the characteristic being measured. A similar procedure is used for constructing categories that represent different levels or intensities of a particular characteristic. Verbal cues (key words and descriptive phrases) have been used, for example, to develop scales that distinguish several levels of such psychological characteristics as hope, depression, and anxiety (Gottschalk and Gelser, 1969; Gottschalk, 1979).

Several strategies may be suggested to aid the nurse in constructing a categorical scheme for content analysis.

1. Carefully read or listen to the available material to develop a sense of the language being used and the divisions into which the data might fall, bearing in mind the conceptual orientation underlying the investigation.

2. Examine existing categorical schemes developed by other content analysts. A number of content dictionaries potentially applicable to nursing have already been developed, and some are available as computer programs. These dictionaries group words with similar meanings under a given conceptual heading (Stone, et al, 1966; Holsti, 1969). The work of Gottschalk and colleagues (Gottschalk and Gelser, 1969; Gottschalk, 1979) has produced several reliable and valid categorical schemes for measuring psychological traits through the content analysis of verbal behavior. An existing scheme or program may be directly relevant to the investigation.

3. After developing a set of categories ask experts in the field of the investigation to evaluate the relevance, clarity, and completeness of the scheme.

STEP 6. DEVELOP EXPLICIT CODING AND SCORING INSTRUCTIONS. These rules embody the criteria for processing the content, that is, for assigning the designated units of analysis to categories. They must be as specific and complete as possible. Accompanying lists of key words and examples should be provided.

STEP 7. PRETEST THE CATEGORIES AND CODING INSTRUCTIONS. The categorical scheme is pretested by applying it, according to the explicit instructions, to small portions of the content to be analyzed. Preferably at least two coders should be asked to analyze the same material so that interrater reliability can be assessed and discrepancies clarified. As a result of the pretesting, categories or instructions may have to be redefined, added, or deleted and the entire scheme re-pretested before use.

STEP 8. TRAIN CODERS AND ESTABLISH AN ACCEPTABLE LEVEL OF RELIABILITY. Careful coder training is an essential step if persons other than the investigator are to be used to perform the analysis. Because subjective perception, which is influenced by culture and experience, plays a role in much content analysis, it is crucial that explicit instructions be provided and several trial runs be carried out before the actual analysis begins. Interrater and intrarater reliability must be assessed throughout the training period and acceptable levels established before training ends.

STEP 9. PERFORM THE ANALYSIS. The data are coded and tabulated according to prescribed procedures established in advance. Each element of the content universe being analyzed (i.e., each document, book, verbal response) is coded using the same procedure. If many content characteristics are being examined, the same content may be processed several times to extract all of the information needed. Because fatigue, boredom, and concurrent experience may influence coding, periodic checks of interrater and intrarater reliability must be performed throughout the coding. The investigator working alone should periodically assess intrarater reliability. Tabulation of content analysis data nearly always involves as a first step a frequency count of the recorded occurrences of each category. The nature of subsequent analyses is determined by the purpose of the investigation.

ADVANTAGES AND DISADVANTAGES

There are several advantages and disadvantages of content analysis as a technique for nursing measurement. Major advantages include the following:

1. The technique allows use of existing information that is available and easily accessible at relatively low cost. Available information can be used for multiple purposes.

2. Characteristics of individuals and groups can be studied unobtrusively, that is, without requiring subjects to do anything out of the ordinary or even making them aware that they are being studied.

3. Information produced for nonscientific purposes can be made usable for scientific inference.

4. Available data sources cover long time frames, thereby allowing study of trends not otherwise amenable to analysis.

5. Computerized approaches are available which greatly simplify difficult categorization and coding procedures.

Major disadvantages are as follows:

1. The procedure is very time consuming.

2. Many materials have been prescreened or edited by others, and hence, are subject to incompleteness or bias.

3. Data in the original sources may not have been compiled systematically. When doubt exists about the accuracy or completeness of a data source, it is recommended that either multiple sources be content analyzed or content analysis be combined with other techniques.

4. Judgment is required in order to interpret the meaning of another's communication; thus, there is a risk of subjectivity on the part of the coder or analyst.

5. Legal or ethical problems may be encountered regarding the use of information that was gathered for another purpose.

INTERVIEW

The interview is a *face-to-face,** *verbal* interchange in which one individual, the interviewer, attempts to elicit information from another, the respondent, generally by means of direct questioning. It is the method that nurses employ most frequently in their practice to obtain information from others. Within the context of this book, the interview is considered to be a measurement instrument designed to yield data to accomplish specified purposes and subject to the same considerations of reliability and validity as other measurement tools.

The interview is used for a variety of purposes in nursing. The most frequent use is to obtain factual (as perceived by the respondent) information about the respondent and events, situations, or persons within the respondent's awareness. Examples are interviews to gather health history or employment history data or data about an individual's past and current health habits and health problems. Because of its potential flexibility, the interview is particularly useful for gathering factual information from respondents who may have difficulty recalling specific events or may be attempting to explain complex processes or situations. Interviews may also be used to elicit an individual's attitudes, opinions, level of knowledge, intentions about future actions, and definitions of standards (i.e., what should be) and to determine the reasons for or influences on particular actions, attitudes, or beliefs (Polit and Hungler, 1978, pp. 331-332).

Although other types of measurement instruments such as questionnaires or projective techniques (discussed in later sections of this chapter) can be used to gather the same types of information, the interview is frequently the method of choice, because it allows opportunity to identify misinterpretation and clarify communication, identify inconsistency, probe for additional information, and pursue selected topics in depth and with greater detail than other methods allow. It is uniquely suited for gathering information from those who are unable to read or complete written documents. Many such populations (e.g., young children, the very ill, the elderly, the blind, the illiterate) are of interest in nursing practice and research.

Because of the diversity of purposes for which it is applicable, the interview is a very useful measurement instrument in nursing practice and research. Certain of its characteristics do, however, place limits on its utility. Because it involves face-to-face interaction, the respondent is always aware that information is being sought and is always influenced, at least to some degree, by perceptions of the interviewer, the questions being asked, and the setting. Thus, the interview may be of little utility in situations in which complete anonymity is desirable or required (e.g., when information about highly sensitive or personal topics is desired or when the respondent may fear retribution). If it is apparent that willingness to respond and truthfulness of response would be compromised by a personal method of gathering information, then an impersonal method would be preferred. In some

---

* In some instances interviews are conducted by telephone and there is no face-to-face interaction.

situations the interview itself (because of the respondent's awareness of being studied and that information of a particular kind is being sought) might markedly alter a natural course of events that was to be examined as such. In such cases, an unobtrusive method of gathering information in which the respondent is unaware of the information-gathering process would be preferable to an interview. Specific advantages and disadvantages of the interview as a measurement instrument are detailed in a later portion of this section.

TYPES OF INTERVIEWS

Interviews are typically classified according to the degree of standardization involved. As discussed in Chapter 8, standardization varies in degree and refers to the control that is exercised regarding the development, content, administration, scoring, and interpretation of a measure. Interviews vary greatly in the degree to which their content, the procedures for administration, and recording and scoring responses are prescribed and embody control. It is possible, therefore, to envision a continuum ranging from highly standardized (structured) to unstandardized (unstructured) interviews. The types of interviews representing the two ends of the continuum are described below and their advantages, disadvantages, and optimal uses presented.

STRUCTURED (STANDARDIZED) INTERVIEW. The structured interview is one in which the wording and sequence of all questions are predetermined and fixed; thus, the interview is presented in the same form to all respondents. An example is the interview conducted by the U.S. Census Bureau. In this, as in other structured interviews, the interviewer is not at liberty to change the wording or order of any question; however, in some instances, alternate wordings are specified for use should a respondent have difficulty understanding what is asked. For example, lay terms for the names of body parts or diseases might be suggested as alternatives to medical terminology. Probes (questions, phrases, or words added to the original question in order to encourage additional or more complete responses) may be included in the standardized interview; however, they are specified in advance and are generally not left to the discretion of the interviewer.

Denzin (1978, pp. 113–114) notes that several assumptions are inherent in the standardized interview. First, it is assumed that since each respondent is presented with identical verbal stimuli, those stimuli will elicit the same range of meanings for each respondent. Second, it is assumed to be possible to find a uniform wording for all questions that will be equally meaningful to each respondent. Third, it is assumed that if the meaning of each stimulus is to be identical for each respondent, then the context (which includes the preceding questions) must be identical; thus, the sequence of questions presented to each respondent must be identical. Finally, it is assumed that by careful development and pilot testing, an interview schedule (list of questions and responses) can be developed that is congruent with the first three assumptions. Denzin goes on to note that these assumptions are often erroneous and, at best, can be met only when respondents have similar characteristics and experiences, so that they will be likely to interpret the meanings of questions from the same frame of reference.

The standardized interview is designed to assure comparability across respondents, thereby allowing one to conclude that any differences found are attributable to variation in response, rather than in the instrument or the way it is administered. The structured interview generally has higher reliability than less standardized forms. Since all questions are prescribed, there is less likelihood of *interviewer bias* than with less standardized interviews. Interviewer bias refers to systematic differences that occur from interviewer to interviewer in the way questions are asked and responses are elicited and recorded (Selltiz, et al, 1959, pp. 583–585). The structured interview also has the advantage that it does not require extensive training of interviewers, because the questions are predetermined. The primary disadvantage of the structured interview is its inflexibility. If an interviewer perceives that a respondent misunderstands a question, nothing can be done to rectify the situation except within the limits specified in the interview schedule. The validity of the interview and the comparability of responses may be seriously compromised if the meaning of the questions is unclear to respondents.

The structured interview is most appropriately used when identical information is needed from all respondents, when comparisons are to be made across respondents, respondents are relatively homogeneous in background and experience, and large or geographically dispersed samples are used. The structured interview is often used in hypothesis-testing research and when rigorous quantification of information is required.

UNSTRUCTURED (UNSTANDARDIZED) INTERVIEW. The unstructured interview is one in which the wording and sequence of the questions are not prescribed but are left to the discretion of the interviewer. An interview schedule or specific set of questions generally is not provided; however, a list of suggested questions may be developed as an aid to the interviewer. Frequently, the interviewer works from a listing of the information needed or topics to be covered, and these are guided by the purpose of the interview. However, the phrasing of questions and the order in which they are asked is changed to fit the characteristics of each respondent. The interviewer has freedom to pursue various topics to different degrees with each respondent. Unstructured interviews are often used in clinical history taking and assessment and in applicant selection interviews. In these instances the interviewer has a listing of topics about which information is needed but is free to phrase and order the questions differently for each respondent.

According to Denzin (1978) a very different set of assumptions underlies the less structured interview. First, it is assumed that ". . . if the meaning of a question is to be standardized it must be formulated in words familiar to those interviewed" (p. 115). In other words, it is not assumed that identical words have identical meanings to different people. Rather, it is desirable to change words to fit respondents, in order to assure the meaningfulness of questions. The second assumption is that no given sequence of questions is satisfactory for all respondents. Instead, the best sequence is determined by the respondent's willingness and readiness to discuss a particular topic. Third, if the interviewer is working from a list of topics to be covered and, in fact, covers them, then it can be asserted that even though the questions are not identical, each respondent is exposed to the same general set of stimuli. Obviously, this assertion is not valid if the interviewer does not have such a list or does not cover all topics during the interview.

The primary advantage of the unstructured interview is its flexibility in allowing the questioning to be geared to fit the interpretation of the respondent and in allowing the interviewer to go beyond a given response to probe its meaning in depth. The main disadvantages of the unstructured interview are inability to make systematic comparisons across respondents, difficulty in establishing reliability, heightened probability of interviewer bias, and the requirement that interviewers be extensively trained. It is a desirable type of interview to use when respondents differ enough in their backgrounds to prevent consistent meaning interpretation; when extensive, in-depth information is needed from each respondent; and when the respondent's meanings and definitions of the situation are important data. The unstructured interview is often used in descriptive and exploratory research directed toward increasing understanding of how particular factors are operating in a given situation.

TYPES OF QUESTIONS OR ITEMS

The basic element of the interview is the question or item. There are two major types of questions included in the interview: the fixed-alternative or closed-ended question and the open-ended or open question. The *closed-ended question* is one that supplies the respondent with a response set containing two or more specified alternative responses from which to choose. Dichotomous, multiple-choice, and scale items (those to which the subject responds by indicating degrees of agreement or disagreement on a fixed scale, Kerlinger, 1973, p. 485) are included in this category. Examples of these types of questions are provided in Chapter 4. The *open-ended question* has no specified alternative responses, and the subject is free to word the response. The structured interview includes either closed- or open-ended items or a combination of the two types. The unstructured interview generally includes open-ended questions but may include both types, for example, when the interviewer asks a question requiring either an affirmative or negative reply. Examples of open-ended questions are as follows:

What is your opinion about the care you received while you were a patient on this floor?

Please describe your head nurse's most outstanding leadership quality.

What is the first thing you remember hearing or seeing as you awoke from the anesthesia?

From a measurement perspective the two types of questions have strengths and weaknesses. The closed-ended question provides uniformity, thus increased reliability. Although it is easy to code, it is more difficult to construct, because the question writer must determine in advance the full range of alternative responses. There exists the possibility that some may be overlooked; however, this problem can often be minimized by subjecting the questions to experts for review and by including one open-ended category in the response set (e.g., other). Closed-ended questions are most appropriately used when the range of possible alternative responses is known, limited, and clear-cut. Since the question writer determines the possible responses available to the respondent, the closed-ended question helps establish the respondent's frame of reference, thereby avoiding responses that are irrelevant or incomparable. On the other hand, since responses are predetermined, they may not be valid indicators of a particular respondent's view. Validity may also be compromised when a subject is enabled (or forced), by virtue of a provided response set, to address a subject on the basis of little or no knowledge. The inclusion of *filter* questions may help eliminate this problem. A *filter question* is used to determine an individual's level of information about or experience with a given topic before proceeding to other questions about it. For example, a question such as "Have you ever been hospitalized?" might be used as a filter to prevent asking those who have no first-hand knowledge of the hospitalization experience specific questions regarding their views on the subject. Generally speaking, closed-ended questions are more efficient to administer and score than open-ended questions. More closed- than open-ended questions can be asked in a given period of time. Closed-ended questions are particularly useful for addressing sensitive topics about which respondents may be reluctant to talk at any length or to provide information. A respondent, for example, may be more likely to indicate annual income by choosing the appropriate category from a provided list than to state the amount in response to an open-ended question.

The open-ended question is relatively easy to construct, but responses are difficult to record and analyze reliably. Because the response is provided verbally and may be complex, it is difficult to record accurately unless a tape recorder is used. The complex procedures of content analysis must be employed in order to code and score responses. Since these procedures are employed after the data have been collected, there is danger that the responses may be misinterpreted by the analyst. Because the open-ended question provides only the frame of reference or context to which the respondent replies, the response may be irrelevant to the purpose for which the question was asked. In an unstructured interview, the question can be reinterpreted by the interviewer. In the structured interview, it is often desirable to develop orienting sentences or to *funnel* questions to help orient the thinking of the respondent. A funnel is a list of questions concerning a given topic, which are arranged in order of decreasing generality. Including broad questions initially allows the respondent to express views without being influenced by subsequent questions. The open-ended question allows the respondent to express responses using his own words. This feature enhances validity not only by enabling the interviewer to detect misunderstanding and ambiguity, but also by reducing bias, since the open-ended question allows the respondent to supply answers that might not have been anticipated by the question developer. Generally, open-ended questions are most appropriate when complex issues or processes are being examined, when relevant dimensions of responses are unknown, and when it is necessary to know how the respondent perceives an issue (Selltiz, et al, 1959, p. 262).

PROCEDURE FOR DEVELOPING THE INTERVIEW SCHEDULE

The following is the procedure recommended for developing an interview schedule. A brief overview of each step is provided. The reader desiring more detailed information about designing interview questions and conducting an interview can consult one of the many excellent resources available: for example, Selltiz et al (1959), Gordon (1980), Richardson, et al (1965), Institute for Social Research (1976), and Bradburn, et al (1979).

STEP 1. DETERMINE THE INFORMATION TO BE SOUGHT. The first step in designing an interview is to decide what information is needed from the respondent. The decision is based on the objectives for the investigation, the questions that the investigation is designed to answer, or the variables and hypotheses that have been identified. It is desirable to develop a blueprint or table of specifications that lists all of the types or categories of information needed and the relative emphasis that is to be given to each category. This allows the interview developer to estimate the number of questions needed to cover each category and to be sure that less important categories are not given more attention than those that are more essential. A sample content outline developed for study of help-seeking behavior is shown in Chapter 2. The categories represent the major topics about which information will be collected and serve as the basis for developing a table of specifications.

STEP 2. DEVELOP THE QUESTION OR ITEMS. After the needed information has been delimited, the next step is to draft the questions and the alternative responses if any are to be provided. This is not an easy task. It involves both translating the purposes into questions that will yield the needed information and motivating the respondent to provide the information. A decision must be made regarding the use of open-ended or closed-ended questions (or a combination of the two) in the light of the strengths and weaknesses of each type and the kind of information that is needed. The wording of each question is crucial, since the meaning must be clear to the respondent and must be precise enough to convey what is expected without biasing the content of the response. Several guidelines are suggested.

1. Be sure that the wording used accurately conveys the meaning intended.

2. Keep sentences and phrases short.

3. Use simple terminology that can be understood by the least educated respondent; if complex or technical terminology is necessary, clearly define each such term before asking the question.

4. Include only one idea per question.

5. Avoid words that have ambiguous interpretations or could be interpreted in more than one way.

6. Avoid terms that are emotionally laden or that might trigger biased responses.

7. Do not ask leading questions; that is, questions that suggest an answer.

8. Avoid personal or delicate content that the respondent may resist answering; if it must be included, word the question as nonoffensively as possible. Sensitive questions are best placed at the end of the interview.

9. If a closed-ended format is being used, clearly define the alternative responses for the respondent. This may be done verbally as part of the question or may be done by writing possible responses on a card or booklet that is shown to the respondent.

10. Attempt to minimize the effect of social desirability by avoiding questions that lead respondents to express socially desirable sentiments, that is, those that imply approval of things generally considered good or indicate behaviors that are expected by society.

11. Use filter questions to be sure that respondents are not being asked to provide answers about topics with which they are unfamiliar.

It is often desirable to provide introductory information to set the stage for a series of questions and communicate to the respondent the context in which they are to be interpreted. This is particularly helpful when one is shifting from one topic to another in the interview. For example, before beginning a series of questions about the nurse's perception of the degree of autonomy (independent decision making) that the job permits, a statement such as the following might be provided.

> You have just told me about the aspects of your job that you find most rewarding. Now I am going to ask you about several kinds of patient-care situations about which you may be expected to make decisions on the job. Some will be situations in which you are able to make decisions on your own. Others will be situations in which you are not able to make decisions by yourself but must consult your coworkers or supervisors. Others will be decisions in which you do not participate at all. After I read a situation to you, tell me whether you think you would be able to make the decision independently, with assistance from others, or not at all.

This statement alerts the respondent to a change in topic and serves to set the stage for a series of situations, varying in the degree of independent decision making which they allow, to which one of three responses is requested.

STEP 3. DETERMINE THE SEQUENCE FOR THE QUESTIONS. Once the questions have been designed, an appropriate sequence must be developed. The main criterion for determining the sequence of questions is that they be arranged in a logical and realistic fashion so that they make sense to the respondent. The order that is generally suggested to elicit the highest degree of cooperation from respondents is as follows. Begin with questions that are most likely to capture the interest of the respondent and increase motivation to cooperate. Less interesting questions and those that may be difficult to answer should come later in the interview. Sensitive or personal questions should be asked near the end of the interview. A respondent who is offended by them may terminate the interview at that point. Traditionally, socio-demographic information is requested at the end of the interview.

In order to make the interview more logical and less confusing to the respondent, it is desirable to cluster questions concerning a given topic.

Within clusters, open-ended should precede closed-ended questions and general questions should precede more specific ones. The reason for this ordering is to avoid earlier questions suggesting responses to those which follow, thus minimizing bias in the response. Two exceptions to the general-to-specific ordering can be suggested. First, some scales require questions to be randomly ordered. Second, when asking the respondent to recall events occurring in the past or to describe a complex process, initial specific questions may help to trigger recollection.

STEP 4. SUBJECT THE QUESTIONS TO REVIEW. After the questions have been written and arranged, they should be submitted to measurement and content experts for review. Measurement experts can often spot ambiguous wording, unclear or imprecise statements, or questions that are unlikely to yield the desired response. Content experts are able to evaluate the clarity of wording, appropriateness of the question to the content area, and the inclusiveness of the response set. It may be helpful at this stage to have individuals who are unfamiliar with the content of the interview review the questions for clarity of meaning and use of readily understandable terminology. Such individuals may also suggest additional responses to consider. The questions are revised on the basis of input received.

STEP 5. DRAFT THE INTERVIEW SCHEDULE. The interview schedule contains not only the questions to be asked but also an introductory statement and explicit instructions for the interviewer and the respondent and a closing statement. Introductory information to be read to the respondent should address the purpose for the interview, what will be done with the information obtained and who will have access to it, risks (if any) and benefits to the respondent and others, an estimate of the time involved, and an orientation to the interviewing and recording procedure. It is appropriate to terminate the interview with a statement of appreciation for the respondent's cooperation.

Instructions to the respondent should be explicit. New instructions are required at each point in the interview when there is a change in format, that is, when different kinds of responses are being requested. Instructions to the interviewer must also be detailed and precise. These should include such matters as indication of whether or not questions may be repeated or reworded, listings of probes for each question in which they are to be used, and instructions about how to record the response. A particularly important aspect of interview instructions in nursing, particularly in research-related interviews, is whether or not the interviewer is permitted to provide any assistance or health-related information to the respondent during or after the interview. Nurse interviewers often find it difficult not to intervene with a respondent who has an obvious problem.

STEP 6. PRETEST THE INTERVIEW. An interview is pretested with individuals who have characteristcs and experiences that are identical to those for whom the interview is designed. The pretest provides the opportunity to detect problems with the wording of instructions or questions, assess the time involved, and assess the reliability and validity of the instrument. The interview schedule may be revised based on input from the pretest results.

STEP 7. TRAIN INTERVIEWERS. Because the interview is an interpersonal interaction, it is essential that interviewers be carefully selected and thoroughly trained before contacting respondents and administering the schedule. The selection of appropriate interviewers must take into account the nature of the anticipated respondents and the complexity of the interview situation. Considerable research has shown that the sex, social class, intelligence, experiential background, and appearance of the interviewer influence the nature of information received from respondents in the interview situation (Gordon, 1980). In general, the more congruent the characteristics and experiences of interviewer and respondent, the more likely is the respondent to cooperate and the more valid are the responses obtained. Once selected, interviewers must be trained. The training period may vary in length from a few hours to several weeks, depending on the complexity and degree of structuring of the interview and the prior experience of the interviewers. Training generally includes not only instruction and practice regarding administration of the questions and the recording or scoring of responses, but also consideration of verbal and nonverbal communication skills, appropriate appearance and dress, control of distracting elements in the interview setting, and techniques for securing cooperation and motivating respondents. Acceptable levels of interrater and intrarater reliability must be established before training can be considered complete.

Adequate training is imperative from a measurement perspective, because the interviewer controls, to a considerable degree, the information obtained. As noted above, interviewer bias can be a substantial threat to reliability and validity. It may occur because of inter- or intra-interviewer differences in the way questions are asked, differences in the way responses are elicited and recorded, differences in the way respondents perceive interviewers, differences in the interviewers' perceptions of the respondents, or differences among situations or settings in which the interviews are conducted (Selltiz, et al, 1959, pp. 538-585).

With a highly structured interview schedule, in which considerable control is built into the instrument itself, it must be assured that the interviewer understands that it must be administered and responses recorded consistently across all respondents in order to achieve reliable and valid results. With unstructured interviews, the interviewer holds considerable discretionary power; thus, thorough understanding of the purposes for the interview and considerable communication skill are essential if the purposes are to be achieved. Regardless of the degree of structuring, personal characteristics and behaviors of the interviewer have been shown to influence the responses obtained. For example, subtle differences in gestures, posture, facial expression, and verbal intonation on the part of the interviewer can convey very different messages to the respondent regarding the attitude toward and interest in the responses (Gordon, 1980). Such factors may systematically influence the reliability and validity of the interview, and a key to minimizing such sources of interviewer bias is advance training.

STEP 8. ADMINISTER AND CODE THE INTERVIEW. The final step in the interview procedure is to administer the interview and record and score responses. The degree to which identical administration, recording, and scoring procedures are consistently employed across all respondents is a function of the degree of structuring embodied in the interview schedule. In addition to the interpersonal factors noted above, several elements in the interview situation itself may influence reliability and validity. For example, the duration and scheduling of the interview in relation to the other demands on a respondent's time or other events may influence the information obtained. A respondent who feels rushed to complete the interview quickly because of time pressures or one who is preoccupied by an anticipated problem may be unwilling or unable to supply accurate information. In determining an optimal setting for the interview it is necessary to take into account convenience to the respondent, possible distractions, degree of privacy required, and the potential influence of the setting on the content of response. A respondent might reply very differently to questions eliciting level of satisfaction with nursing care in a hospital setting than in a home setting.

The means used to record responses also influence reliability and validity. Reliability is generally higher for closed-ended than open-ended questions, because responses are recorded in a straight-forward manner on a precoded schedule. Open-ended questions require that the interviewer take notes or that a tape recorder be used. The advantages and disadvantages of both techniques are discussed by Gordon (1980). In general, the more complex the information, the more rapid the information flow, and the greater the likelihood of unanticipated responses, then the more preferable is the use of the tape recorder, despite the increased time and cost involved in transcription. In order to increase reliability and validity, open-ended interview data should be transcribed and coded as soon after the interview as possible. Ideally the transcription and coding should be done by (or at the very least with clarifying input from) the interviewer.

During the administration phase of the interview, it is necessary to make periodic checks of interrater reliability. This may be done by having one other person accompany the interviewer and record and code responses or by tape recording the interview for another individual to code. Reliability coefficients are then computed using the two sets of scores.

RELIABILITY AND VALIDITY

Throughout the discussion of the interview it has been maintained that reliability and validity are crucial considerations. However, the assessment of reliability and validity of interviews has often been neglected because of the time and effort entailed. Reliability assessment includes consideration of interrater reliability (determined at the time of pretesting the interview schedule, during interviewer training, and periodically throughout use of the interview with respondents) and reliability of the instrument itself. The latter assessment generally is carried out using the procedures of test-retest reliability, wherein the same respondent is interviewed more than once using the same schedule, and results are compared. Because this is a time-consuming procedure, which makes considerable demands on the respondent, it is often carried out only during the pretesting phase of instrument development. However, it is advisable to compute test-retest reliability on a small sample of interviews during the administration phase as well. Parallel forms reliability assessment may also be employed for structured interviews; however, split-half reliability is generally not appropriate.

Validity of interview information is a complex issue. Denzin (1972, pp. 136-137) notes that major sources of invalidity in the interview include (1) lack of commonly comprehended meanings; (2) differences in situations and settings; (3) reactive effects of the interview itself, in which respondents modify their responses simply because of being interviewed; (4) demand characteristic effects; and (5) reverse demand characteristic effects. Demand characteristic effects refer to respondents' deliberately monitoring responses to fit perceived demands. Reverse demand characteristic effects occur when the interviewer develops an interpretation of the instrument and attempts to convey that meaning to the respondent. Careful instrument design, with attention to the wording of questions and the input of experts, can minimize some of these sources of invalidity, as can on-going evaluation of tape recordings to monitor possible bias.

A major problem with interviews is assessing the validity of factual information reported by respondents, that is, assessing the degree to which the respondent is telling the truth. In most instances it must simply be assumed that the responses are valid; however, this assumption may be problematic when sensitive issues are involved, when a given response may cast an unfavorable light on the respondent, and when there is difficulty with recall of information. There are ways in which the validity of self-report information can be assessed. For example, within the context of the interview itself the interviewer can observe whether the respondent is disturbed by certain questions or hesitates to answer. Such observations should be noted, so that they can be taken into account in interpreting the information. Inconsistencies in response can also be noted, carefully called to the respondent's attention, and clarified in order to increase validity. Likewise, inconsistencies between self reports and behavior can also be noted by the interviewer. For example, a parent may verbally report a very permissive attitude toward discipline and behave very differently in the presence of the interviewer. Validity may also be assessed by gathering information external to the interview situation in order to check the accuracy of responses. The report that an individual was hospitalized for a given length of time, for example, could be checked against hospital records. The reports of more than one individual (e.g., two or three members of a family or group) can also be compared. Other measurement instruments (e.g., questionnaire, observation) can also be employed in conjunction with the interview as a means for assessing concurrent validity.

EXAMPLE

Alexander and her associates (1982) used a structured interview to measure factors associated with hospital staff nurses' perceptions of autonomy in the work situation. The 30-minute interview was administered to 789 nurses on the clinical unit of employment at the staff nurses' convenience by a staff of trained professional interviewers.

The interview schedule contained questions about the nurse's background and demographic characteristics, perception of the job, and unit and job satisfaction. Measures of personal characteristics included level of education, whether or not this was the nurse's first hospital position, length of employment at the study hospital, and locus of control. The latter variable was operationalized as the summed score of five items (selected on the basis of high item-to-total correlations) selected from those on a 29-item scale developed by Rotter. Perceived job-related characteristics included (1) the staff nurse's attitudes toward the head nurse's leadership style (measured on a five-item scale); (2) the nurse's perception of the frequency with which inappropriate assignments were delegated by physicians; and (3) the nurse's perception of the adequacy of time to devote to professional development. The perceived autonomy variable was measured using a four-item scale developed by Quinn and Shepard and selected on the basis of its relevance, stability, and widespread use. This interview, therefore, contained a combination of items developed by the authors and scale items developed by others. Although reliability and validity data for the interview as a whole were not reported, the internal consistency reliability of the five-item Head Nurse Scale developed by the authors was 0.89 (Cronbach's alpha).

ADVANTAGES AND DISADVANTAGES

The interview has advantages and disadvantages as a measurement tool for use in nursing. Major advantages are its flexibility and its ability to provide on-site clarification of meaning and identification of misunderstanding, to pursue requests for complex information, and to explore particular topics in depth. Because the interviewer is present, the opportunity is provided to use interpersonal skills in establishing rapport and cooperation and setting the stage for the information request. These factors result in a higher response rate and more complete responses than those that result from the use of impersonal measures. The interviewer's presence also provides the opportunity to gather additional information simultaneously through observation and to appraise the validity of the response as it is being given. The interview also provides access to certain populations from which written responses simply cannot be obtained.

The major disadvantage of the interview is its cost in money, effort, and time. Considerable costs are incurred when interviewers must be hired and trained and when responses must be transcribed. The time commitment on the part of the interviewer and respondent may be extensive. Scheduling constraints may result in inconvenience to the interviewer, often necessitating evening or weekend work. The face-to-face interview is generally impractical for large-scale projects involving numerous, widely dispersed respondents; however, a telphone interview may be a possible alternative. (For information about the advantages and disadvantages of the telephone interview, see Simon, 1978 and Dillman, 1978.) Other disadvantages of the interview include inability to provide anonymity, difficulty in achieving uniform administration conditions across respondents, and potential for interviewer bias. Such disadvantages can be minimized through careful instrument construction and interviewer training.

QUESTIONNAIRE

The questionnaire is a form or document containing questions or other types of items to which the subject supplies a written response. The questionnaire, unlike the interview, is self-administered by the respondent. Since it does not entail verbal interchange, a questionnaire can be mailed or simply handed to a respondent. The questionnaire is therefore considered more impersonal than an interview. Whereas interviews vary in the degree to which they are predefined and structured, the questionnaire is always structured, in that the questions or items and their order are predetermined and fixed. Although it is structured, the questionnaire can be quite versatile. Either closed- or open-ended questions can be included, as can a variety of types of scale items including checklists, semantic differential, Likert and Guttman scales, and sociometric measures.

Like the interview, the questionnaire is a relatively direct method of obtaining information. It is used to elicit factual information, attitudes, beliefs, opinions, intentions, and standards, and to assess level of knowledge. Because no personal interaction is required for its use, the questionnaire is often the method of choice for large-scale research projects and for eliciting information and opinions about sensitive or controversial topics. On the other hand, this feature renders the questionnaire less useful than the interview for eliciting complex opinions or gathering information about complex processes or events that the respondent may have difficulty remembering. Because it is structured, the questionnaire is useful in situations in which a high degree of consistency is required for descriptive or comparative purposes. The printed format of the questionnaire makes it ideal for scales involving underlying spatial assumptions which are more accurately portrayed by print or graphics than verbally (e.g., the assumption of equal scale intervals) and for questions that require the respondent to rank or compare numerous items or to select responses from a long or complex response set. Examples of uses of questionnaires in nursing include research studies of the knowledge, attitudes, and behaviors of patients, families and nurses; patient opinion surveys in nursing homes or hospitals; health-history and health-habit assessments carried out in conjunction with physical examinations; student and peer evaluation of courses and programs in schools of nursing; and surveys to assess the health resource needs of certain groups and communities.

PROCEDURE FOR DEVELOPING THE QUESTIONNAIRE

The procedure for developing the questionnaire is very similar to that for developing the interview (see previous section of this chapter), and many of the considerations for each step are identical. Consequently, the only elements of the procedure that will be detailed below are those that are specific to the questionnaire. For detailed information about constructing questionnaires, the reader is referred to Oppenheim (1966), Bradburn, et al (1979), and Dillman (1978).

STEP 1. DETERMINE THE INFORMATION TO BE SOUGHT. This step is identical to the interview, in that objectives must be specified and a blueprint or table of specifications developed.

STEP 2. DEVELOP THE QUESTIONS OR ITEMS. In developing questions or items to be included in a questionnaire it is important to consider clarity of meaning, the understandability of the language used, the ability of the respondent to answer, and the potential for biasing response. The guidelines suggested for writing interview questions apply equally to questionnaire items. Since there is no individual present to assist the respondent to understand what is being asked or to clarify misperceptions, it is even more crucial in questionnaire construction to word each item clearly, avoid ambiguous terms, define terms with which the respondent may be unfamiliar, and provide explicit instructions about how the responses are to be recorded. For example, for closed-ended questions it is necessary to specify the number of responses that may be chosen (e.g., one, all that apply) and the way in which the respondent is to indicate the chosen responses (e.g., circle the response, check the response, fill in the appropriate space on the response sheet). For open-ended questions it may be helpful to include a list of suggested topics, examples, or subquestions in order to cue the respondent about the kind of information expected or the aspects of the question to consider in formulating a response. In general, it is best to avoid open-ended questions that demand a complicated, detailed, or long response on questionnaires. Instead, a series of questions, each of which has a narrower scope, should be substituted. With a questionnaire one cannot draw on the interpersonal skills of an interviewer to motivate or encourage response. Consequently, the question itself must be worded in a way that facilitates a correct interpretation and willing response. A number of techniques can be used to personalize questionnaire items; for example, using conversational sentence structure, using the first and second person pronouns, and italicizing or underlining words that are to receive emphasis. Because of inability to rectify misinterpretation, it is important to use introductory phrases or sentences to supply the context for interpreting questions.

Since the questionnaire is printed or typed, the format for questions and response sets is an important consideration. Clarity, ease of reading, and ease of following instructions are key criteria. Response sets are typically separated from the question and are usually aligned vertically. Filter questions, which direct the respondent to different portions of the questionnaire depending on the response selected, are often difficult for respondents to handle without confusion. A frequent pattern is to indicate following the question or next to each alternative response the next step for the respondent to take (Polit and Hungler, 1978). For example:

      _____ yes   (Continue to question 2)
      _____ no   (Skip to question 3)

A less confusing format is to draw arrows to the next question that the respondent should answer. An example is provided.

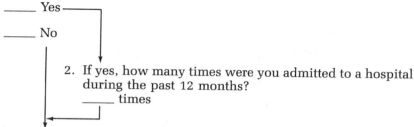

1. Have you been hospitalized during the past 12 months?

_____ Yes

_____ No

    2. If yes, how many times were you admitted to a hospital during the past 12 months?

      _____ times

3. Have you visited an outpatient clinic during the past 12 months?

_____ yes

_____ no

The format, appearance, or sequence of responses may inadvertently bias or unintentionally cue the respondent. For example, the space provided for the response to an open-ended question indicates the approximate length of the response expected. If one response in a set is substantially longer or shorter than the others, the respondent may perceive it to be the expected response.

STEP 3. DETERMINE THE SEQUENCE FOR THE QUESTIONS OR ITEMS. Guidelines for sequencing questionnaire items are identical to those for the interview.

STEP 4. SUBJECT THE QUESTIONNAIRE TO REVIEW. As with the interview, the opinions of measurement and content experts, as well as persons unfamiliar with the content, should be sought in order to assess the clarity and completeness of questions and response sets. It is generally desirable to compile a preliminary draft of the questionnaire for review, so that it can be examined as a whole and the format evaluated. Revisions are made on the basis of input received.

STEP 5. DRAFT THE QUESTIONNAIRE AND COVER LETTER. The questionnaire is compiled into the form that will be used for respondents. Explicit instructions about how it is to be self-administered and how responses are to be recorded should be included on the questionnaire. This means that prior decisions must be made about how the data are to be handled. For example, use of optical scanning sheets may be preferable to having the responses recorded on the questionnaire itself if the instrument is to be used with a large sample. The format for the questionnaire should be clear, legible, and uncrowded, since a questionnaire that is difficult to read or follow is likely to arouse frustration in the respondent and may be discarded or returned incomplete.

If the questionnaire is to be mailed, a cover letter must be drafted. The cover letter is designed to introduce to the respondent the purpose for the questionnaire and its intended uses. Information is also included about the risks and benefits to the respondent and others, confidentiality, an estimate of the time required for completion, and explicit instructions about what the respondent is to do with the questionnaire when it has been completed. Since the cover letter replaces personal contact, it must be worded carefully and in a manner that is likely to motivate the respondent to reply. If the questionnaire is to be handed to the respondent rather than mailed, a script is prepared for an introductory verbal statement containing the same kind of information as a cover letter.

The decision about whether to mail a questionnaire or distribute it via personal contact is primarily based on the nature of the population or sample of respondents that is to receive the questionnaire. If the respondents can be easily reached by personal contact, it is generally preferable to use personal rather than mail distribution, because response rates are likely to be higher. Personal distribution by the investigator or other cooperating individuals is feasible for many nursing applications of the questionnaire, for example, those that involve patients or staff in local hospitals or health agencies or intact community or student groups. For large or geographically dispersed samples, mail distribution may be the only practical approach, despite the problems involved. The primary problems are low response rates and the increasing costs of postage. Strategies for increasing response rates for mailed questionnaires are addressed below. Mailing costs must be weighed against the costs incurred in personal distribution, that is, expenditures of time and possibly money for travel. When sensitive topics are being addressed, either mail distribution or a combined approach using personal distribution with a mailed return is generally preferable, because anonymity can be guaranteed.

STEP 6. PRETEST THE QUESTIONNAIRE. The questionnaire is pretested with individuals who are similar to those for whom the instrument is designed. The pretest may be conducted by mail; however, it is generally preferable to distribute the questionnaire to the pretest sample in person, then to follow the administration with an interview in which the respondents are asked to indicate their reactions to the questions and format, identify any portions of the questionnaire with which they had difficulty, and suggest improvements. The personal approach to pretesting also allows validation of the estimated time needed to complete the questionnaire. Item analysis and reliability and validity assessments are computed following the pretest and necessary revisions are made.

STEP 7. ADMINISTER AND SCORE THE QUESTIONNAIRE. Once a final version of the questionnaire has been prepared, decisions must be made about the administration procedure. One of the key characteristics of the questionnaire is its standardization, which allows one to make the assumption that all respondents are presented with identical stimuli. If the information from the questionnaire is to be used for comparison across respondents, it is essential that the conditions of administration be as standard as possible. In the case of a personally distributed questionnaire it would be important to maintain as much consistency as possible in the individuals distributing the questionnaire to respondents, the types of settings in which it is distributed and completed, and the way in which the questionnaire is introduced and cooperation secured. For example, if nursing administrators in each of several hospitals were to distribute a questionnaire to staff nurses, it would be important to select administrators who were in identical positions and to instruct each one to read the predefined introductory statement in the same way to all potential respondents in a predesignated type of setting. If one administrator distributed the questionnaires and asked the respondents to complete them during a staff meeting and another distributed the questionnaires on the patient units and asked respondents to complete them at home, the different conditions of administration could potentially influence the results and render the two sets of data incomparable.

Mailed questionnaires should be packaged identically and sent to similar settings (e.g., either work address or home address, but not a combination of the two) in order to standardize administration conditions as much as possible. It should be noted that with a mailed questionnaire the investigator has no control over the specific conditions under which the respondent chooses to self-administer the instrument. Considerable variation can occur in the degree of input or help that is sought from others, the order in which the questions are answered, the setting in which the instrument is answered, and the amount of distraction that may occur. Thus, complete standardization is impossible to achieve.

One of the major problems with a mailed questionnaire is the likelihood of a low response rate. The result is not only a diminished sample size, but also a set of responses that may be atypical of the sample as a whole, since nonresponse is not a random process (Oppenheim, 1966, p. 34). Several techniques can be suggested to improve response rates with mailed questionnaires. These include (1) supplying a self-addressed and stamped return envelope; (2) following up the original administration with mailed or telephone reminders; and (3) offering incentives or rewards (e.g., small amounts of money or inexpensive gifts) either in advance or upon receipt of the completed questionnaire. Strategies already mentioned, such as careful wording of the cover letter to establish rapport and providing a clear and attractive questionnaire, also enhance response rates. A number of experiments have been conducted to determine the effects on response rates of specific variables such as paper color, type of envelope and stamp, type of letterhead, typed versus written address, initiatives, and timing and type of follow-up on response rates. The findings are inconclusive, however.

Since response rates are predictably problematic with mailed questionnaires it is helpful to make provision at the time of administration for estimating the nonresponse bias that may exist because of systematic differences between those who respond and those who do not. For example, a record should be kept of the date when each questionnaire is returned, because late respondents have been found to be similar to nonrespondents (Oppenheim, 1966, p. 34). Early and late responses can be compared to detect bias. If data are available about some characteristics of the entire sample to whom questionnaires were sent, then the characteristics of those who returned questionnaires can be compared with those of nonrespondents to determine differences and with the sample as a whole to determine representativeness. Once the degree of potential bias is assessed, it can be taken into account in interpreting the information obtained.

The coding and scoring procedures for questionnaires with closed-ended questions are straightforward but do require prior decisions about how to handle unanswered questions, unclear or unreadable responses, or misinterpretation of instructions (e.g., checking multiple responses instead of one for each question). The important point is that all questionnaires should be treated identically. Coding and scoring open-ended questions is more complex and time consuming, requiring application of content analysis techniques to the responses.

Once the data have been obtained from the questionnaire, reliability and validity are assessed using the approaches detailed in Chapters 5 and 7. Some of the cross-checking procedures described for the interview can also be employed to assess the validity of factual information provided on the questionnaire. Examples include checking responses against external sources of information such as hospital or clinic records and including consistency checks within the questionnaire itself, whereby the same information is requested in more than one way.

EXAMPLE

A questionnaire was used in a study by Markowitz, et al (1981) to compare nurses', physicians', and pharmacists' knowledge of the hazards of medications. The instrument contained a brief introduction, an assurance of anonymity, instructions plus a sample question, personal questions about the practitioner's position and background, and 25 examination questions (p. 368).

After a meeting between the researcher and all prospective respondents, personal distribution of the tool was accomplished with assistance from selected administrative personnel. Completed questionnaires were collected in a ballot-type box. The total sample size was 216, reflecting a response rate of 98 percent.

In order to develop the 25 items designed to measure level of knowledge, a multistep procedure was carried out. First, 50 multiple-choice and true-false questions were generated using information in pertinent references. The questions covered information about hazards associated with prescribing, dispensing, and administering commonly used medications. The questions were reviewed by a panel of six experts who were asked to validate correct answers to the questions and to rate each question on a four-point scale for its relevance to the study. The 25 questions that received the highest total ratings were used on the final instrument. No reliability assessment was reported.

The personal information items addressed number of years of practice, hospital service affiliation (for nurses and physicians), and for nurses, the type of nursing program from which they graduated. A closed-ended multiple-choice format was used. Personal questions were kept to a minimum to preserve anonymity.

ADVANTAGES AND DISADVANTAGES

The questionnaire has several advantages as a measurement instrument. Major advantages are its cost efficiency and convenience, particularly when access to geographically dispersed respondents is desired, and time and funds are limited. The questionnaire is more time efficient and convenient than the interview, not only for the investigator, but also for the respondent, who is often able to plan the self-administration time, pace, and setting independently. Another advantage is that its impersonal and standardized format assures that all respondents are exposed to uniform stimuli. Such a feature increases reliability, facilitates comparison across respondents, and removes the threat to validity that results from interviewer bias. The questionnaire also allows complete anonymity to be preserved, a feature that is believed to increase the validity of response, especially to sensitive issues and personal questions.

The disadvantages of the questionnaire include low response rates, high rates of missing data, inability to rectify respondents' misunderstandings, inability to adapt questions and their wording to respondents' individual needs and styles, inability to probe complex issues in depth, and, for mailed questionnaires, inability to control the conditions of administration. Problems related to clarity of meaning may not be identified until after the fact of data collection; however, this disadvantage can be largely eliminated through careful pretesting. The questionnaire can be used only by literate respondents, a factor that limits its use for many populations that are salient for nursing practice and research.

DELPHI TECHNIQUE

The Delphi Technique is usually employed to quantify the judgments of experts, to assess priorities, or to make long-range forecasts. In addition, Linstone and Turoff (1975) suggest the following variety of applications for the Delphi:

1. gathering current and historical data not accurately known or available;
2. examining the significance of historical events;
3. evaluating possible budget allocations;
4. exploring planning options;
5. planning program and/or curriculum development;
6. collating the structure of a model;
7. delineating the pros and cons associated with potential policy options;
8. developing causal relationships in complex economic or social phenomena;
9. distinguishing and clarifying real and perceived human motivations;
10. exposing priorities of personal values and/or social goals (p. 4).

In its conventional form, the Delphi Technique, also referred to as the Delphi Exercise, is used in the following way.

1. A panel of experts on the topic of interest is identified. Selection of this panel of experts proceeds with care and concern that a variety of personalities, interests, perceptions, demographics, and the like are represented by those chosen to participate in order to avoid biases as a result of panel membership.

2. Each expert who agrees to participate is then asked to complete a questionnaire designed to elicit opinions, estimates, or predictions regarding the topic. In no instances do participants meet or discuss issues face to

face, and in most instances they are geographically remote from one another. The format usually, but not always, is a paper-and-pencil, structured, formal questionnaire, constructed by the investigator, participants, or both, that may be administered by mail, in a personal interview, or at an interactive online computer console. The questionnaire is accompanied by a set of instructions, guidelines, and ground rules and contains a series of items using quantitative or qualitative scales concerned with study objectives. Some questionnaires may include open-ended requests for information as well. The questionnaire is constructed using the principles and practices outlined in the previous section of this chapter.

3. Responses when received are tabulated, summarized, and returned to the experts. Statistical feedback usually includes a measure of central tendency, a measure of dispersion, and, in some instances, the complete frequency distribution of responses for each item. The reliability and validity of the questionnaire is also assessed using the appropriate procedures discussed in Chapter 5 and the previous section of this chapter. The anonymity of individuals' responses to items is preserved, but the investigator may list respondents' names and office locations as part of the study. In some cases those providing extreme responses (i.e., outliers) may be asked by the investigator to provide written justification for their responses.

4. Using the combined information of all members of the panel, as reflected in the primary round, each expert again predicts, comments, and responds to the new information in another questionnaire, which is returned to the investigator for analysis.

5. This process is repeated until the resulting data reflect a consensus of opinions, predictions, or beliefs among all the experts on the panel. It should be noted that when an interactive computer is employed, the procedure is often referred to as a *Delphi Conference*. By programming a computer to administer and compile panel results it is often possible to eliminate the delay and, hence, reduce the cost accrued in summarizing each round of the Delphi.

Linstone and Turoff suggest the following as circumstances in which the Delphi is most appropriately employed:

When:
. . . the problem to be addressed does not lend itself to precise analytical techniques but can benefit from subjective judgement on a collective basis,
. . . the individuals needed to contribute to the examination of a broad or complex problem have no history of adequate communication and may represent diverse backgrounds with respect to experience or expertise,
. . . input is needed from more individuals than can effectively interact in a face-to-face exchange,
. . . time and cost make frequent group meetings infeasible,
. . . disagreements among individuals are so severe or politically unpalatable that the communication process must be refereed and/or anonymity assured,
. . . the heterogeneity of the participants must be preserved to assure validity of the results, i.e., avoidance of domination by quantity or by strength of personality ("bandwagon effect") (p. 4).

The Delphi technique is appealing because of its adaptability to a variety of data collection settings. Experts are usually those individuals who are most involved in a variety of undertakings, are busy, and are located in varied and scattered geographical locations. Hence, this approach affords an opportunity to gain input from experts without the difficulties inherent in gaining personal access to such a population. Similarly, experts need not adjust their busy schedules to attend a meeting, be subject to influence by other experts, or relinquish their anonymity, all factors tending to further minimize biases in the resulting data. Another advantage of the method stems from the fact that it provides for condensing the opinions of many and varied experts on a topic into a few precise and clearly defined statements.

Critics of the method assert that results represent opinions of experts and may or may not be consistent with reality. Attention to variance in the selection of the panel members as well as precision and care to avoid overgeneralization in reporting of findings can do much to minimize this concern. Two other disadvantages of the method relate to economy. The procedure is costly in materials and services (e.g., postage, multiple data, analysis and processing, printing a number of questionnaires) and in terms of the time requirement for the collection of data (i.e., since subsequent questionnaires cannot be designed and distributed until the responses from the preceding one are received and tabulated, the collection of data is dependent upon a speedy response by busy experts). For these reasons, the use of the Delphi Technique in nursing is perhaps best limited to those instances in which the benefits to be gained from the effort outweigh the actual cost.

Several authors have noted potential pitfalls to be avoided when using the Delphi Technique. These include but are not limited to:

1. overstructuring of the Delphi by the investigator, thus disallowing the respondents an opportunity to contribute other perspectives related to the problem;

2. excessive vagueness of the Delphi, reducing the information produced by respondents;

3. using inadequate techniques for summarizing and presenting group responses;

4. ignoring and not exploring disagreements so that discouraged dissenters drop out and an artificial consensus results;

5. underestimating the demands on respondents to participate and failing to properly compensate them for their time if the Delphi is not an integral aspect of their job function;

6. overgeneralizing results;

7. taking inadequate care to obtain a large, representative sample of experts (Linstone and Turoff, 1975, p. 6; Linstone, 1975, pp. 573-586; and Sackman, 1975, pp. 5-27).

In some cases, modifications of the Delphi Technique, if undertaken with an eye to preserving the basic integrity of the method, may be more desirable than the specific steps of the coventional procedure outlined. For example, Turoff(1975) points out that the Delphi as originally designed was intended to deal with technical topics and to obtain consensus among homogeneous groups of experts. When employed for delineating the pros and cons associated with potential policy options, the Delphi instead seeks to generate the strongest possible opposing views on the potential resolutions of a major policy issue. He asserts that a policy issue is one for which there are no experts, only informed advocates and referees. Hence, in this case the expert is redefined as an advocate for effectiveness or efficiency and must compete with the advocates for concerned interest groups within the society or organization involved with the issue. Furthermore, the Policy Delphi rests on the premise that the decision maker is not interested in having a group generate his decision, but rather, in having an informed group present all the options and supporting evidence for his consideration; that is, the Policy Delphi is a tool for the analysis of policy issues and not a tool for making a decision, it is a decision-analysis tool versus a decision-making tool. Hence, generating consensus is not the prime objective and in some cases the design of the Delphi may be altered to inhibit consensus formation (pp. 84-101). Those interested in an example of how the Delphi Technique has been employed in the area of health policy formulation will find an article by Moscovice and associates (1978) useful.

Examples of the use of the Delphi Technique in nursing are limited perhaps because of the economics of its use. In 1975, Lindeman reported in *Nursing Research* the results of a Delphi Survey of Priorites in Clinical Nursing Research obtained from a panel of 433 nurse and nonnurse experts. Potential panel members were sought through correspondence to nursing organizations, military officials, allied health organizations, funding agencies and foundations, personal contact, and review of published rosters and membership lists. Expert was operationally defined as a person knowledgeable about clinical practice as well as one who had an appreciation for research. The Delphi procedure in this study consisted of four survey rounds:

Round I: Identification of burning questions about the practice of nursing.

Round II: Respond to a 150-item questionnaire answering the following questions:

a. Is this an area in which nursing should assume primary research responsibility?

b. How important is research on this topic for the profession of nursing?

c. What is the likelihood of change in patient welfare because of research on the topic?

Round III: Response to the same questionnaire with statistical summary of Round II responses.

Round IV: Response to same questionnaire with statistical summary of Round III response and minority report (p. 436).

The scale underlying responses to the 150-item questionnaire ranged from 1 to 7 with the higher number referring to the greater value or impact of the question. Statistical summaries provided during Rounds III and IV included for all three questions and for each item: the individual panel member's response, the median for the total panel, the response range, and the interquartile range. In Round III respondents were asked to comment on statements for which they answered outside the interquartile range and then Round IV included a 79-page minority report of all the comments of respondents who were outside the interquartile range in Round III of the study. The first round of the study began March 1974, and the final input was completed by September 1974. The report of this study provides numerous examples of questionnaire items and procedures that would be worthwhile reading for those readers interested in employing the Delphi method.

Another example of the use of the Delphi Technique in nursing appeared in the 1981 *Journal of Nursing Administration*. In this instance, Ventura and Walegora-Serafin reported on the results of a Delphi survey of 347 nursing administrators, clinical nursing staff, and nursing researchers in Veterans Administration hospitals nationwide in order to identify priorities for nursing research specifically related to the care of the veteran. Potential participants in this study were identified by letters sent to the chiefs of nursing service in 170 VA Medical Centers and Independent Clinics. The Delphi procedure included three rounds. During Round I each nurse willing to participate submitted three questions related to the nursing care of the veteran believed to warrant study. A group of three nurses then classified the questions into general topic areas and then developed 73 statements related to the care of the veteran patient. In Rounds II and III, nurse participants reviewed and rated each of the 73 statements using a 1 to 7 scale in terms of the question, "What would be the magnitude of the impact on the care of the veteran patient if increased knowledge was available in this area?" A rating of 1 indicated the least impact and 7 the greatest impact. In addition, during Round III respondents reviewed feedback consisting of their own individual rating and the group median for each of the 73 statements from Round II (p. 31).

Other examples of the use of the Delphi procedure in nursing can be found in the works of Oberst (1978), Hope (1977), and McNally (1974).

PROJECTIVE TECHNIQUES

Projective techniques encompass those measures that are based on the assumption that people interpret and react to ambiguous and unstructured situations in ways that reflect underlying motives, needs, desires, attitudes, values, and personality characteristics. Since people are believed to project aspects of themselves into their perceptions and interpretations, inferences can be made about their cognitive and affective characteristics by examining responses to stimuli, particularly those for which there is no commonly accepted meaning. These responses are believed to reflect fundamental aspects of psychological functioning (Anastasi, 1976, p. 558). The less structured and more ambiguous the stimulus, the more likely is the individual to project into it personal interpretations, thereby revealing personal characteristics.

TYPES OF PROJECTIVE TECHNIQUES. The term projective techniques is used to encompass many different measurement tools, devices, and strategies including those in which the individual responds verbally or in writing to visual or verbal stimuli and those in which the individual is encouraged to exhibit self-expression through the handling of materials, construction of products, play activities, or role playing. Kerlinger (1973, pp. 515-520) has identified four major types of projective techniques: association, construction, completion, and expressive. Characteristics and examples of each type are presented in Table 9-1. Procedures for administration and scoring, reliability and validity estimates, and reported uses of

TABLE 9-1 Types of projective techniques

I. Association Techniques
Characteristics

A. Subject is exposed to one or more pictorial or verbal stimuli and is asked to respond with the first word or idea that comes to mind.
B. Stimulus pictures or word sequences are typically ambiguous in meaning.
C. The underlying purpose for the measure is generally not apparent to the subject.

Example	Procedure	Use	Reliability/Validity	Comments
Rorschach Inkblot Test	Subject is shown 10 symmetrical inkblots and, for each, is asked to tell what is seen. Examiner keeps a verbatim record and notes the content of the response, use of whole vs. part of the image, injection of movement into the inkblot, use of colored and white spaces, position in which cards are held, remarks, and facial expressions. The most common scoring categories are location, determinants, and content. The major content categories include human figures, human details, animal figures, animal details, anatomic diagrams, and inanimate objects.	Use is widespread. Interpretation is generally related to personality variables such as impulsiveness, sensitivity, and emotional stability. A number of modifications have been developed. Originally, it was developed and normed for adults, but norms have been developed for children.	Reliability is characteristically low. Validity as a personality measure is questionable (Eysenck, 1959); it may be a more promising measure of cognitive style and perceptual organization (Anastasi, 1976).	Time consuming to administer. Special training is required for scoring and interpretation. Response productivity (total number of responses) varies and is related to age, intelligence, and education. Verbal aptitude influences the score (Anastasi, 1976, pp. 561-562).

Holtzman Inkblot Test	Subject is shown 45 cards, each containing inkblots. Some are achromatic and some are colored; some inkblots are asymmetric. Subject is asked to say what is seen, but responses are limited to one per card. Administration and scoring are standardized, with scores being obtained for 22 response variables. Scores are interpreted by reference to published norms.	Used for adults and children for measuring personality variables, hostility, anxiety, and pathognomonic verbalization. Guides for scoring and interpretation are available.	Interrater reliability is satisfactory. Split-half and alternate-form reliability are acceptable. Considerable validity data have been accumulated and are promising (Anastasi, 1976, pp. 564-565).	A group form of the instrument has been designed for intact groups, such as classes.
Word Association	Subject is presented with a verbal or printed series of disconnected words and is asked to add to the series the first words which come to mind. Scheme for scoring the word or sequence should be predetermined. Some word association tests are interpretable with reference to published norms (e.g., the Kent-Rosanoff Free Association Test).	Used in research to study thought processes, creativity, interests, verbal behavior, and attitudes, and in marketing research.	Higher reliability than many other projective techniques, because number of responses is generally limited. Reliability is highest for tests with standard scoring procedures.	Easy to administer. Neutral and/or emotionally tinged words may be included. If both are used, neutral terms are interspersed.

TABLE 9-1 Continued

II. Construction Technique
Characteristics

A. Subject is presented with a stimulus situation and asked to construct a product in response.
B. Stimulus is characteristically ambiguous and subject to any number of interpretations.
C. Focus is on the product rather than on the process used to produce it.
D. Reliability and validity are characteristically low or unexamined.
E. A standard stimulus is generally used consistently across subjects.

Example	Procedure	Use	Reliability/Validity	Comments
Murray's Thematic Apperception Test (TAT)	Nineteen cards, each containing a picture of an interaction situation, are shown to the subject one at a time. The subject is asked to tell a story that describes the event pictured, what led up to the event, how the characters are feeling, and the outcome that will result. Then subject is shown a blank card and is asked to describe a scene and construct a story about it. Responses are content analyzed according to a defined procedure. Four sets of overlapping cards are available for boys, girls, men over 14, and women over 14. Clinicians seldom administer over 10 cards to a respondent (Anastasi, 1976, p. 566).	Originally developed to measure motives and is most commonly used in that way, e.g., to measure achievement motivation, need for affiliation, fear of success. Also used to measure creativity, attitude toward authority figures and minority groups, and elements of parent-child relationships (Polit and Hungler, 1978, p. 384). Also used to identify environmental factors that interfere with need satisfaction.	Reliability and validity are low, although quantitative scoring schemes have yielded acceptable scorer reliability. Responses are sensitive to temporary conditions such as hunger, fatigue, and social frustration (Anastasi, 1976, p. 567).	Can be administered to groups or individuals. Several modifications have been developed using different pictorial stimuli; similar procedures are used, although the subject may be asked to write, rather than tell, the stories.

Test	Description	Purpose/Use	Evaluation
Machover's Draw-A-Person Test (D-A-P)	Subject is given a paper and pencil and asked to draw a person. After completion, the subject is asked to draw a person of the opposite sex. The response is interpreted on the basis of position, size of the person drawn, degree of completeness of representing body parts, shading, etc. Questions may be asked about the persons drawn. Interpretation is qualitative.	Frequently used with children and in studies of self-image, body image, and sexual attitudes.	Reliability and validity are low. The interpretative guide is stated in terms of generalizations with no supporting evidence. Drawing ability of the subject appears to influence interpretation (Anastasi, 1976, pp. 575-576). It is often assumed that the drawing represents the subject's self-image.
Rosenzweig Picture-Frustration Test (P-F)	Subject is presented with a set of cartoon drawings, each containing two characters. Dialogue for one of the characters is provided in a balloon in the drawing; the other balloon is blank. The subject is asked to construct the response that would be given by the second character. Responses are content analyzed in terms of type and direction of aggression or other type of characteristic expressed.	Originally designed to depict frustrating situations, and responses were evaluated in terms of aggressiveness. Forms exist for children and adults. Subsequent modifications have been used to measure many psychological concepts and attitudes.	Since this measure is relatively structured, scoring procedures are relatively objective and reliability is acceptable. This measure is relatively structured; scoring procedures are relatively objective. Norms have been established.

TABLE 9-1 Continued

	Procedure	Use	Reliability/Validity	Comments
Bender Visual Motor Gestalt Test	Subject is presented with a card on which designs are drawn, and a piece of paper and pencil, then is asked to copy the designs. Scoring takes into account omission, distortion, and rotation of figures.	Has been used for diagnosing perceptual problems and assessing personality traits.	Predictive validity has been established with respect to reading failure, perceptual difficulty, and some types of brain damage; but validity has not been established with respect to personality characteristics.	

III. Completion Techniques
Characteristics

A. The subject is presented with an incomplete verbal or written stimulus and is asked to complete it.

B. The stimulus may be worded in first or third person, and evidence is inconclusive regarding which is preferable.

C. Stimuli may be worded to encourage expression of own views or those of "most people." The latter form may not elicit feelings of the subject but interpretation of belief about others' feelings.

D. Responses are generally less complex, thus simpler to score and interpret, than those from other types of projective techniques.

Example	Procedure	Use	Reliability/Validity	Comments
Sentence Completion	The subject is presented with a series of incomplete (partial) sentences and is asked to complete them. Generally a time limit is imposed to encourage spontaneous response. Responses are content analyzed according to a predetermined coding scheme.	Most often used to measure attitudes toward a particular object, experience, or group. Also has been used in marketing research and clinical practice.	Reliability varies with the type of stimulus used and specificity of the coding scheme.	An advantage is its flexibility; however, some standardized sentence completion measures have been published, e.g. the Rotter Incomplete Sentence Blank with 40 sentence stems, which is used as a measure of adjustment. Related procedures are story, argument, or discussion completion.

IV. Expressive Techniques
Characteristics

A. Subject is presented with a stimulus situation and raw material (which may include other people) and is asked to construct a product.
B. Focus is on the *process* of construction rather than on the content of the product.
C. Expressive techniques are based on the assumption that people express their needs, emotions, and motives through manipulation of materials (Kerlinger, 1973, p. 518).
D. Expressive techniques are used in combination with observational methods and techniques.
E. Expressive techniques have been characteristically employed as therapeutic devices, as well as diagnostic or assessment measures.

Example	Procedure	Use	Reliability/ Validity	Comments
Play Techniques	Subject is given raw material, usually dolls or other toys such as trucks or weapons or art materials, and is asked to play with or arrange them. The stimulus situation may be completely unstructured or some structuring may be provided by setting the scene for the play. For example, the subject may be told the dolls represent a family that has just experienced the death of a pet dog. Responses are observed and often coded according to a predetermined scheme, with choices of objects, verbal and emotional expressions, and manipulation of objects being observed.	Frequently used for measuring characteristics (e.g., fear, aggressiveness, hostility) and attitudes of children. However, the technique has been modified for adults (e.g., asking subjects to arrange doll-like figures on a board to depict social or spatial arrangements). Has been used for therapy and research.	Reliability varies with degree of situation structuring and specificity of coding scheme.	Particularly useful with children. Flexible, since a number of different raw materials may be used.

TABLE 9-1 Continued

Role-playing	Subject is presented with instructions describing a stimulus situation (usually a simulated social interaction) and is instructed to act out a role as though it were a real life situation. Subjects may be asked to act out roles either as themselves (psychodrama) or someone else (sociodrama). The behavior is observed and either recorded for later analysis or coded immediately. Videotaping may be used.	May be used to examine attitudes, motives, personality characteristics, and interpersonal skills. Frequently is used in conjunction with training programs and in individual or group therapy with clients.	Reliability varies with situation structuring, standardization of instructions, and coding schemes. Validity is highly dependent on subject's definition of the situation.	Instructions to the subject(s) structure the situation to encourage manifestation of the variable to be measured. Observational scheme should be predetermined to assure that relevant variables are identified and coded. It is generally helpful to set a time limit on the role-playing episode.

specific tests can be found in the compendia of measurement tools described in the Appendix.

All projective techniques share several common characteristics. First, they involve presenting the subject with a stimulus that is unstructured and ambiguous. This feature is commonly cited as the defining characteristic of projective techniques. The techniques listed as examples in Table 9-1 differ somewhat in the degree to which stimuli are ambiguous and unstructured (e.g., Rorschach inkblots are more ambiguous than some incomplete sentences or role-play stimuli); however, all use stimuli that are considerably less structured than those employed in most other measurement instruments such as questionnaires and interviews. In contrast with questionnaire and interview items (stimuli), which are worded as clearly as possible to assure that all subjects interpret them in the way that the investigator intends, the projective technique stimulus is intentionally ambiguous in order to encourage the subject to interpret it freely. The more unstructured the stimulus, the more open it is to interpretation by the subject and the more likely it is to elicit a wide variety of different responses. This characteristic of projective techniques increases their flexibility and the likelihood that the subject's unique perspective will be displayed in the interpretation; however, it generally precludes systematic comparison across subjects.

Second, projective techniques are characteristically indirect, in that they do not ask the subject to reveal information directly. Rather, inferences are made on the basis of responses to stimuli which do not clearly indicate to the subject what is being measured or how responses will be interpreted. Unlike the more direct approaches to measuring attitudes, values, motives, and personality characteristics, projective techniques do not rely on the subject's candor, self-insight, or willingness to reveal specific personal information. This feature decreases the likelihood that the subject will become defensive, manipulate the response, deliberately provide false information, or refuse to reveal personal characteristics. It makes the techniques well suited for examining issues that are sensitive or emotionally charged or situations in which social desirability is likely to influence response, and for eliciting information from individuals who are unwilling or unable to reveal information about their internal processes. These techniques are regarded as being effective in revealing covert or unconscious aspects of personality.

A third characteristic of projective techniques is that they allow the subject free response. There are no right or wrong answers, nor are potential responses constrained or limited by a predefined response set. This feature allows focus on the subject's perceptions without imposing restrictions or interpretations. As a result of the free format, however, there is a risk that responses may be irrelevant to the purpose for which the measure is being administered and/or highly inconsistent from subject to subject. Given the degree of variability in responses, they are difficult and time consuming to analyze, and there are often problems achieving acceptable levels of interrater reliability.

Finally, projective techniques are characterized by their high level of dependence on the subjective processes of the investigator, observer, or examiner to interpret responses (Nunnally, 1978, p. 570). Rather than taking responses at their face value, responses are ". . . interpreted in terms of some preestablished psychological conceptualization of what . . . responses to the specific test situation mean." (Selltiz, et al, 1959, p. 282) Considerable inference is required to link subjects' responses to the internal characteristics which they are presumed to indicate. This feature of projective techniques has given rise to questions about their objectivity, since different observers of the same response may interpret it very differently.

UTILITY

Projective techniques were initially developed for use in clinical psychology and psychiatry as measures to aid in diagnosis and treatment of patients with emotional problems. They have been used subsequently in both clinical and research contexts to gain better understanding of personality, attitudes, values, prejudices, motivation for behavior, fears, and anxieties. Their use, although widespread, has been subject to considerable controversy, largely in relation to their questionable reliability and validity. These issues are discussed in detail below.

The use of projective techniques in nursing has been limited, with some types being used more frequently than others. Some of the measures developed primarily for psychological and psychiatric practice, such as the Rorschach Inkblot Test and the Thematic Apperception Test (TAT), require considerable background and extensive training to administer and interpret. Only those nurses with special training and expertise in the use of these measures should attempt to employ them. The projective techniques most frequently used in nursing practice are expressive techniques such as role-playing. Role-playing is used in nursing education, leadership training, evaluation, and group and individual therapy, often to allow subjects to gain insight into their own attitudes and interpersonal skills or to develop more effective interpersonal strategies. It also has been used as a means for evaluating the ability of subjects to apply knowledge and skills gained during training sessions or continuing education programs by presenting them with hypothetical stimulus situations that simulate those that might be encountered in the practice environment. Play techniques have been employed in clinical nursing practice and have proven particularly useful with children, as a means for introducing them to hospital routines or assessing such characteristics as their aggressiveness, perceptions of parents, siblings, and peers, or fear of hospital procedures. Their use in research has been limited, the most frequent uses being in studies of children (Mencke, 1978; Porter, 1974) and communication patterns, and in research evaluating the effectiveness of specific educational experiences. Because of their flexibility, projective techniques have potential utility for therapy and skill and insight development and some assessment purposes in clinical and educational settings. However, because of problems related to their reliability and validity they are not well suited to research applications nor to assessment or evaluation situations in which objective and precise measurement is desired.

RELIABILITY AND VALIDITY

Although they have been used extensively and considerable effort has been devoted to evaluating and improving their psychometric properties, projective techniques have been severely criticized by measurement experts because of their low reliability and validity (Eysenck, 1959, pp. 276-277; Nunnally, 1978; Anastasi, 1976; Jensen, 1965; Molish, 1972; Stanley and Hopkins, 1972). Problems of reliability stem from (1) a general lack of precise rules and procedures; (2) the high degree of subjectivity involved in administering, scoring, and interpreting the measures; and (3) difficulty in defining the domain of content to be measured (Nunnally, 1978). Because stimuli are characteristically unstructured, there is difficulty achieving consistency in the way the measures are administered, and the quality of responses generated is frequently a function of the tester's skill and personality. Since there is a high degree of inference involved in linking a subject's response with the characteristic being measured and wide diversity exists in the aspects of responses from which inferences may be drawn, it is often difficult for raters to agree about scoring and interpretation. Reliability coefficients have characteristically been lower for highly unstructured projective techniques than for those, such as sentence completion or word association, which involve more structured stimuli and more limited response possibilities. Some improvement in the reliability of the former type of projective techniques has resulted from developing explicit procedures and scoring rules and modifying the original techniques somewhat to assure more consistency and focus responses to a greater degree. However, even with relatively objective scoring procedures the interpretation of the data from many of the projective techniques depends on the clinical experience, theoretical orientation, and skill of the examiner.

A number of steps may be taken to improve the reliability of projective techniques. These include the following:

1. Standardizing instructions and stimuli given to subjects;
2. Developing homogeneous criteria and scales for scoring responses;
3. Developing explicit and detailed instructions for use;
4. Limiting measurement to a single dimension or trait;
5. Limiting the number (or length) and focus of possible responses by structuring the stimulus situation;
6. Providing explicit and rigorous training for those who will be administering and scoring the measure;
7. Carefully assessing the degree of interrater reliability prior to and throughout use of the measure and during interpretive phases; and
8. Using established norms for interpretation.

Anastasi (1976, p. 586) cautions, however, that elaborate quantitative scoring systems may create an illusion of objectivity that is unfounded. Nunnally (1978, pp. 571-574) advocates developing alternative forms of projective measures, a procedure that requires careful definition of the domain of content. He notes that the most appropriate measure of reliability for projective techniques is the correlation of alternative forms administered and scored by different examiners.

The validity of projective techniques, particularly those purporting to measure global aspects of personality, is open to considerable question. There simply has been insufficient evidence to support the construct, predictive, or discriminative validity of most projective measures. Many of the validation studies that have been carried out for projective techniques have serious methodological problems. The methodologically sound empirical investigations have tended to suggest that there is no relationship between the results of projective measures of attitudes, motives, and personality characteristics and the results of independent diagnostic assessments or more objective measures of the same constructs or traits. It has been shown that projective measures do not discriminate between ill and healthy subjects or between those known to differ with respect to various traits or behavior patterns, nor are they successful predictors of specific behaviors (Eysenck, 1959, pp. 276-277; Anastasi, 1976). These problems in establishing validity may at least in part be attributable to the many extraneous factors and temporary states that have been found to affect subjects' responses to projective measures. These findings call into question the fundamental assumptions underlying the measures, that is, that responses to ambiguous stimuli reflect enduring psychological characteristics. Although some measures have acceptable validity for specific purposes (see Table 9-1), serious problems of reliability and validity exist for most projective measures and should not be underestimated. Thus, a very thorough reliability and validity assessment should accompany the use of any projective technique. Those measuring global aspects of personality are most appropriately subjected to estimates of construct validity. For those measuring more specific attitudes, discriminate validity and construct validity may be examined using the procedures described in Chapters 5 and 7.

Projective techniques are currently increasing in popularity, particularly in clinical practice with children. Given their present state of development, it is recommended that nurse clinicians and researchers exercise caution in their use. For research purposes the authors recommend that they be used only in conjunction with other measures of the same variables. In those instances in which no better alternatives exist, every effort should be made to establish acceptable levels of reliability and validity of the instrument before its use, and to evaluate and report its reliability and vaidity in the context of the study in which it is used, in order to assist consumers of the research to interpret and evaluate the results.

ADVANTAGES AND DISADVANTAGES

Projective techniques have several advantages, which include (1) their flexibility and adaptability to a variety of situations and special populations; (2) their relative insusceptibility to subjects' faking responses; (3) their lack of dependence on subjects' self-insight and willingness to reveal information about themselves; (4) their presumed ability to probe dimensions of the unconscious; and (5) their open acknowledgment of the importance of subjective perception and interpretation. They also use an approach that is highly compatible with the holistic perspective advocated by many nursing theorists and practitioners. Projective techniques, because they present the subject with an interesting task, are often used to help establish rapport and help the subject feel at ease. They are useful with special populations, such as young children, the illiterate, and those with language handicaps. However, their utility is primarily as qualitative clinical aids, rather than as measurement instruments yielding quantitative information.

Their primary disadvantages are the problems of reliability and validity which result from their subjectivity and general lack of standardization and precision. Other disadvantages include the time, effort, and level of specialized expertise that are required to score and interpret the information obtained and the general lack of normative data, particularly for relevant subgroups. From a measurement perspective, the disadvantages outweigh the advantages and projective techniques should be employed only as clinical aids by highly skilled clinicians.

Q-SORT

The Q-Sort is a norm-referenced technique for the measurement of affect that is usually employed in order to (1) assess the degree of similarity between different subjects' or different groups of subjects' attitudes, expectations, or perceptions at a given point in time; or (2) determine the change in subjects or groups of subjects' attitudes or perceptions over time. For example, in regard to the first purpose, one might be concerned with the question of how Nurse A's attitudes toward the gerontological patient compared with those of Nurse B. Do they agree? Disagree? To what extent are their attitudes the same? On what basis do they disagree? Similarly, comparisons might be made between responses by any two relevant subjects' or groups of subjects' Q-Sort, for example, Nurse A might be compared with Physician A or staff nurses as a group might be compared with gerontology patients' families as a group. Examples of questions addressed by the second purpose are: (1) How does Nurse A agree with his or her own responses to the Q-Sort when it is administered a second time after his or her attendance at an inservice program on the elderly? Or (2) Do attitudes of families who are having difficulty coping with an elderly member change as a result of counseling? In this case the Q-Sort is generally used as a measure of the effectiveness of various methods or treatments designed to change attitudes.

The Q-Sort technique usually proceeds in the following manner.

1. A subject is presented with 25 to 75 3 × 5 inch index cards, each of which contains a descriptive statement. The statements or items may be derived in a variety of different ways, for example, from personality inventories, case histories of patients with similar health problems, statements recurring in the course of nurse-client interactions, or statements emanating from a particular theoretical or conceptual framework.

2. The subject is asked to sort a specified number of cards into a predetermined number of different categories or piles, usually 9 to 11 according to the study purpose.

3. Summary statistics (e.g., mode, median, and mean rank, interquartile range) are determined for each item. The similarity of responses is examined by correlating item scores for two or more subjects.

Although this procedure, on the surface, appears relatively straightforward and simple to employ, several factors need careful consideration when it is used. More specifically, attention needs to be given to (1) how items are selected; (2) the type of response required; (3) the arrangement of piles; (4) scoring, analysis, and interpretations that can be made on the basis of the measure; and (5) reliability and validity.

ITEM SELECTION

The Q-Sort is an ordinal scaling technique conceptually based on small sampling theory. The study population consists of traits, characteristics, and attitudes for a small number of subjects. It is generally assumed that the universe or domain to be sampled from is known and finite. To facilitate comparison of the items with each other, the Q-Sort is particularly useful when the universe is greater than 25 items but less than or equal to 75 (Fox, 1976, p. 235). The identification of the items to be rated is an especially important consideration; hence, the development of the cards is an extensive and very critical undertaking. The most important concern in the selection of items for the Q-Sort is that those selected be truly representative of the universe to be measured, thus providing a reliable and valid measure of the variable of interest.

The results obtained by the use of the Q-Sort will vary widely with the nature of the universe of statements from which items are selected. Mowrer (1953, pp. 358-359) exemplifies a potential problem in this area likely to result if one selects items from the domain of what he refers to as "universally applicable" and "universally inapplicable" statements. Such statements for a population of normal subjects might be: "I usually walk in an upright position," "I eat recurrently," "I frequently hold my breath for as much as ten minutes." By selecting such items for a Q-Sort and using a dichotomous distribution, one could insure the finding that different persons correlate highly, that is, are quite homogeneous. On the other hand, he points out, if one selects "idiosyncratic" characteristics such as "place and date of birth," "address of present residence," and "full name of spouse" as items, one could insure the finding that the correlation between persons would be very low, that is, that persons are very heterogeneous. Similarly, by selecting characteristics that fall in the middle range of universality, one could insure results that would group individuals into societies or into special roles (e.g., professions, political parties).

Mowrer suggests as one solution to this dilemma the selection of items that refer to state characteristics, that is, those with respect to which the subjects are likely to change, rather than trait characteristics that are stable over time and not amenable to change. After the item universe is thus defined, the items selected should be pretested to ascertain that they are understandable, representative, and workable.

Stephenson (1953) proposed that items for incusion in the Q-Sort be selected in the following manner. First, *all* statements that by some operational criterion fall within the chosen domain be collected and listed. Then from this exhaustive list a sample of items be selected at random to serve as statements for inclusion in the Q-Sort. In his own research of Jungian types Stephenson aggregated approximately 2000 statements used by Jung in discussing introverts and extroverts and then selected, strictly at random, samples of items which then served as the Q-sets in subsequent research.

In nursing, Freihofer and Felton (1976) used a similar selection approach in their study of nursing behaviors in bereavement. More specifically the nursing behaviors for the Q-Sort were obtained from nurse experts and an exhaustive review of the professional and lay literature on loss, grief, and crisis intervention. In this manner they compiled a list of 125 descriptive statements appropriate for use as helpful nursing behaviors toward the bereaved. From these areas a three-tier classification system was derived to order client-oriented nursing behaviors: (1) promoting patient comfort and hygiene; (2) indicating understanding of patient emotional needs; and (3) indicating understanding of grief, grieving, and loss of the bereaved. From the total 125 items generated, 88 were selected for the Q-Sort and assigned to one of the three specified categories. Items were pretested prior to their use in the study.

The advantage of this type of selection method stems from the fact that the procedure is clearly specified, consequently replicable, and the Q-sets derived are truly representative of the delimited universe (i.e., successive sampling from the universe results in comparable Q-sets). A primary disadvantage results from the cost involved in delimiting all items in the universe. Another disadvantage cited by Block (1961) is that the method fails to consider the nature of the universe it samples. He contends that when a universe is operationalized to render it concrete, there is no guarantee that the resulting aggregate will properly express the underlying abstractly defined universe. The consequences of this purely empirical approach to item selection may be redundancies in the coverage of certain portions of the domain and inadequate coverage of others, resulting in a Q-Sort that does not adequately represent the true universe. This of course is a danger whenever a measure is solely empirically derived and highlights the importance of a conceptual framework to guide the operationalization of a phenomenon.

Yet another approach to the problem of selecting a representative set of items for inclusion in the Q-Sort was employed by Block (1961) and his associates in developing the California Q-Sort. The California Q-Sort (CQ) is a standardized measure designed to provide a description of individual personality in terms of the relative salience of personality dimensions. Initially, in an attempt to comprehensively delimit the personality domain as measured by contemporary clinicians, 90 personality variables were expressed in item form. A number of these items were adapted from an established Q-Sort derived earlier for use by assessors in a study of Air Force officers (MacKinnon, 1958). Block notes, in discussing this process, that this initial item collection represented and was somewhat biased by the personal theoretical preferences of the item writers.

For this reason, these 90 items were then subjected to scrutiny by two psychologists and a psychoanalyst who attended to each item's clarity and psychological importance and its implications for the sufficiency of the total item set. This step of the process according to Block took approximately 60 hours of meetings. Next, the item choices of the 3-person group of experts were submitted to a larger group of practicing clinical psychologists who again scrutinized the items from their own perspectives in the same manner as the group of experts. The 108-item Q-set resulting from these efforts was then empirically tested via research over a 14-month period of time. Revisions were then made on the basis of the findings from the pilot research resulting in another revised CQ set consisting of 115 items. The 115-item CQ set was then used in research and clinical practice over a period of three years before it was revised by incorporating suggestions accumulated during that time. In addition the measurement properties of all of the CQ sets were empirically investigated at the same time, and the present form containing 100 Q-items resulted.

Other approaches to Q-Sort item selection are suggested by the work of Dunlap and Hadley (1965) and Whiting (1955). Dunlap and Hadley, using

Q-Sort methodology in self-evaluation of conference leadership skill, derived their items from two major sources: (1) program objectives and (2) responses to pre- and post-self-conception instruments used in the first year of their three-year program. Whiting, using the Q-Sort to determine the way in which nurses' duties, functions, and interpersonal relationships are perceived by nurses themselves and by others outside of nursing, derived items for his Q-Sort on the basis of available empirical findings in his area of concern.

In summary, there are a number of varied approaches to identifying appropriate items for the Q-Sort. The utility of a given approach is largely a function of the probability that it will lead one to comprehensively identify and include in the Q-Sort items that are truly representative of the domain or universe to be measured.

The rubric Q-Sort is applied to a number of different types of sorts that require subjects to respond in different ways. In fact, the literature on Q-Sort is abundant with arguments regarding what can legitimately be referred to as a Q-Sort and what cannot. For this reason, it is important when applying the technique to be aware of the various types of sorts referred to in the literature, to be clear regarding the purpose for the measure in the context of a particular situation, and to insure that what the subject is asked to do in the way of sorting is consistent with the measurement purpose.

The *S-sort*, also referred to as the *S-procedure* and *self-sort*, requires the subject to arrange the items in terms of how he or she views them at a given point in time. The *ideal-sort* asks the subject to sort the cards according to his or her ideal of the best possible in regard to the attitude being measured. The subject usually is asked to sort the cards in terms of their applicability to other persons, social stereotypes, or the like. When a variation of this type of sort, called a *self-ideal-sort*, is used, the respondent is directed to answer in terms of how he or she would like to be.

Self- and ideal-sorts are often obtained from the same individual or group and correlated to determine agreement. The *prediction-sort* asks the subject to sort the cards according to the manner in which he or she predicts another subject will make the sort. The prediction-sort is often compared with the self-sort of the other subject, for example, having the nurse complete a prediction-sort and then comparing the results with the self-sort of a patient may be used as an index of how well the nurse understands the patient's expectations and is personally sensitive to the patient's views. The term, *before and after treatment sorts*, is used to refer to those instances in which a sort is obtained prior to the implementation of a particular treatment geared to changing attitudes and then is compared with one obtained post treatment. Self-sorts are often employed as before and after sorts.

THE ARRANGEMENT OF PILES

The Q-Sort differs from the more frequently encountered rating scale technique in that it requires the subject to order or rank a set of items in clusters rather than singly as in the case of the rating scale. In most instances, the sorting into clusters or piles is prespecified in such a way that the resulting distribution is normal in shape. For example, suppose a Q-Sort is developed to determine what subjects believe to be the most important to the least important characteristics of a nurse practitioner. One hundred statements each describing one characteristic from the universe of nurse practitioner attributes are typed on cards and presented to the subject. The subject is then asked to sort the 100 items into 9 piles according to the following scheme.

. . . In Pile 1, on the extreme left, place the one item which you feel is the least important characteristic of a nurse practitioner.

. . . In Pile 9 on the extreme right, place the one item you feel is the most important characteristic of a nurse practitioner.

. . . Next, in Pile 2, place the 4 next least important items and in Pile 8, place the 4 next most important items.

. . . Then in Piles 3 and 7, place the 11 next least and most important items, respectively.

. . . In Piles 4 and 6, place 21 items each in terms of their being less or more important.

. . . In Pile 5, place the remaining 26 cards that you believe are of medium importance.

Hence, in this manner, the subject is forced to arrange the statements into an approximately normal curve illustrated in Figure 9-2, beginning with consideration of the extremes and moving toward the middle. This example illustrates only one of many possible item-pile arrangements that will lead to an approximately normal distribution of results.

It is obvious from this example that the phrasing of directions to the subject is both a difficult and important task. Reliability and validity of Q-Sort data are endangered if directions are not clearly specified in a manner that is readily understood and followed by the subject. For this reason, users of the Q-Sort have tried a variety of approaches to simplifying this task. For example, Freidofer and Felton (1976) combined written instructions with a video cassette demonstration tape of how to do the Q-Sort, making both available to subjects for reference during the entire sorting period.

Critics of the Q-Sort technique note that the greatest precision in the sorting occurs at the extremes, while discriminations between middle piles are generally less precise. This, they contend, permits only the study of extremes (for example, most and least important) and provides little or no information regarding the items in between. Whiting (1958) attempted to introduce more precision into his sorting, and hence, minimize this disadvantage, by changing instructions concerning sorting from one step of sorting 9 piles of varying numbers of items to 4 steps of sorting items into 3 different piles; that is, first the subject was asked to sort 100 cards into three piles of high, medium, and low, the high and low containing 16 cards each, and the medium pile 68. Then subjects were asked to sort the 16 cards in the high pile into three piles containing 1,4, and 11 items each, with the highest item going into the first pile, and the remaining 11 into the third pile. The same procedure was carried out for the cards in the low pile. Then the medium pile of 68 cards was separated into 3 piles of 21, 26, and 21 cards. The first pile containing 21 items was considered slightly greater than medium, the second 26 items neither high nor low, and the third 21 items slightly less than medium (p. 72).

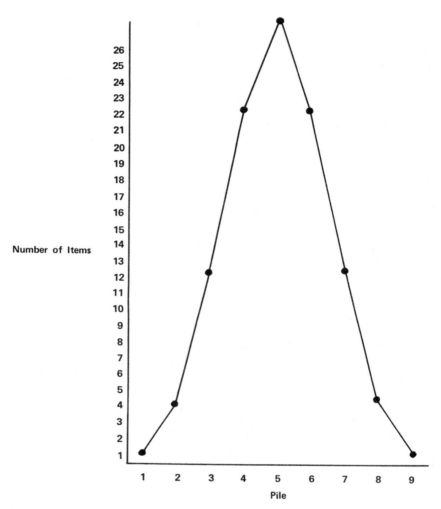

FIGURE 9-2. One alternative for sorting items into a normal distribution.

An important consideration in sorting relates to the optimal number of piles or categories. Although studies indicate that subjects can reliably discriminate up to 20 points on a rating scale, most users of the Q-Sort have found 9 to 11 to be the optimal number. Another factor often overlooked is that although the desired distribution shape is usually a normal curve, depending upon the purpose for the measure, other distributions may be prescribed as well. In addition to the normal distribution, other symmetric distributions of interest might include:

1. A unimodal distribution in which there is piling of items in the middle categories.
2. A rectangular distribution in which there are an equal number of items in each of the categories.

3. A U-shaped distribution in which the bulk of the items is placed in the extreme categories with few in the middle.

A debate in the literature on Q-Sorts that should be noted here relates to whether sorting should be forced, as in the preceding discussion, or unforced, as when the number of piles or items to be placed in piles is left to the subjects' discretion. Block (1961) empirically investigated the alternative consequences of the forced and unforced sorting procedures and found that:

1. Forced sorting permits a clearer assessment of the degree of similarity between sorts than does unforced;
2. Unforced sorting tends to provide fewer discriminations than the forced sort and consequently is more susceptible to the Barnum effect (Meehl, 1956), that is, the tendency to say very general and very generally true things about an individual;
3. Unforced sorting, contrary to its advocates' claims, is not likely to be more reliable than forced;
4. Unforced sorting does not, as some argue, provide more information not also and as easily accessible via the forced sort;
5. Unforced sorting provides data that are often unwieldy and at times impossible to work with, while forced sorting provides data in a convenient and readily processed form (p. 78).

In summary, in most nursing situations, it is our belief that the Q-Sort has its greatest utility in norm-referenced measurement situations and hence that forced sorting in order to obtain an approximately normal distribution is the most desirable approach.

SCORING, ANALYSIS, AND INTERPRETATION

After the sorting, each item is usually assigned a score corresponding to the pile into which it was placed; that is, if a particular item was placed in pile 4, it would be assigned a score of 4, while one placed in pile 9 would be scored 9. Each subject's sort for each item is thus computed. Summary statistics including measures of central tendency, variance, and standard deviation are determined to examine each item's placement across all subjects. For example, a mean for each statement might be calculated and the statements ranked according to their mean. The standard deviation for each item is examined to assess those items in which scores were more diversified (higher standard deviation) and those in which there was less variance in how individual subjects viewed them. To determine similarity between subjects' rankings of statements the Spearman rank-order correlation (Siegel, 1956) or Pearson Product-Moment Correlation Coefficient (Waltz and Bausell, 1981) is computed.

For example, if the concern is with determining the similarity between one subject's self-sort and the same subject's ideal-sort, the correlation would be determined using the arrangement in Figure 9-3.

It should be noted for Figure 9-3 that the items or cards column contains each statement included in the Q-Sort and that the self-sort and ideal-sort columns contain numbers that correspond to the pile or category into which the item was placed. Using the Pearson Correlation Coefficient as an index of similarity, if an $r = 0.70$ was obtained, one could say that there

Item (Card)	Self-Sort (Number of pile in which item sorted)	Ideal-Sort (Number of pile in which item sorted)
A	9	2
B	5	4
C	8	7
D	1	9
etc.		

FIGURE 9-3. An example of setting up the correlation between one subject's self-sort and an ideal-sort.

was moderate agreement between the self- and ideal-sort, and equivalently by squaring r, that is, 0.70×0.70, that 49 percent of the variance in the self-sort was explained by the ideal-sort and vice versa.

It should be noted that the Q-Sort provides information regarding ordering and therefore permits conclusions only about ordering, that is, results enable one to draw conclusions regarding the relative position of every item within the universe of items. Too frequently, overinterpretations are made on the basis of Q-Sort results. The reader who wishes a more in-depth discussion of approaches to the analysis and interpretation of Q-Sort data is referred to Chapter VII of Block (1961, pp. 89-115).

RELIABILITY AND VALIDITY

Intrarater reliability is of concern when the same individual is asked to sort the same set of items on two or more occasions. As with all cases when this type of reliability is employed it is important to ascertain that nothing occurred in the interval between the sortings to influence responses. Interrater reliability is paramount when two or more subjects respond to the same items at one or more points in time. Specific procedures for determining these two types of reliability are discussed in Chapter 5.

Because of the concern with the selection of items that adequately represent the domain or universe of interest, the determination of content validity is paramount when the Q-Sort technique is used. Depending upon the purpose for the measure, construct or criterion-related validity may be of equal concern. Specific procedures for determining these types of validity are addressed in Chapter 5.

ADVANTAGES AND DISADVANTAGES

From the preceding discussion, it should be apparent that the Q-Sort technique, if properly employed, has utility for the measurement of significant phenomena in a variety of nursing situations, especially in clinical settings. In this vein, the reader who is interested in exploring further the variety of possibilities that exist for the use of the Q-Sort in nursing will find the following references very helpful: Bourque (1960), Cornell (1974), DeWolfe and Governale (1963), Englehardt (1971), Fuhrer and Ware and Scott (1978), Gorham (1958), Gorham (1962), Green and Stone (1972), Hanson and Beech (1963), Hayes and Swenson (1963), Irwin and Meier (1973), Shannon (1973), MacAndrew and Elliott (1959), Miller (1966), Miller

(1965), Moore, White, and Willman (1962), Olson (1968), Redman (1968), Stone and Green (1975), Verhonick (1960), Whiting (1959), and Whiting and Murray (1961).

In addition to the flexibility it affords, the fact that the Q-Sort has as its unit of analysis items rather than subjects renders it more amenable to experimental control than other methods, such as interviews and rating scales. Because subjects' responses are structured, less social desirability comes into play and the problems of missing data, and not applicable and mid-point, undecided, or neutral responses are virtually nonexistent. Fewer subjects are required than with most other methods, and once the Q-Sort is developed and tested, it tends to be less time consuming and less costly to adminster than most other methods for the measurement of attitudes. In fact, the control inherent in the method, its adaptability to a variety of measurement concerns, and the relative simplicity with which it can be administered renders it particularly useful for making interorganizational comparisons (e.g., comparisons between hospitals). In addition to being complete, the data resulting from application of the Q-Sort procedure tend to be relatively simple to handle and analyze and tend to demonstrate high reliability.

Disadvantages stem from the fact that the Q-Sort, depending upon its scope, can be time consuming to administer. Similarly, if sufficient attention is not given to item selection, validity may suffer. In addition, critics have argued that when subjects are forced to place a predetermined number of closely related items into distinct piles, they may make mechanical rather than conceptual choices simply to complete the procedure. This danger may be minimized, however, by using a 4-step procedure such as the one developed by Whiting (1955) or by ensuring that directions are clearly specified and that the subject understands and accepts the importance of the study.

SUMMARY

This chapter focused on specific strategies and techniques for the design of physiologic and observational measures, content analysis, interviews, questionnaires, Delphi technique, projective techniques, and Q-sort methodology. These tools and procedures were selected from the wide variety of available methods and devices because of their frequent use or misuse in nursing or on the basis of their potential utility for use in nursing measurement. Although content emphasized steps to be taken in developing such methods, concern was given as well to the essential considerations to be made in selecting such measures in instances in which nurses choose to employ existing tools and procedures rather than developing their own.

REFERENCES

PHYSIOLOGIC MEASUREMENT

BAUER, JD, ACKERMANN, PG, AND TORO, G: *Clinical Laboratory Methods*, Eighth Edition. C.V. Mosby, St. Louis, 1974.

CROMWELL, L, WEIBELL, FJ, AND PFEIFFER, EA: *Biomedical Instrumentation and Measurements*, Second Edition. Prentice-Hall, Englewood Cliffs, NJ, 1980.

FERRIS, CD: *Guide to Medical Laboratory Instruments*. Little, Brown and Company, Boston, 1980.

KAGAWA-BUSBY, KS, HEITKEMPER, MM, HANSEN, BC, HANSON, RL AND VANDERBURG, V.V.: "Effects of diet temperature on tolerance of enteral feedings." *Nursing Research* 29 (5):276-280, 1980.

POLIT, D AND HUNGLER, B: *Nursing Research: Principles and Methods*. J.B. Lippincott Company, Philadelphia, 1978, pp. 273-298.

WEISS, MD: *Biomedical Instrumentation*. Chilton Book Company, Philadelphia, 1973.

WIDMANN, FH: *Clinical Interpretation of Laboratory Tests*. F.A. Davis Company, Philadelphia, 1979.

OBSERVATIONAL METHODS

ALTMANN, J: "Observational study of behavior: Sampling methods." *Behaviour* 49:228-267, 1973.

ANDERSON, CJ: "Enhancing reciprocity between mother and neonate." *Nursing Research* 30(2):89-93, 1981.

DENZIN, NK: *Sociological Methods: A Sourcebook*. McGraw-Hill Book Company, New York, 1978a.

DENZIN, NK: *The Research Act: A Theoretical Introduction to Sociological Methods*. McGraw-Hill Book Company, New York, 1978b.

GLASER, BG AND STRAUSS, A: *The Discovery of Grounded Theory*. Aldine, Chicago, 1967.

HOLADAY, B: "Maternal responses to their chronically ill infants' attachment behavior of crying." *Nursing Research* 30(6):343-348, 1981.

HURLEY, PM: "Communication patterns and conflict in marital dyads." *Nursing Research* 30(1):38-42, 1981.

JOHNSON, SM, CHRISTENSEN, A, AND BELLAMY, GT: "Evaluation of family intervention through unobtrusive audio recordings: Experiences in 'bugging' children." *Journal of Applied Behavior Analysis* 9:213-219, 1976.

JOHNSON, SM AND LOBITZ, GK: "Parental manipulation of child behavior in home observation." *Journal of Applied Behavior Analysis* 7:23-31, 1974.

KAZDIN, AE: "Direct observations as unobtrusive measures in treatment evaluation." *New Directions for Methodology of Behavioral Science* 1:19-31, 1979.

MERCATORIS, M AND CRAIGHEAD, WE: "Effects of nonparticipant observation on teacher and pupil classroom behavior." *Journal of Educational Psychology* 66:512-519, 1974.

POLIT, D AND HUNGLER, B: *Nursing Research: Principles and Methods*. J.B. Lippincott Company, Philadelphia, 1978, pp. 299-324.

ROBERTS, RR AND RENZAGLIA, GA: "The influence of tape recording on counseling. *Journal of Counseling Psychology* 12:10-16, 1965.

SURRATT, PR, ULRICH, RE, AND HAWKINS, RP: "An elementary student as a behavioral engineer." *Journal of Applied Behavior Analysis* 2:58-92, 1969.

WHITE, GD: "The effects of observer presence on the activity level of families." *Journal of Applied Behavior Analysis* 10:734, 1977.

CONTENT ANALYSIS

BALES, RF: *Interaction Process Analysis: A Method for the Study of Small Groups*. Addison-Wesley, Reading, MA, 1951.

BERELSON, B: "Content Analysis." In LINDZEY, G (ed): *Handbook of Social Psychology*. Addison-Wesley, Reading, MA, 1954.

BUDD, RW, THORP, RK, AND DONOHEW, L: *Content Analysis of Communications*. Macmillan, New York, 1967.

CARNEY, TF: *Content Analysis: A Technique for Systematic Inference from Communication*. University of Manitoba Press, Winnipeg, 1972.

GOTTSCHALK, LA AND GELSER, G: *The Measurement of Psychological States Through the Content Analysis of Verbal Behavior*. University of California Press, Berkeley, 1969.

GOTTSCHALK, LA: *The Content Analysis of Verbal Behavior*. SP Medical and Scientific Books, New York, 1979.

HOLSTI, OR: *Content Analysis for the Social Sciences and Humanities*. Addision-Wesley, Cambridge, MA, 1969.

JOHNSON, WL AND HARDIN, CA: *Content and Dynamics of Home Visits of Public Health Nurses. Part I*. American Nurses' Foundation, New York, 1962.

JOHNSON, WL: *Content and Dynamics of Home Visits of Public Health Nurses. Part II*. American Nurses' Foundation, New York, 1969.

KERLINGER, FN: *Foundations of Behavioral Research*, ed. 2. Holt, Rinehart and Winston, New York, 1973.

MARKOFF, J, SHAPIRO, G, AND WEITMAN, S: "Toward the integration of content analysis and general methodology." In HEISE, D (ed): *Sociological Methodology 1975*. Josey-Bass, San Francisco, 1977, pp. 1-58.

STONE, PJ, DUNPHY, DC, SMITH, MS, AND OGILVIE, DM: *The General Inquirer: A Computer Approach to Content Analysis*. MIT Press, Cambridge, MA, 1966.

INTERVIEWS

ALEXANDER, CS, WEISMAN, CS, AND CHASE, GA: "Determinants of staff nurses' perception of autonomy within different clinical contexts." *Nursing Research* 31(1):48-52, 1982.

BRADBUM, NM, SUDMAN, S, et al: *Improving Interviewing Method and Questionnaire Design*. Josey-Bass, San Francisco, 1979.

DENZIN, NK: *The Research Act*. McGraw-Hill, New York, 1972.

DENZIN, NK: *The Research Act*, ed. 2. McGraw-Hill, New York, 1972.

DILLMAN, DA: *Mail and Telephone Surveys: The Total Design Method*. John Wiley, New York, 1978.

GORDON, RL *Interviewing: Strategy, Techniques and Tactics*, ed. 3. Dorsey Press, Homewood, IL, 1980.

INSTITUTE FOR SOCIAL RESEARCH. *Interviewer Training Manual*. University of Michigan, Ann Arbor, 1976.

KAHN, R AND CANNELL, C: *The Dynamics of Interviewing*. Wiley, New York, 1957.

KERLINGER, FN: *Foundations of Behavioral Research*, ed. 2. Holt, Rinehart and Winston, New York, 1973.

POLIT, D AND HUNGLER, B: *Nursing Research: Principles and Methods*. J.B. Lippincott, Philadelphia, 1978.

RICHARDSON, SA, DOHRENWEND, B, AND KLEIN, D: *Interviewing: Its Forms and Functions*. Basic Books, New York, 1965.

SELLTIZ, C, JAHODA, M, DEUTCH, M, AND COOK, S: *Research Methods in Social Relations*. Holt, Rinehart and Winston, New York, 1959.

SIMON, J: *Basic Research Methods in Social Science*, ed. 2. Random House, New York, 1978.

QUESTIONNAIRE

BRADBURN, NM, SUDMAN, S, et al: *Improving Interview Method and Questionnaire Design*. Josey-Bass, San Francisco, 1979.

DILLMAN, DA: *Mail and Telephone Surveys: The Total Design Method*. John Wiley, New York, 1978.

MARKOWITZ, JS, PEARSON, G. KAY, BG, AND LOEWENSTEIN, R: "Nurses, physicians, and pharmacists: Their knowledge of hazards of medications." *Nursing Research* 30(6):366-370, 1981.

OPPENHEIM, AN: *Questionnaire Design and Attitude Measurement.* Basic Books, New York, 1966.

POLIT, D AND HUNGLER, B: *Nursing Research Principles and Methods.* J.B. Lippincott, Philadelphia, 1978.

DELPHI

HOPE, G: "An Empirical Investigation to Identify Continuing Education Needs for Nurses in a National Health Agency." Unpublished Doctoral Dissertation, Catholic University of America, Washington, DC, 1977.

LINDEMAN, C: "Delphi Survey of Priorities in Clinical Nursing Research." *Nursing Research* 24(6):434-441, 1975.

LINSTONE, H: "Eight Basic Pitfalls: A Checklist." In LINSTONE, H. AND TUROFF, M (eds): *The Delphi Method Techniques and Applications.* Addison-Wesley, Wellesley, MA, pp. 573-586.

LINSTONE, H AND TUROFF, M: *The Delphi Method Techniques and Applications.* Addison-Wesley, Wellesley, MA, 1975.

MCNALLY, JA: "Toward Anticipating Possible Needs for Nursing Services that Might Emerge From Anticipated Social and Technological Development: A Demonstration of a Use of the Delphi Method." Unpublished Doctoral Dissertation, Columbia University, New York.

MOSCOVICE, I, ARMSTRONG, P, SHORTELL, S, AND BENNETT, R: "Health Services Research for Decision-Makers: The Use of the Delphi Technique to Determine Health Priorities." *Journal of Health Politics, Policy and Law* 2:388-409, 1978.

OBERST, M: "Priorities in Cancer Nursing Research." *Cancer Nursing* 1(4):181-190, 1978.

SACKMAN, H: *Delphi Critique: Expert Opinion, Forecasting, and Group Process.* Lexington Books, D.C. Heath and Co., 1975.

TUROFF, M: "The Policy Delphi." In LINSTONE, H AND TUROFF, M (eds): *The Delphi Method Techniques and Applications.* Addison-Wesley, 1975, pp. 84-101.

VENTURA, M AND WALEGORA-SERAFIN, B: "Setting Priorities for Nursing Research." *The Journal of Nursing Administration,* June, 1981, pp. 30-34.

PROJECTIVE TECHNIQUES

ANASTASI, A: *Psychological Testing,* ed. 4. Macmillan, New York, 1976, pp. 558-587.

ANDERSON, HH AND ANDERSON, GL: *An Introduction to Projective Techniques and Other Devices for Understanding the Dynamics of Human Behavior.* Prentice Hall, Englewood Cliffs, NJ, 1951.

EYSENCK, JJ: "Rorschach review." In BUROS, OK (ed): *The Fifth Mental Measurements Yearbook.* Gryphon Press, Highland Park, NJ, 1959, pp. 276-278.

JENSEN, AR: "Review of the Rorschach." In BUROS, OK (ed): *The Sixth Mental Measurement Yearbook.* Gryphon Press, Highland Park, NJ, 1965.

KERLINGER, FN: *Foundations of Behavioral Research,* ed. 2. Holt, Rinehart and Winston, New York, 1973, pp. 514-521.

LINDZEY, G: "On the classification of projective techniques." *Psychological Bulletin* 56:158-168, 1959.

MENKE, EM: "Game to identify hospitalized children's perception of stress." In *Instruments for Measuring Nursing Practice and Other Health Care Variables. Volume I.* USDHEW (DHEW Publication No. HRA 78-53), Washington, DC, 1978, pp. 187-188.

MOLISH, HB: "Projective methodologies." In MUSSEN, P AND ROZENZWEIG, M (eds.): *Annual Review of Psychology.* Vol. 23, Annual Review, Palo Alto, CA, 1972.

NUNNALLY, JC: *Psychometric Theory,* ed. 2. McGraw-Hill, New York, 1978, pp. 568-575.

POLIT, D AND HUNGLER, B: *Nursing Research: Principles and Methods.* J.B. Lippincott, Philadelphia, 1978, pp. 384-387.

PORTER, CS: "Grade school children's perceptions of their internal body parts." *Nursing Research* 23:384-391, 1974.

STANLEY, JC AND HOPKINS, KD: *Educational and Psychological Measurement and Evaluation.* Prentice-Hall, Englewood Cliffs, NJ, 1972, pp. 396-402.

ZUBIN, J, ERON, LC, AND SHUMER, F: *An Experimental Approach to Projective Techniques.* Wiley, New York, 1965.

Q-SORT

BLOCK, J: *The Q-Sort Method in Personality Assessment and Psychiatric Research.* Charles C Thomas, Springfield, IL, 1961.

BOURQUE, EJ: "The Construction and Evaluation of An Instrument Based on Q-Methodology Which Measures the Relative Importance of Self-Perceived Needs of the Tuberculous." Unpublished Ed.D. dissertation, Boston University School of Education, Boston, 1958. Abstracted in *Nursing Research* 9(2):95, 1960.

CORNELL, SA: "Development of an Instrument for Measuring the Quality of Nursing Care." *Nursing Research* 23(2):108-117, 1974.

DEWOLFE, AS AND GOVERNALE, CS: "Fear of Tuberculosis and Prior Psychiatric Experience." *Nursing Research* 12(3):175-180, 1963.

DUNLAY, MS AND HADLEY, BJ: "Quasi Q-Sort Methodology in Self-Evaluation of Conference Leadership Skill." *Nursing Research* 14(2):119-125, 1965.

ENGELHARDT, K: "Faculty Time Study." *Nursing Research* 20(1):74-77, 1971.

FOX, DJ: *Fundamentals of Research in Nursing.* Appleton-Century-Crofts, New York, 1976.

FREIHOFER, P AND FELTON, G: "Nursing Behaviors in Bereavement: An Exploratory Study." *Nursing Research* 25(5):332-337, 1976.

FUHRER, MJ, WARE, KE, AND SCOTT, RW: "The Nursing Attendant's Role in a Rehabilitation Setting: Conceptions and Attitudinal Correlates." *Nursing Research* 17(4):343-348, 1978.

GORHAM, DR: "An Evaluation of Attitude Towards Psychiatric Nursing Care." *Nursing Research* 7(2):71-76, 1958.

GORHAM, WA: "Staff Nursing Behaviors Contributing to Patient Care and Improvement." *Nursing Research* 11(2):68-79, 1962.

GREEN, JL AND STONE, JC: "Developing and Testing Q-Cards and Content Analysis in Group Interviews." *Nursing Research* 21(4):342-347, 1972.

HANSON, RC AND BEECH, MJ: "Communicating Health Arguments Across the Cultures." *Nursing Research* 12(4):237-241, 1963.

HAYES, JE, SR. AND SWENSON, WM: "The Effect of a Three-Months Educational Experience in Psychiatric Nursing on the Self-Concept of a Group of Nursing Students." *Nursing Research* 12(2):113-116, 1963.

IRWIN, BL AND MEIER, JS: "Supportive Measures for Relatives of the Fatally Ill." *Communicating Nursing Research: Collaboration and Competition* 6:119-128, 1973.

MACANDREW, C AND ELLIOTT, JE: "Varying Images of the Professional Nurse: A Case Study." *Nursing Research* 8(1):33-35, 1959.

MACKINNON, DW, et al: "An Assessment Study of Air Force Officers: Part I. Design of the Study and Description of the Variables." Lackland Air Force Base, Texas: Personnel Laboratory, Wright Air Development Center, 1958 (*Technical Report*; WADC-TW-58-91, Part I, ASTIA Document No. AD 152-040).

MEEHL, PE: "Wanted—A Good Cookbook." *American Psychologist* 11:263-272, 1956.

MILLER DI: "Characteristics of Graduate Students in Four Clinical Nursing Specialties." *Nursing Research* 14(2):106-113, 1965.

MILLER, DI: "Characteristics of Graduate Students Preparing for Teaching or Supervision in a Nursing Specialty." *Nursing Research* 15(2):168-171, 1966.

MOORE, L, WHITE, GD, AND WILLMAN, MD: "Factors Influencing the Behavior of Students in Nursing." *Nursing Research* 11(2):97-99, 1962.

MOWRER, OH: *Psychotherapy: Theory and Research.* Ronald Press, New York, 1953.

OLSON, ME: "Comparison of Head Nurse and Staff Nurse Attitudes Towards Various Aspects of Nursing Care." *Nursing Research* 17(4):349-352, 1968.

REDMAN, BK: "Nursing Teacher Perceptiveness of Student Attitudes." *Nursing Research* 17(1):59-64, 1968.

SHANNON, AM: "Critique of Supportive Measures for Relatives of the Fatally Ill." *Communicating Nursing Research: Collaboration and Competition* 6:129-135, 1973.

SIEGEL, A: *Nonparametric Statistics for the Behavioral Sciences.* McGraw-Hill, New York, 1956.

STEPHENSON, W: *The Study of Behavior: Q Technique and Its Methodology.* University of Chicago Press, Chicago, 1953.

STONE, JC AND GREEN, JL: "The Impact of a Professional Baccalaureate Degree Program." *Nursing Research* 24(4):287-292, 1975.

VERHONICK, PJ: "A Plan for Field Experience in Nursing Service Administration for Army Nurse Corps Officers." Unpublished Ed.D. dissertation, Teachers College, Columbia University, New York, 1958. Abstracted in *Nursing Research* 9(2):84, 1960.

WALTZ, C AND BAUSELL, RB: *Nursing Research, Design, Statistics and Computer Analysis.* F.A. Davis, Co., Philadelphia, 1981.

WHITING, JF: "Q-Sort: A Technique for Evaluating Perceptions of Interpersonal Relationships." *Nursing Research* 4(2):70-73, 1955.

WHITING, JF: "Patients' Needs, Nurses' Needs, and the Healing Process." *American Journal of Nursing* 59(5):661-665, 1959.

WHITING, JF AND MURRAY, MA: "Toward a Theory of Hospital Structure Based on Objective, Quantitative Data." Association of American Medical Colleges, Evanston, IL, 1961. Abstracted in Nursing Research 10(4):234, 1961.

10

ISSUES
IN NURSING MEASUREMENT

As nurses have become more involved in the development and use of devices for measuring nursing phenomena, several issues and problems have emerged which require careful consideration. For the most part, these concerns can be classified into two major categories: those that deal with linking conceptualization of phenomena with measurement, and ethical issues in measurement. The first part of this chapter addresses the most commonly encountered measurement situations in which linking conceptualization and operationalization is of central concern. These include the selection and use of existing instruments, measuring state and trait characteristics, and process and outcome measurement. The last part of the chapter deals with ethical issues in measurement in terms of the responsibilities of the nurse during the measurement process to human subjects and to the profession. In most cases answers to the issues are available if measurement principles are carefully followed and if the nurse is sensitive to the demands that a particular measurement procedure can place on subjects.

SELECTION AND USE OF EXISTING INSTRUMENTS

An issue that nurses frequently confront in clinical practice, education, administration, and research activities is whether to use instruments developed by others or develop new instruments to measure the variables of interest. On the one hand, it is generally much less costly and time consuming to use pre-existing instruments than to expend the effort necessary to develop and adequately test a new measure. In addition to the pragmatic advantages, the use of existing instruments is beneficial from a knowledge-building perspective. It allows systematic comparisons to be made across time and space and among different populations, because the characteristics are being measured in the same way. Use of existing tools and devices provides an ever-increasing data base for evaluating the properties of the instruments themselves and allows the accumulation of information about a particular concept or variable and its relation to others as it is measured and used in different contexts. On the other hand, nurses often discover after extensive search of the literature that no instruments have been developed to measure a particular concept or variable. This is particularly true of instruments specific to nursing care interventions (Ventura, et al, 1981). They may find that existing instruments simply are not adequate because of their conceptual basis, psychometric properties, inapplicability to nursing settings, or inadequate testing. In such instances, it is necessary to develop a new instrument or substantially modify an existing one. There is clearly a need for nurses to develop sound measurement tools for use in nursing. High priority is currently being placed on tool development in the profession (Ventura, et al, 1981); thus, a marked increase is expected in the number of instruments available that are appropriate for nursing measurement.

It is our position that when instruments appropriate for the intended purpose already exist, they should be used in preference to developing new ones. However, determining the adequacy of existing instruments, using them, and reporting their use appropriately are vitally important activities which involve careful consideration of a variety of factors. The following treatment of the evaluation, use, and reporting of existing instruments is intended to summarize and reinforce recommendations set forth in previous chapters.

EVALUATING EXISTING INSTRUMENTS

Regardless of the intended purpose for which measurement is being undertaken, a necessary activity is to determine the extent to which instruments may already exist that measure the variables of interest. Sources and examples of available instruments are included in the Appendix. Once potential instruments have been located, they must be carefully evaluated in light of the purpose for which they are to be used. This is a process which requires sophistication in the concepts of measurement and cannot be conducted superficially or with strong disciplinary bias. For example, an instrument's availability, previous widespread use, and purported ability to measure a concept or variable of interest are not sufficient conditions for legitimating its use for a given nursing measurement activity. Likewise, the fact that an instrument has been developed within the context of another discipline does not automatically preclude its applicability to nursing questions.

Evaluation of the adequacy of any existing instrument requires that consideration be given to its purpose, conceptual basis, development, and psychometric properties. It is critical that the potential borrower or user of the instrument obtain the information necessary to evaluate these features. Such information may not be readily available and may require active search by the potential user, including personal contact with the instrument's developer and others who have used it. Although time consuming, obtaining such information before selecting an instrument helps to prevent problems and dilemmas that result from the use of inappropriate or psychometrically inadequate measures and that cannot be rectified after the measure has been employed. Major areas requiring attention when evaluating existing tools for use in nursing measurement are considered briefly in the next sections. They serve to highlight the information that tool developers have a responsibility to provide about their work in the literature.

PURPOSE. Every measurement instrument is developed for a purpose, whether or not it is explicitly stated by the developer. The purposes for which the tool was originally developed need not be identical to those for which its use is being evaluated, but they should be congruent. For example, a tool developed to measure the climate of an organization for research purposes might be employed subsequently by nursing service administrators to assess the characteristics of a hospital, provided that organizational climate is an attribute of interest and provided that the instrument addresses dimensions of climate that are meaningful in a hospital setting. An instrument developed to measure the climate of an industrial organization may not be relevant to a hospital, because the structures, levels, and responsibilities of personnel and goals of the two types of organizations differ considerably. To cite another example, assume nurses working in the coronary care unit of a hospital wish to assess the coping ability of women whose spouses have been admitted to the unit. While several instruments have been developed to measure women's coping behaviors, it would be important for the nurses to determine whether the instruments were designed to measure coping in acute problem situations and whether the wording of the items would be acceptable to women facing the possibility of a spouse's death. Since the purpose for which an instrument is developed is inherently linked to its content and format, it is important that the instrument as a whole and individual items be scrutinized carefully in light of the intended use in particular settings and for particular populations.

When evaluating existing measures to assess the degree of fit between the purpose for which they were developed and that for which they are being considered, several features must be taken into account. The instrument itself and literature describing situations in which it has been employed must be examined to provide information about the following features.

Stated Aim of the Measurement Tool. Instruments are developed with one of several goals in mind (e.g., description, diagnosis, screening, selection, or prediction). Each requires different information. For example, a tool developed to provide descriptive information about applicants to a nursing education program may be too imprecise to supply the data for decision making.

Norm- Versus Criterion-Referenced Mode. As detailed in Chapters 4 through 7, norm- and criterion-referenced measures are developed and interpreted differently for different purposes and should not be used interchangeably. Availability of norms for the former type of measure is an important consideration in instrument selection.

Population. A measure is developed for a particular population and is specific to individuals or groups with given characteristics such as age, educational level, culture, previous life experiences, and health status (including specific pathologic conditions), and often cannot be used for other populations without considerable modification. It is also necessary to determine whether the target population for an instrument is composed of individuals or intact groups.

Setting. Often an instrument is designed for use in a particular setting such as a hospital, school, industry, or home, and cannot easily be transferred to another context. This is particularly true of physiologic and observational measures, but it is also an important consideration in other types of measures such as interviews and questionnaires that require the subject to take a given setting or context into account in formulating responses. Since nursing is practiced in highly diverse settings, assumptions inherent in an instrument about the nature of the context or setting may not be valid even in a seemingly similar situation.

Time Perspective. All instruments have an inherent orientation with respect to time. Some take only the present into account, while others require recall of past events or projection into the future. In nursing it is also important to ascertain the extent to which a given instrument may be oriented toward short- versus long-term conditions or situations.

CONCEPTUAL BASIS FOR THE INSTRUMENT. When evaluating an existing instrument for potential use it is vital to ascertain the conceptual basis for its development. Inherent in every instrument are assumptions about the nature of the entity being measured. These may be explicitly stated by the developer or may have to be inferred. In either case, it is crucial to remember, as detailed in Chapter 2, that every instrument reflects a particular perspective and conceptual mapping which must be evaluated in terms of its congruence with the views of the potential user. Many instruments useful in nursing measure complex concepts, such as stress, anxiety, social support, coping, competency, communication, role, and health, which have been conceptualized from many different theoretical perspectives. Depending upon the perspective being used, the instruments developed to measure the same concept may differ considerably in the dimensions that are highlighted. (For example, see discussions by Norbeck et al, 1981 and Brandt and Weinert, 1981, regarding the development of instruments to measure social support systems.)

The major consideration in evaluating an existing instrument is the degree of fit between the current conceptualization and that which guided the development of the instrument. In addition to ascertaining that underlying assumptions are compatible, important points in assessing the degree of fit include the following: (1) whether the entity to be measured is conceptualized as static or dynamic; (2) whether the entity is conceptualized objectively, subjectively, or both; and (3) the extent to which the original conceptualization includes those aspects or dimensions of meaning that are deemed essential in the situation for which it is being evaluated. As noted in reviews of published nursing research by Batey (1977), Waltz and Strickland (1982), and others, a common problem is that the instrument chosen to measure a given concept often is not conceptually congruent with the investigator's perspective and theoretical definition of that concept, so validity is compromised and findings cannot be interpreted adequately. The only way to eliminate this problem is to define the meaning domain explicitly and evaluate the domains of existing instruments in that light. Information concerning the conceptual basis and domain of an existing instrument is often available in works written or cited by the developer, in compendia that describe measurement tools, and in review articles and texts that compare theoretical perspectives related to a given concept.

PSYCHOMETRIC PROPERTIES. Reliability and validity are fundamental considerations when evaluating an existing instrument for potential use, a point which has been emphasized repeatedly throughout this book. Given the importance of these properties, it is essential that information about the reliability and validity of any instrument be obtained and evaluated before it is selected for use. A thorough assessment requires that the potential user take into account the procedures that were used to develop the instrument, as well as those that were used to assess its psychometric properties, not only at the time of development but in subsequent applications. Attention must be given to the types of reliability and validity assessed and to the specific populations and administration conditions for which data have been reported, recognizing that psychometric properties may change under different conditions. Important considerations in evaluating the psychometric properties of an instrument include (1) the number and recency of reliability and validity estimates; (2) the diversity of conditions for which estimates have been reported; (3) the nature of the samples from which reliability and validity data were obtained; (4) the degree of similarity between the situation for which the instrument is being evaluated and those for which psychometric data are available; and (5) the appropriateness of the procedures used to assess reliability and validity, given the type of instrument and its intended use. All of the above considerations must be viewed in light of the specific requirements of the purposes for which the instrument will be used, including the degree of precision and accuracy that is necessary. For example, considerably more measurement error can be tolerated in an exploratory study to describe patients' level of satisfaction with emergency room facilities than is acceptable in an epidemiologic investigation to identify the causes of an increased nosocomial infection rate in the same hospital.

Despite the importance of applying basic measurement principles and practices to instrument selection, a recent review of published research reports (Waltz and Strickland, 1982) revealed little evidence of rigorous evaluation. In a majority of instances reliability and validity were either not reported or not investigated concurrently. There was heavy reliance on content validity, with little cognizance of the import of construct and criterion-related validity. These findings highlight the need for increased attention to using rigorous criteria in tool selection.

Psychometric properties, conceptualization, and purpose are three major features that provide a basis for evaluating and comparing existing instruments. Also important are pragmatic considerations related to (1) the cost, time, and any special requirements or arrangements involved in purchase, administration, and scoring; (2) the demands made on potential subjects; and (3) whether it is possible to secure permission to use the instrument for the intended purpose. After careful review of the above features it is often possible to identify one or more existing tools that are acceptable. If more than one instrument appears to be satisfactory, then, all else being equal, the one with higher reported reliability and validity should be selected. In some instances existing tools require minor modifications (e.g., wording changes, shortening) for use in a particular nursing situation. To modify an existing instrument is generally more efficient than to develop a new one; however, it must be emphasized that changing an instrument in any way, in essence, creates a new tool. Thus, previous estimates of properties and previously established norms are inapplicable.

USE AND REPORTING

The use of existing instruments entails considerable responsibility on the part of the user. Permission to use a given instrument for a specific purpose must be secured from the developer or publisher, preferably in writing. Any instructions or conditions specified by the developer must be followed; these may involve specifications regarding subjects, procedures for administration, scoring, and interpretation, or requirements for sharing information obtained or problems encountered. The importance of adhering to predetermined procedures in the use of standardized instruments was emphasized in Chapter 8. Adherence to specified procedures is equally important in the use of nonstandardized measures if comparisions are to be made across the results of several administrations or in reference to established norms.

Although previously gathered reliability and validity data may have been secured regarding an existing instrument, its reliability and validity for a different sample is essentially unknown. Thus, it is necessary to assess the psychometric properties of the instrument with each sample. In instances in which the sample or setting differs considerably from previous applications, it is advisable to pretest the instrument and calculate reliability and validity statistics prior to use. The latter should be recalculated concurrently with use of the instrument and reported. Failure to address current reliability and validity estimates is a common problem, as noted above.

Considerations related to reporting the use of existing instruments concern reports to the developer as well as to the scientific and professional community as a whole. Even when the developer does not require feedback following use of the instrument, it is desirable to communicate the results of having used it. Particularly important is the communication of (1) any difficulties encountered in administration, calibration, scoring, and interpretation; (2) the results of reliability and validity testing; and (3) any suggestions for modification or future applications. Such feedback is vital to the improvement of the instrument and its ultimate utility.

Given the desirability of accumulating knowledge and building on the work of others, the user of an existing instrument has responsibility to disseminate information regarding its properties and potential utility to the scientific community by publishing reports of its use. Several important points need to be made in this regard. First, any modifications must be detailed explicitly and resulting psychometric data shared. Second, reporting the use of measurement tools should include but not be limited to the research literature. Many instruments developed for research can be employed fruitfully in nursing administration, education, and practice settings if their existence, strengths, and weaknesses are known. Third, information about instruments that measure variables of interdisciplinary interest is appropriately shared with relevant nonnursing audiences and frequently serves as the basis for fruitful collaboration. Finally, failures as well as successes are important. The finding that an instrument demonstrated low reliability or validity when applied to a particular population or in a particular setting or the observation that problems were experienced during its use would be vital to preventing future problems. Such information is as crucial to share as evidence that an instrument was used successfully.

MEASURING STATE AND TRAIT CHARACTERISTICS

Most attributes that are measured are conceptualized as stable or exhibiting little variation over time, given the same measurement circumstances. However, in the real world a number of attributes can and do vary from moment to moment and day to day. Those attributes that are conceptualized as being stable with little variability are referred to as *trait* characteristics. *State* attributes are conceptualized as dynamic and changeable over relatively short periods of time and from one situation to another.

TRAIT ATTRIBUTES

A trait description provides a statistical summary of the attribute of interest over many situations. Scores on a trait measure for an attribute represent the probability that an individual will react in a defined way in response to a defined class of situations or stimuli (Cronbach, 1970). For example, if assertiveness is conceptualized as a trait, one would be interested in the typical or usual assertiveness level. If a trait measure of assertiveness indicated that a nurse is assertive, this does not mean that the nurse is assertive in all situations. No one is 100 percent assertive or 0 percent assertive. It only implies that the nurse is assertive in most situations. The nurse might be very nonassertive in interactions with her supervisor, and this score would not reflect this difference in assertiveness level for this particular situation.

Conceptualization of attributes of individuals as traits is deeply embedded in Western languages. Most adjectives that are used to characterize people are descriptive traits, for example, honest, happy, shy, thrifty, liberal, healthy, hypertensive, or hyperactive. Three assumptions underlie trait conceptualizations (Cronbach, 1970):

1. Behavior is habitual within individuals. A person tends to exhibit consistent reactions over a range of similar situations.
2. Different individuals vary in the frequency and degree of any type of behavior or response.
3. Personalities have some degree of stability.

Traits, therefore, economically describe broad characteristics of phenomena. Measurement of trait attributes focuses on significant variation in general behavior over a wide range of situations and does not consider specific behaviors or responses in specific situations.

Since the 1960s there has been concern about the lack of emphasis on situational specificity in measurement (Anastasi, 1976). In the area of personality assessment, much criticism has been leveled regarding the conceptualization of attributes as general, ubiquitous styles. There has been a tendency to reject personality description in terms of broad traits (Bandura, 1979; Goldfried and Kent, 1972; Mischel, 1969, 1973). This type of criticism has been provided with regard to all traits; however, there is higher cross-situational consistency and temporal stability of cognitive as compared with noncognitive attributes (Anastasi, 1976).

Individuals exhibit situational specificity for many attributes. A particular situation may elicit a specific attribute or behavior quite differently than another situation. For example, a person might be calm during a physical examinination if there has been no indication of potential problems, but may on another occasion be highly anxious during a physical examination if there are signs of illness. Similarly, a person who cheats on income taxes might be scrupulously honest in money matters with business associates. Hence, there is a person by situation interaction in the exhibition of many attributes, because a person may exhibit an attribute differently in different situations.

STATE ATTRIBUTES

State attributes reflect the variability of phenomena over rather short periods of time and from situation to situation. A nurse may have good reason for wanting to measure how an attribute changes from time to time or from one situation to another. For example, a nurse might want to know under what circumstances a patient's blood pressure increases or decreases or whether it changes in response to treatment. Within this context, blood pressure would be conceptualized as a state attribute. Many physiologic variables that are observed within nursing clinical settings are conceptualized as state characteristics, since such variables are measured to assess responses to illness or treatment over time. Nurse researchers often study state attributes within the realm of their investigations. There may be an interest in studying the effects of a mood-altering drug on the anxiety and depression levels of clients, for example. Hence, the focus of measurement of state attributes is on the nature of a particular attribute at a particular point in time or in a particular situation. Phenomena are perceived as possessing the potential for having an affinity to time and situation, and the aim of measuring state attributes is to detect the state of phenomena at a given moment or in a given situation.

A specific concept may be conceptualized either as a trait or state. The manner in which the concept is conceptualized and used will determine whether it should be measured as a trait or state.

IMPLICATIONS FOR MEASUREMENT

Conceptualization of an attribute as either a trait or state has implications for how a measurement tool is constructed, how a measurement procedure is conducted, how a device is used, and how reliability and validity are assessed. Consider that state characteristics are conceptualized as dynamic and changeable, while trait attributes reflect typical responses. A device designed to measure a state attribute must possess the sensitivity and precision to detect changes over time. On the other hand, a tool designed to measure a trait attribute should consistently measure the attribute over long periods of time given the same measurement circumstances.

The usual trait inventory is phrased in a manner to obtain information about a person's life style or typical behavior, and it does not elicit information regarding present state or state at a particular moment. When tools are constructed to obtain information on a subject's state, questions are framed in terms of the present moment or the time of interest: "Are you tense?" This same question framed in terms of a trait attribute would be: "Are you usually tense?" The way in which items are framed on a tool affects the information obtained by altering the response set (Cronbach, 1970).

Zuckerman and Lubin (1965) have developed the Multiple Affect Adjective Check List which measures trait and state mood, specifically, anxiety, depression, and hostility. This questionnaire was developed in two forms: general and today. The general form measures trait mood and the today form measures state mood. The only difference between the two forms is in the directions to the respondent. The subject is instructed to respond to the general form according to how he generally feels. On the today form the subject is instructed to respond according to how he feels at the moment. The adjective checklists for both forms are identical and are scored by the same keys to arrive at scores for anxiety, depression, and hostility. Retest reliabilites for the trait scale were satisfactorily high; but this was not the case for the state scale, for which temporal stability is not expected. The internal-consistency reliabilities on both forms of the tool at a single testing were high.

For the most part, physiologic phenomena are highly variable, even within the same individual, and often are conceptualized as state attributes. However, there are times when determining whether a physiologic measurement is reflective of trait or state is important. For example, in the case of blood pressure one would not want to initiate long-term treatment for hypertension unless the client is typically hypertensive. Therefore, it would be important to have a good estimate of the individual's typical or trait blood pressure. If the nurse took the client's blood pressure while he was unusually anxious, the blood pressure reading might be unusually high due to his present emotional state. Hence, the results of the measurement would be a state measurement instead of a trait measurement. The nurse must be clear about the purposes for which a specific physiologic variable is being measured, understand under what conditions such measurements are likely to be most stable and variable, and obtain measurements at times and in situations that will provide the type of data that are most useful.

Since state attributes are changeable and trait attributes are considered relatively stable, this must be given consideration in the assessment of reliability. Although test-retest reliability would be preferably high for a tool that measures a trait attribute, this would not be expected for a tool that measures a state attribute. Since state attributes are changeable, test-retest reliability has little usefulness in the assessment of tools that measure states. Preferable measures of reliability for a state measure would be internal-consistency or parallel forms reliability, and where appropriate, interrater reliability.

When validity is assessed, the approaches that are useful for assessing tools that measure trait attributes also are useful for assessing state measures. Hypothesis testing as a means of construct validation often is employed to support the validity of state measures. For example, a group of subjects might be administered the measure at a time when or in a situation in which the state attribute would be expected to be low and at another point in time when it would be expected to be significantly higher. If significant differences were found between the measurements over time or from one situation to another, this would support the validity of the tool. During validity assessments of the Multiple Affect Adjective Check List, college students scored significantly higher on the today form of the tool on examination days than on nonexamination days (Winter, Ferreira, and Ransom, 1963; Zuckerman, 1960; Zuckerman and Baise, 1962; Zuckerman, Lubin, Vogel, and Valerius, 1965).

INTERPRETING STATE AND TRAIT MEASUREMENTS

As noted previously, when tools are selected to measure an attribute, care should be taken that the conceptual orientation of the tool is consistent with the purpose for which the tool is used. This is particularly important in terms of whether a state or trait characteristic is the focus of measurement. A nurse would not want to use a tool that measured trait anxiety, for example, when the purpose is to measure state anxiety, or vice versa. Whether state or trait attributes are measured will influence the type of interpretations that can be validly made about the results. If a nurse is interested in the long-term effects of a particular phenomenon, it would be more appropriate to employ a trait measure. The reason for this would be that the nurse is really interested in making interpretations about the influence of the phenomenon on the general responses or behaviors of the subject in terms of that attribute, that is, on the trait expression of the attribute. If, on the other hand, the concern is with the changes that occur within a relatively short time period or in a particular situation, then a state measure would be employed. One cannot assume that changes reflected by a state measure are long lasting. Neither can one assume that lack of change in scores obtained by a trait measure also indicates lack of situational or short-term fluctuations in the attribute. The interpretations that can be appropriately made about trait and state characteristics are directly linked to the nature of the measurement tool and the circumstances under which the measurements are made.

PROCESS AND OUTCOME MEASUREMENT

Process and outcome measurement has become very popular and highly valued in nursing. This trend has come about because of an increased emphasis on investigating the worth of nursing programs and activities in clinical and educational settings, and because nurses have become more interested in understanding the relationship between nursing activities and practice outcomes. Pressures external to the nursing profession also have contributed to nursing interest and activity in this area. The passage of the Professional Standards Review Organization (PSRO) legislation (P.L. 92-603) in 1972 further encouraged interest in process and outcome measurement. This legislation mandated that the quality of medical care financed by federal funds be monitored. Although the legislation was primarily aimed at physicians, it did not exclude other health care providers. Nurses increased their activity in the area of monitoring the quality of nursing care, and this required that measurement of processes and outcomes in nursing be given special attention. In addition to its impact via PSRO legislation, the federal government also stimulated interest in process and outcome measurement by requiring that educational and health care programs that receive federal funding be evaluated. As part of the evaluation of the processes for implementing such programs, nurses were required to focus on measurement of process and outcome variables.

With all of this activity, process and outcome measurement has not proven to be a simple matter. Issues have been raised regarding frameworks that should be used, the approaches to process and outcome measurement, and the meaning of findings. This section will address such issues. However, before focusing specifically on measurement of process and outcomes, per se, it is necessary to provide definitions of these terms.

DEFINITIONS

Process is the manner or approach by which a program or provider delivers services to clients. *Outcomes* are the outputs or results of the program or the activities of the provider. It is noteworthy that one should be careful not to confuse process/outcome measurement with process/outcome research and evaluation. *Process/outcome research* involves investigating relationships between process variables or outcome variables in order to make decisions regarding statistical hypotheses and inductive inferences concerning the probable truth or falsity of a research hypothesis. Process/outcome research is conducted primarily to build theory and to add to the knowledge base in an area. *Process/outcome evaluation* is a decision-making process by which one examines the manner in which a program or provider delivers services or their outputs and makes judgments about what is done or how well objectives are met. Evaluation of processes and outcomes can be expected to lead to suggestions for action to improve effectiveness and efficiency. Nursing quality of care assessment and nursing audit are examples of process/outcome evaluations. *Process/outcome measurement* relates to how a specified process or outcome is operationalized, that is, quantified or classified. Measurement is a part of the research process and the evaluation process but is not synonymous with either.

PROCESS MEASUREMENT

The term process by its very nature is dynamic, and it projects a sense of movement and fluidity. This quality makes the measurement of a particular process quite challenging. However, the approach to operationalizing a process follows the same basic principles as for measurement of most other variables. Since measurement should be based on how a variable is conceptualized, this indicates that the measurement of process must consider its dynamic quality. The specific process that is the focus of measurement should be clearly defined in a manner that captures the essence of its characteristics. The determination of a conceptual framework for the process is one of the first essential steps in the development of a reliable and valid measurement approach. Since most processes are not unitary phenomena, a number of concepts may be required for the formulation of a sound definition (Horn, 1980). Each concept in the framework must be defined and the relationships between key variables identified. Specification errors in the conceptual framework can lead to an invalid measurement procedure. When formulating a conceptual framework for the process, specification errors can arise from three sources: (1) underspecification (missing key variables) or overspecification (including extra variables); (2) inaccurate or incomplete definitions of the key variables; and (3) inaccurate identification of the relationships among the key variables (Atwood, 1980, p. 105; Blalock, 1964).

Once the conceptual framework of the process has been delineated, the blueprint or specific approach to measurement is developed. The measurement approach should address the key variables that are included in the conceptual framework; therefore, several variables or dimensions may be included in the measurement. If the nursing process model were used as the conceptual framework for measuring the process of nursing care, one would include assessment, planning, implementation, and evaluation as key components in the measurement.

Two popular nursing care process tools are Phaneuf's (1976) Nursing Audit and Wandelt and Ager's (1974) Quality Patient Care Scale (QualPaCS). Phaneuf conceptualized nursing by its legal definition and delineated seven categories for which criteria were derived: execution of nursing process, teaching, execution of physician orders, observation of symptoms, supervision of patients, supervision of others, and reporting and recording. The conceptual basis of QualPaCS is the interaction of the nurse and patient in the following areas: psychosocial individual, psychosocial group, physical, general, communications on behalf of the patient, and professional implications. For the most part, measurement of process in nursing has been approached conceptually in two ways: by focusing on the services or care provided by the nurse, and by focusing on the services or care received by the client (Bloch, 1975).

When process measurement is conducted during process evaluation, criteria or standards are specified which describe the nature and, when appropriate, the events that should occur in the process and the expected interaction of activities and participants involved in the process. The criteria serve as the basis for making judgments regarding the adequacy of the process. In developing criteria, one seeks to specify the important aspects of the process in measureable terms. For example, the process criteria for nursing care on a specified nursing unit might include the following:

Comatose patients will be repositioned every two hours.

Each patient having an alteration in body image will be assessed by a psychiatric nurse specialist (Lang, 1976, p. 22).

Process criteria for a nursing education program might include:

Admission criteria and procedures are closely followed.

Students are provided opportunities to evaluate the curriculum.

Faculty members involve students in their research activities.

Several types of measurement methods are amenable to measuring processes and included among these are observation, interviews, diaries, record audit, and questionnaires. Tools that employ the branching technique are particularly useful when the nature of the process involves several interrelated steps that are dependent upon each other, such as with measurement of the process of decision making. The branching technique provides several options or choices along the way at various stages of the process. The option selected will determine other situations or options that will be presented to the subjects. Hence, the various available options, if selected, subsequently provide different situations or options in a sequential manner similar to the branches of a tree.

Because of the complexity of the nature of most processes and the number of key variables that may be involved, multiple measures can increase the reliability and validity of results. Therefore, use of multiple measures in process measurement is encouraged.

A major concern related to process measurement is that the act of measuring the process may alter the process and, thereby, the subsequent findings. This issue might not be crucial during process evaluation in which information obtained may be intentionally used for making decisions for change. Clearly, process measurement can give clues to corrective action and provide a means for elucidating consequences of certain actions. However, this problem could be a severe limitation to research studies that require the measurement of process variables. In any case, efforts should be made to conduct measurements as unobtrusively as possible.

OUTCOME MEASUREMENT

A major issue for nurses regarding outcome measurement is that of selecting appropriate outcomes for study. In a given situation, a wide array of variables may be appropriate for outcome measurement. As with process measurement, in most instances there is no single concept that is likely to adequately represent the outcomes of a particular intervention or process. Therefore, the outcomes selected must be based on and be consistent with the conceptual framework that is being considered. In other words, the outcomes selected must be meaningful to the focus of the investigation. If the focus of the study is concerned with health state, then the appropriate outcome variables should relate to health state. If the basic problem is conceptualized in terms of cognitive phenomena, then appropriate cognitive outcomes should be selected (Bloch, 1975).

Clinical outcomes that are discussed in the general nursing literature frequently are limited to the consideration of disease status, symptoms, and function. Clinical outcomes in the research literature often deal with a single psychosocial variable rather than including several psychosocial, cognitive, and physiologic variables. Review of the research literature in terms of outcome variables included in studies indicates that nurses tend to select those outcome variables that are more easily obtained or are convenient (Waltz and Strickland, 1982). Donabedian (1970) suggests that outcome measurement should include a variety of client states and behaviors, such as level of satisfaction with care, knowledge of illness, and compliance with the prescribed health regimen. Since nursing views humans as biopsychosocial beings, then key outcome variables in those areas should be selected which relate to the framework under consideration. The study of several key outcome variables and their relationships with each other and the intervention will provide more information and will more likely further develop the knowledge base regarding the phenomenon of interest than a single outcome variable.

When the interest is on evaluating the outcomes of a process such as an educational program or health care program, the focus might be on assessing outcomes of provider behaviors, on the influence of the program on provider and client attitudes, or the impact of the program's services within a specified geographic area. When programs are assessed, the objectives or goals of the program are the primary outcome criteria. Outcome criteria are used to make judgments regarding the effectiveness of a process or program. An outcome criterion or standard can be considered valid if it is an accurate statement of the following (Bloch, 1980, p. 71):

(a) Something that should or should not occur in the status of the patient (or client),
(b) The level at which it should occur,
(c) The point in time at which it should occur, and
(d) Something that is expected to occur in good measure as a result of the care (or process) which is to be assessed.

Patient care goals should be formulated in a manner that they can serve as the outcome criteria for assessing the quality of the process of nursing care provided to an individual patient (Inger and Aspinall, 1981). Examples are:

The patient will care for colostomy without assistance prior to discharge.

The patient will lose 10 pounds within six months.

Another issue that causes concern about the selection of outcomes is that most outcomes are influenced by many factors beyond those that are the focus of study. A client's attitudes, behaviors, health state, or knowledge may be influenced by care or services received from other providers. It is difficult to select outcomes that can be solely attributed to any one factor, such as nursing care or a particular health care program or educational program. However, in most instances it is possible to select outcomes that can be related temporally to the intervention or process that is the focus of investigation. Temporally relating variations in outcomes to the expected sources of such changes supports the validity and usefulness of the outcome selected. Thus, timing of measurements is important. Outcomes are selected that are expected to respond to the type of action, intervention, or process that is conducted. The prevention and healing rate of decubitus ulcers is an example of an outcome that would be expected to respond to nursing care. Another related issue is that nursing addresses, to a great extent, subtle psychosocial problems. The impact of nursing on the client's state may be difficult to measure, because psychosocial variables often are difficult to measure.

As with the measurement of process variables, the use of multiple measures of outcome variables can provide more support for reliability and validity. Interviews, questionnaires, record audit, direct observation, and use of laboratory data are among the various approaches that may be employed for the measurement of outcomes. However, it should be noted that record audit will not provide reliable and valid indicators unless measurement or the method of recording data is reliable and valid. Whereas certain information on a record, such as temperature readings or results of laboratory tests, may be highly reliable and valid, others, such as behaviors learned by the client for self care, may not be adequately documented.

ETHICAL ISSUES IN MEASUREMENT

Concern with ethical dimensions of practice and research is one of the hallmarks of a profession. In recent years nursing, like many other professions, has focused increased attention on these matters and established standards, codes, and guidelines designed to assure ethical practice and protection of patients and subjects. Examples include the American Nurses' Association's *Human Rights Guidelines for Nurses in Clinical and Other Research* (Beneoliel and Berthold, 1975) and *Code for Nurses* (1975) and the Royal College of Nursing's publication entitled *Ethics Related to Research in Nursing* (1977). Despite the existence of such guidelines, a complex set of issues must be confronted by nurses engaged in measurement, whether in the context of research, clinical practice, administration, or education.

The purpose of this section is to call attention to some of these issues, recognizing that there are no simple solutions. While an exhaustive discussion is beyond the scope of this book, responsibilities of the nurse to clients or subjects, to colleagues, and to the scientific and professional community will be highlighted.

ETHICAL ISSUES RELATED TO MEASUREMENT OF HUMAN SUBJECTS

Most of the ethical issues regarding measurement of human subjects have been addressed in connection with biomedical and social research. Following World War II and the Nuremberg trials, which called attention to abuses in human experimentation, there has been ongoing activity to assure ethical and humane treatment of human and animal subjects in research. Guidelines are provided in such well-known documents as the Nuremberg Code and the Declaration of Helsinki; in the codes of professional organizations such as the American Nurses' Association, American Medical Association, American Dental Association, American Psychological Association, American Sociological Association, American Hospital Association, American Political Science Association, American Anthropological Association, and American Personnel and Guidance Association (see Bower and de Gasparis, 1978, for information about these guidelines and Beauchamp and Walters, 1982, for reprints of some of these codes); and in published requirements for research funded by the U.S. Department of Health and Human Services. The guidelines address multiple aspects of research, and hence include, but are broader in scope than, measurement considerations that represent the focus of the following discussion. They should be consulted and followed by any nurse proposing to engage in research involving human subjects.

Although the research context has given rise to many of the ethical issues surrounding measurement of human subjects, all nursing measurement activities involve similar ethical considerations. Generally, measurement issues and guidelines specific to nonresearch contexts have not been elaborated as extensively as for research. However, one example of standards that include ethical considerations is the *Standards for Evaluations of Educational Programs, Projects and Materials* (Joint Commission on Standards for Educational Evaluation, 1981). The following discussion is primarily oriented toward ethical issues and recommendations in the research context, since these are the most restrictive and, in most instances, are applicable in other situations. However, special considerations specific to other contexts for nursing measurement will also be addressed.

Rights of subjects must be recognized and preserved in measurement activities. The rights most commonly considered in discussions of research ethics are the rights to informed consent; refusal to participate or withdrawal without recrimination; privacy; confidentiality and anonymity; and protection from harm. Measurement-related issues and responsibilities for each of these areas will be addressed in the next sections.

INFORMED CONSENT. The principle of informed consent has two components according to Hayter (1979:110): "recognition of self determination and thorough understanding of the proposed participation." Adherence to this principle requires that the subject must be fully informed of and comprehend what is involved and must agree freely to participate before measurement can be carried out. The information provided to the potential subject includes description of the procedures that will be carried out and their purposes, the time and energy required, the way in which information will be handled and used, and any discomforts, risks, and benefits which can be expected. In research contexts the subject is also given explicit instruction that withdrawal from participation is possible without prejudice (Bower and de Gasparis, 1978, p. 36-37). It should be noted that the provision of information does not necessarily ensure comprehension by potential subjects. The latter can be heightened by careful wording of the information provided and asking subjects to voice their understanding and interpretation of what will be required before consent can be assumed to be secured.

Although the right to informed consent has been universally accepted, it raises a number of issues. The most difficult dilemma is that providing information to potential subjects about the measurement activity may serve to alter the outcomes of the measurement. For example, if a subject is aware in advance that behavior will be observed for a given purpose, modification of behavior during the observation period is likely. The measurement procedures for which informed consent is most likely to compromise validity are observation, content analysis, unobtrusive measures, and projective techniques.

Proposed solutions to the problems are themselves issue-laden. One suggestion is to provide the required explanation in a debriefing session immediately after data are gathered; however, ex post facto information does not really provide for informed consent and subjects can become embarrassed and angry. Another suggestion is to provide only general information to subjects initially, eliminating detailed explanations until after measurement is complete. While some reactivity to measures may be eliminated in this way, the information provided before measurement should be sufficient to provide a basis for decision making, and the elements of voluntary participation and free withdrawal stressed. Deception and coercion must be avoided.

Another difficult issue surrounding informed consent is ensuring the rights of individuals who have limited ability to comprehend or who are unable to do so. Examples include children, the mentally retarded, the mentally ill, and the unconscious patient. Although consent has generally been secured from a relative or guardian, a number of questions have been raised regarding these populations that need vigilant protection. Positions that have been taken regarding the appropriateness of securing parental approval for children's participation in research, for example, are described by Hayter (1979). Parents or guardians must be informed of the implications of participation, and a signed release or permission should be secured. Permission to conduct measurement activities with these potentially vulnerable subjects should never be assumed simply because the relative or guardian does not raise specific objections (Joint Commission on Standards for Educational Evaluation, 1981, p. 82).

Other individuals whose rights to informed consent can be easily compromised are those who are members of captive audiences. The examples most frequently encountered in nursing are patients, particularly those who are hospitalized, students, and employees. The major problem is that these individuals may perceive pressure to comply with requests to participate in measurement activities or research and may acquiesce even though they do not really wish to do so. The perceived pressure may be due to status and power differentials between potential subject and the investigator, the promise of rewards, or concern that failure to participate will jeopardize the subject's condition or position. Dilemmas exist regarding whether such captive subjects should even be asked to participate and whether, even if they are told that a genuine choice exists, they will perceive participation to be completely voluntary. In the measurement contexts other than research, there may be instances in which the individual may accurately perceive limited freedom of choice regarding measurement activities. For example, once having signed a general consent form, the hospitalized patient is often assumed to be willing to acquiesce to a considerable number of measurement activities, including invasive laboratory procedures, only the most potentially dangerous of which usually require special consent assurance. The American Hospital Association's *Patient's Bill of Rights* (see Beauchamp and Walters, 1982, pp. 127-128) indicates that the patient has the right to receive information necessary to give informed consent before the start of any procedure or treatment; however, the extent to which such information is actually communicated for relatively routine procedures is questionable. Similarly, the student who has voluntarily enrolled in an educational program is the recipient of many measurement activities undertaken to evaluate mastery of content and skills and the educational program. Such activities are a routine part of the educational environment, and failure to participate may have negative consequences for the student. In the research, clinical, and program evaluation contexts, it is essential to provide a genuine choice, to provide as complete information as possible, and to avoid applying subtle pressures to which captive subjects are susceptible. In the educational and administrative contexts, at the very least, potential subjects should be informed before entering the situation (i.e., before enrolling in an educational program or taking a position) of the measurement-related expectations and the consequences of nonparticipation.

The purpose of any measurement activity should be explained before it is carried out, and the extent to which choice is possible should be communicated. The right to informed consent is often problematic in content analysis of client, student, or employee records for research or program evaluation purposes. Consent to use recorded information for a purpose other than that for which it was originally obtained ideally should be secured from the individual about whom the information is recorded; however, this is not always possible. Questions have been raised regarding the extent to which such information should be accessible, by whom, and who has the authority to approve access to information in records if the individual subject's approval cannot be secured, as is frequently the case in retrospective record reviews. At present these questions have not been answered; however, research-related practices are becoming more restrictive, preventing data collected for one purpose or study to be used for others without securing consent.

REFUSAL OR WITHDRAWAL. A generally accepted ethical position is that research subjects should be free to refuse to participate or to withdraw from participation without recrimination or prejudice. As noted previously, potential subjects should be informed of this right at the time their informed consent is solicited, and subtle pressures to participate should be avoided. Special attention is required to ensure that no negative consequences stem from refusal or withdrawal from research-related measurement activities. This includes actions to prevent negative attitudes being directed toward the subject. In the clinical, educational, and administrative

328

contexts, the individual has a right to refuse or withdraw from measurement activities; however, there may be negative consequences to this action. The individual should be informed of the consequences before the decision is made whether to participate.

PRIVACY. The right to privacy has many implications for measurement. Although defined in a variety of ways, the right to privacy asserts essentially that an individual should be able to decide how much of himself (including thoughts, emotions, attitudes, physical presence, and personal facts) to share with others. Measurement activities are designed to yield information about individuals or groups and involve at least some intrusion into an individual's life and activities. As such, they are in potential violation of this basic right unless care is taken. Three major points regarding the right to privacy should be borne in mind. First, individuals and cultural groups differ in the extent to which they are willing to divulge specific kinds of information, to whom, and under what conditions. For example, a client may be willing to reveal information about sexual behavior to a nurse or physician in a one-to-one interview in a therapeutic context, but unwilling to answer the same questions on a survey research questionnaire or in a group setting. Similarly, a nursing student might be more willing to allow a stranger collecting research data than a faculty member responsible for evaluating the student's progress to administer a personality inventory. Some topics such as drug use, alcohol use, sexual behavior, or family relationships might be willingly discussed by some individuals but not others for a variety of reasons which cannot always be anticipated. Given the social, cultural, and situational relativity with which privacy is defined, it is necessary that every effort be made to understand the social and cultural values of potential subjects and that no prior assumptions be made that a given measurement activity, even a particular question or item on an instrument, will be universally acceptable. Rather, each subject has a right to know in advance what information is to be gathered and how it will be used. In addition, the audiences who have a right to know the information should be negotiated with the subject in advance. Subjects must have the right to refuse to answer any questions or otherwise reveal information which they deem private.

Second, the nurse, by virtue of being an accepted and generally trusted health care provider, often receives information from and about clients which they would not reveal to a nonprofessional. The nurse's unique status in relation to clients should be recognized and care be taken that it is not used to the client's disadvantage. Any intent to share the information with others should be explicitly revealed to the client in advance. Information gathered in a caregiving context should not be used for other purposes (e.g., research) without the client's permission.

Third, measurement procedures differ in the extent to which they are likely to compromise the right to privacy. The most serious questions have been raised about those procedures that allow measurement without the subject's knowledge or active involvement (e.g., unobtrusive measures, observation, or content analysis of records or tape recordings) and those that may encourage the subject to reveal more information than intended (e.g., in-depth interviews, projective techniques, and psychological tests). The former are problematic in that they invalidate the subject's right to decide what to reveal. The latter pose problems because they remove some of the subject's ability to control the content revealed. Coercion (overt and subtle) and deceit should be avoided. Further, data should be handled, interpreted, and shared carefully, with attention to potential privacy violations. Particularly in situations in which the subject may inadvertently reveal more than intended or in which the information gathered might have negative consequences (e.g., cause others to alter their opinion of the subject), it is advisable to check with the individual before sharing any information with others.

CONFIDENTIALITY-ANONYMITY. Closely related to the right to privacy is the ethical principle, reflected in the codes of professional associations, that the anonymity of subjects be preserved whenever possible and that information that would allow identification of the subject be held in confidence by the professional. This right not only protects the subject but also has the important measurement implication of increasing the likelihood that responses will be more truthful and complete (i.e., more valid) than if anonymity and confidentiality cannot be ensured. Complete anonymity of subjects is possible in a few types of measurement activities, such as mailed questionnaires; but even in such instances it may be impractical to promise complete anonymity, because follow-up of nonrespondents is precluded. Generally the principle of anonymity has been operationalized in research as ensuring that subjects will not be identifiable in public reports by name or any other defining characteristics. In nonresearch contexts the right to anonymity may be difficult or impossible to ensure under certain conditions, such as when measurement data about a client are needed for assessment, diagnosis, and intervention, or instances in which data about a particular student or employee are used to evaluate performance. The degree to which anonymity can or cannot be ensured should be made clear to the subject prior to initiating the measurement. Promises of anonymity should never be given unless they can be guaranteed.

The right to confidentiality means that the subject should have the right to assume that information yielded by measurement activities will not be made generally accessible without prior consent. The specific right-to-know audiences who will have access to the information should be specified to the subject. For example, measurement data recorded on a hospitalized patient's record are appropriately available only to those hospital personnel who must have access to the information to provide care and cannot be legitimately obtained by others without the patient's consent or judicial mandate. In addition to highlighting some responsibilities of the nurse regarding informed consent and care in the handling and reporting of data, the right to confidentiality poses some potential ethical issues. First, controversies sometimes arise when access to data collected in research is requested by agency personnel for other purposes. In order to prevent such problems, expectations and procedures for sharing research findings should be mutually defined by the nurse researcher and agency personnel before data are collected, and these procedures should be shared with subjects. Second, a measurement activity may yield information that the nurse feels compelled to share in order to protect the subject's or society's interests. For example, a research subject who has been guaranteed confidentiality may reveal to the nurse in an interview the intention to inflict harm. The nurse must confront the difficult dilemma of whether to violate the subject's rights or potentially jeopardize life by failing to report the incident. Aside from the seemingly obvious but often impossible solution of attempting to secure the subject's consent to share the information with a specified individual or agency, there is no easy or correct answer.

PROTECTION FROM HARM. Nursing as a profession is dedicated to enhancing the health and well being of human beings; it may seem self-evident that professional ethics underscore the importance of preventing or minimizing potential risks to subjects, regardless of the context for measurement. All measurement activities involve possible risks and benefits which, although they may not be fully known in advance, must be anticipated and evaluated before deciding whether to initiate the activity. In assessing risks associated with measurement, it is necessary to consider those that may result from the measurement procedure itself and those that may result from the way in which the results of measurement are used.

The most readily apparent risks of measurement procedures are those that are associated with physical harm. The physiologic measures employed by nurses generally involve little danger to the subject, because they are minimally invasive. This does not preclude the possibility that seemingly routine and innocuous measures may involve possible risks, particularly with subjects who are very ill. For example, withdrawal of blood for a laboratory test may introduce infection; repeated blood pressure monitoring may cause pain or vascular problems; or an improperly maintained or operated ECG recorder could result in an electrical shock. While relatively unlikely and largely preventable, such risks are inherent in some nursing measurement activities and should be acknowledged and minimized.

Less obvious, but equally important, are psychological risks potentially associated with many of the measurement activities commonly employed in nursing. A measurement instrument or activity may inadvertently expose the subject to stress resulting from loss of self-esteem, generation of self-doubt, embarrassment, guilt, disturbing self-insights, fright, or concern about things of which the subject was previously unaware. For example, an instrument measuring parent-adolescent relations may include items that cause the parent to worry about aspects of the relationship or the adequacy of specific parenting behaviors; a measure that requests factual information or recall of specific events may embarrass a subject who is not able to respond; or psychological inventories may provide the subject with insight into aspects of personality which alter previous perceptions and cause distress. A frequently cited example of a stress-producing instrument is one that would suggest or reveal (directly or indirectly) latent homosexual tendencies. While most measurement-related sources of psychological harm are inadvertent, potential measures and items should be assessed carefully in light of their capacity for exposing subjects to psychological risk.

A related consideration that the nurse needs to assess honestly is the extent to which planned measurement activities will make demands on the subject's time and energy. Given the importance of obtaining multiple measures of a given concept, it is easy to lose sight of the time that may be involved in a subject's completing several instruments. Overdemanding time requirements may result in unwillingness to participate in measurement activities, or in withdrawal, fatigue, and anger, which may ultimately compromise reliability and validity. Measurement procedures should be designed to minimize disruption and should be feasible, realistic, and possible to carry out with reasonable effort.

Some measurement procedures, such as measuring heart rate changes after exercise, impose energy requirements that may be risky to some clients. The amount of time and energy required to complete planned measurement activities and the condition and situation of the potential subject should be taken into account, recognizing that different types of measures impose different demands. For example, busy individuals such as employees and mothers of young children may be unable to participate in time-consuming measurement procedures such as in-depth interviews. Subjects who are ill or under stress are particularly vulnerable to risk of fatigue and should not be expected to engage in lengthy sessions or physically demanding activities. Unrealistic or impractical demands on subjects should be avoided, even if it means sacrificing optimal measurement practices. Subjects should always be informed in advance of the time and energy requirements involved and their special needs taken into account in planning and scheduling measurement activities.

Individuals or groups may experience harm that results not from the measurement procedure itself, but from the way in which the results of measurement are interpreted and used. One of the most important risks encountered by subjects is being labeled negatively as a result of measurement. A number of cognitive and personality measures, even some physiologic measures, are designed to produce scores to which labels may be assigned (e.g., normal, abnormal, hypertensive, paranoid, obsessive-compulsive, gifted, neurotic, antisocial, homosexual, other-directed). Some clearly have negative connotations. Whether or not the measurement results and labels are actually communicated to the subject, those that cast an individual or group in a negative light when communicated to others may have deleterious consequences. Information that may jeopardize the self-esteem and reputations of subjects should not be reported without providing them an opportunity to present their perspective.

Use of measurement information to label subjects is problematic, particularly given considerations of measurement error and bias inherent in instruments. Unless individual and cultural differences are expressly taken into account in procuring and interpreting measurement data, a given conclusion or label, whether negative or positive, can be unwarranted. Many frequently used instruments such as intelligence tests, attitude scales, personality inventories, and behavioral checklists are culturally biased and are inappropriate for some subpopulations. For example, instruments measuring mother-infant attachment frequently incorporate behavioral indicators that reflect American, white, middle-class behavioral patterns and have not been sufficiently well tested to establish their validity with other cultural and socioeconomic populations. Even some physiologic measures such as the Apgar measure of the health status of a newborn has questionable validity for nonwhite racial groups. Using unmodified tools and undifferentiated norms for potentially biased measures can result in inaccurate interpretation and erroneous, unjustified interpretations and labels. Full and frank disclosure of measurement information requires that the limitations of tools and procedures be made explicit to aid in interpretation.

In many instances measurement information is used as the basis for decisions that may profoundly influence a subject's life. Examples include admissions decisions in educational programs, employment decisions, and decisions about the desirability or efficacy of a particular nursing intervention. In such instances there is invariably some degree of risk to the subject because of the possibility of inaccurate interpretation. Although it cannot be eliminated completely, risk can be minimized through carefully scrutinizing reliability and validity of measures, using only defensible information sources and disclosing relevant information about their credibility, using multiple indicators, and interpreting scores in the light of measurement error.

Since it is impossible to remove all possibility of risk from measurement activities, it is necessary to evaluate the degree of potential risk in relation to the potential benefits which will accrue to the subject or society as a result of the activity. The *risk-benefit ratio* expresses the relationship of all anticipated risks and human costs to all anticipated and future benefits (Schlenker and Forsythe, 1977). Although there are difficulties computing such a ratio (Diener and Crandall, 1978, pp. 24-26), the premise is that in order to justify a given activity, benefits should counterbalance and outweigh risks. Some potential benefits of measurement activities for subjects include increased understanding of oneself or one's relationships to others, acquisition of new information, increased awareness of options available, opportunity to express one's views or opinions, perceived prestige related to having been selected to participate, and having the opportunity to contribute to a worthwhile undertaking. Some measurement activities result in no potential benefits to the subject directly but are beneficial to society, in that they contribute to knowledge and understanding of health-related phenomena and the ultimate improvement of health care. All known risks and benefits must be communicated to subjects as the basis for informed consent and every effort made to eliminate or minimize risks and maximize benefits. An activity should not be undertaken if benefits do not justify the costs (Joint Commission on Standards for Educational Evaluation, 1981, p. 83).

Discussion of risks and benefits of measurement activities would be incomplete without acknowledging that nurses who engage in measurement may themselves incur some personal risk. The nurse is potentially liable if found to be acting in violation of subjects' rights or inflicting any psychological, social, or physical harm in the process of gathering, interpreting, and reporting measurement data. Peer review of planned measurement activities, accomplished through such mechanisms as institutional review boards, is helpful in identifying potential human rights violations and ensuring that appropriate precautions are taken. Also helpful are guidelines of professional associations and government. Such mechanisms protect not only the subject but also the investigator and should be viewed as a valuable resource.

Personal risk can also be incurred in the process of gathering measurement information from subjects. For example, data collection in some settings (e.g., dangerous neighborhoods, hospital units with a high infection rate) and with some populations of interest to nurses (e.g., drug addicts, combative patients) may result in physical harm unless proper precautions are taken. Psychological problems can result from repeatedly being used as a sounding board for subjects' problems, repeatedly being exposed to depressing situations, or undertaking personally unrealistic time and energy demands related to measurement. While all such risks cannot be eliminated, every effort should be made to minimize them. Clinical agencies that employ nurses are beginning to take steps to acknowledge and protect the rights of nurses who are expected to participate in medical or nursing research by, for example, developing policies that ensure the right to refuse to become involved in any research activity deemed unsafe or unethical, mandating that nurses be included as members of institutional review boards, and defining the procedures to be used in identifying vulnerable subjects and securing informed consent (Hodgman, 1981a,b).

In summary, protecting the rights of subjects is a basic consideration in planning and undertaking any measurement activity. The nurse has the responsibility to become informed about and adhere to existing policies and guidelines that help guarantee those rights. Other responsibilities that have been highlighted in this section include (1) providing potential subjects with sufficient information upon which to base a decision about whether to participate; (2) allowing refusal and withdrawal without recrimination whenever possible (or when impossible, informing subjects of the consequences); (3) allowing subjects the right to withhold information that they do not wish to share; (4) evaluating carefully the extent to which a measure may encourage the subject to reveal private information; (5) avoiding the use of measures and practices that employ deception or coercion; (6) evaluating and communicating all potential risks and benefits associated with a measurement activity; (7) eliminating or minimizing risks to the greatest extent possible; (8) handling data with care to preserve the anonymity and confidentiality of subjects; (9) restricting use of measurement data to the purposes for which permission has been secured from subjects; (10) refraining from using measurement information to assign labels to individuals or groups; (11) employing reliable and valid measures; and (12) employing caution in the interpretation of measurement information. Since many ethical issues related to nursing measurement remain open to considerable controversy, the nurse who is unsure of the ethical and risk-related consequences of a given activity is well advised to consult others before proceeding. Potential resources include ethicists, lawyers, measurement experts, and medical and nursing personnel. Another valuable resource is the growing body of literature in philosophy, nursing, medicine, and other fields which addresses ethical issues. Regan (1980) has pointed out the importance of becoming familiar with the literature of ethics in order to discover the highly nuanced views that exist about most ethical issues. He warns of the danger of trivializing ethical considerations by using insufficient information as the basis for decision making about intricate ethical issues.

ETHICAL ISSUES IN RELATION TO THE SCIENTIFIC AND PROFESSIONAL COMMUNITY

The importance of making available to the professional community information about measurement instruments that have been developed and used and the results of measurement has been addressed in an earlier section of this chapter. Related ethical issues are described below.

Throughout this book, emphasis has been placed on the importance of adhering to sound measurement principles in the development, selection, and use of instruments and devices to measure variables of interest to the nursing community. Ethical problems result when unsound measurement practices are used. Improper use of instruments or use of those with questionable psychometric properties not only poses potential risks to subjects but also represents misuse of subjects' and nurses' time. It also has important consequences for nursing knowledge and practice. Inadequate measurement has the potential to produce useless or erroneous information which, if accepted uncritically as fact, can have a negative impact on practice and, if incorporated into the literature, can have a negative impact on the knowledge upon which it is based. The nurse engaged in measurement has the ethical responsibility to apply sound principles at every stage of the measurement process and to disclose fully any violation of these principles in using or reporting measurement information. Likewise, the consumer of measurement information (i.e., the reader of research reports, the decision maker) has responsibility to scrutinize the procedures used in the light of sound measurement principles and to evaluate and use findings conservatively.

The current dearth of sound nursing measures has been noted and the need for nurses to develop measurement tools and procedures addressed (Ventura, et al, 1981). Development of measures, regardless of how sound and sophisticated they may be, does little to advance professional knowledge and practice, unless information about them is disseminated. Hence, it is argued that it is an ethical responsibility to make instruments and information about them available to others (nurses and nonnurses) via publication and other routes of intra- and interprofessional communication. The developer of an instrument should honestly and accurately report the way in which it was developed, tested, and used, providing all relevant psychometric data and acknowledging its known limitations and flaws, so that potential users can make informed judgments about its defensibility and utility and correctly interpret resulting data. Data about extraneous or confounding variables that may influence subjects' scores should be reported as well.

Questions can be raised regarding the point in the development and testing of an instrument when it is appropriate to share information about it with others. On the one hand, premature reporting before the instrument has been sufficiently well tested to ascertain its properties in different situations may overestimate its potential value and provide insufficient information to allow reasonable evaluation by possible users. On the other hand, inordinate delay in reporting the availability of an instrument precludes its use by others and may impede the accumulation of data about its properties, much of which can be furnished by others using the tool. After a tool has been developed, pretested, and revised, and used at least once, there is generally sufficient information to legitimate reporting its availability, provided the state of its development and testing is made explicit and appropriate cautionary statements are included. The instrument should be neither underrated nor oversold. Rather, the caveat is to provide sufficient data for informed evaluation by others.

As suggested in an earlier section of this chapter, users of existing instruments incur ethical responsibilities. The most obvious requirements, which unfortunately are not always followed, are to obtain permission for intended use of the tool and to give credit to the developer when reporting its use. These requirements should obtain whether an instrument is used in its original form or modified. The user is obliged to report to the developer and others the results of use and any problems encountered.

Instrument development is frequently undertaken as a collaborative activity. Collaboration in which each individual plays an active role based on particular areas of expertise is often necessary to produce a high quality instrument. Nurses frequently collaborate in tool development with measurement experts or statisticians, for example, in order to combine substantive and methodological expertise. In addition to clearly defining roles and responsibilities, collaboration requires that professional ethics and norms be considered in assigning credit for the ultimate product and related publications. Ideally, guidelines for acknowledging contributions and awarding credit should be agreed upon before collaboration begins.

Measurement instruments and activities are important aspects of nursing research, practice, education, and administration. Thus, information about and derived from them constitutes an essential part of nursing knowledge which the nurse has an obligation to share and use according to accepted scientific and professional ethics.

SUMMARY

This chapter has considered several measurement issues that have confronted nurses as they have attempted to improve and, as much as possible, perfect measurement techniques. Most of these concerns are related to the need to link conceptualization of phenomena with their operationalization and the desire to conduct measurement ethically and professionally. There is often difficulty in linking conceptualization with operationalization when existing tools are selected and used, when state and trait characteristics must be differentiated for measurement, or when measurement of processes and outcomes is required.

The use of existing instruments for nursing measurement is advocated for building knowledge. However, an instrument should be selected only if it is congruent with the intended purpose, conceptually consistent with the theoretical and measurement perspectives being employed, and psychometrically sound. Selection of an existing instrument should be based on careful evaluation of those available in the light of specific needs. Once selected, the instrument should be used according to the criteria and specifications set by the developer, and the results of its use communicated to the nursing community.

Attributes that are measured can be conceptualized as dynamic and changeable (state attributes) or as static and consistent over time (trait attributes). Most cognitive attributes are relatively stable and are conceptualized as traits. Physiologic characteristics and affective attributes are often quite variable over time from situation to situation. A number of attributes can be measured as state or trait variables; however, the manner in which the attribute is conceptualized and used should dictate whether it should be measured as a trait or state.

The approaches to measuring processes and outcomes follow the same principles as those that dictate operationalizing other phenomena. Measurement of process is complicated by the dynamic nature of processes and by the fact that most processes include a number of interrelated concepts and steps. Process measurement requires clear definition achieved by specifying and relating key concepts. The measurement approach must be based on the conceptual framework for the process. When process measurement is done during an evaluation procedure, criteria are specified for measuring the adequacy of the process. Process measurement should be conducted as unobtrusively as possible, since measurement itself may alter the process and affect findings.

When the focus of measurement is on assessing outcomes of a particular intervention or process, a large number of variables may be available. However, the selection of outcomes should be based on the conceptual framework that is the focus of the investigation. Several key variables should be selected and measured in a manner consistent with the conceptual framework. When outcome measurement is conducted to facilitate the evaluation of an intervention, process, or program, outcome criteria are delineated. It is often difficult to clearly specify the cause of a particular nursing outcome, because it may be influenced by many factors. Temporal relationships between interventions and measurement of outcomes are important in outcome assessment.

Ethical considerations permeate many aspects of nursing measurement. The rights of human subjects to informed consent, refusal or withdrawal from participation, privacy, anonymity and confidentiality, and protection from harm raise a number of ethical dilemmas and incur responsibilities for the nurse who engages in measurement. The nurse whose activities cross several different contexts may experience difficulties in defining and adhering to a standard set of ethical principles. Hence, the assistance of others with expertise in ethics is frequently required as a basis for decision making when planning and implementing measurement. Ethical dimensions of measurement are not limited to those involving human subjects but extend to the way in which instruments are developed, selected, and used and to the reporting of measurement data.

REFERENCES

AMERICAN NURSES' ASSOCIATION: Code for Nurses. American Nurses' Association, Kansas City, MO, 1976.

ANASTASI, A: Psychological Testing, ed. 4. Macmillan, New York, 1976.

ATWOOD, JR:.''A research perspective.'' Nursing Research 29(2):104-108, 1980.

BANDURA, A: Principles of Behavior Modification. Holt, Rinehart and Winston, New York, 1969.

BATEY, M: ''Conceptualization: Knowledge and logic guiding empirical research.'' Nursing Research 26(5):325-329, 1977.

BEAUCHAMP, TL AND WALTERS, L: Contemporary Issues in Bioethics, ed. 2. Wadsworth Publishing Co., Belmont, CA, 1982.

BENOLIEL, JO AND BERTHOLD, JS: *Human Rights Guidelines for Nurses in Clinical Research.* American Nurses' Association, Kansas City, MO, 1975.

BLALOCK, HM, JR.: *Causal Inferences in Nonexperimental Research.* University of North Carolina Press, Chapel Hill, 1964.

BLOCH, D: "Evaluation of nursing care in terms of process and outcome: Issues in research and quality assurance." *Nursing Research* 24(4):256-263, 1975.

BLOCH, D: "Interrelated issues in evaluation and evaluation research: A researcher's perspective." *Nursing Research* 29(2):69-73, 1980.

BOWER, RT AND DE GASPARIS, P: *Ethics in Social Research.* Praeger, New York, 1978.

BRANDT, PA AND WEINERT, C: "The PRQ—A social support system". *Nursing Research* 30(3):277-280, 1981.

CRONBACH, LJ: *Essentials of Psychological Testing,* ed. 3. Harper and Row, New York, 1970.

DIENER, E AND CRANDALL, R: *Ethics in Social and Behavioral Research.* University of Chicago Press, Chicago, 1978.

DONABEDIAN, A: "Patient care evaluation." *Hospitals,* 44:131ff, 1970.

GOLDFRIED, MR AND KENT, RN "Traditional versus behavioral personality assessment: A comparison of methodological and theoretical assumptions." *Psychological Bulletin* 77:409-420, 1972.

HAYTER, J: "Issues related to human subjects." In DOWNS, FS AND FLEMING, JW: *Issues in Nursing Research.* Appleton-Century-Crofts, New York, 1979, pp. 107-147.

HORN, BJ: "Establishing valid and reliable criteria: A researcher's perspective." *Nursing Research* 29(2):88-90, 1980.

HODGMAN, EC: "Research policy for nursing services: Part 1." *Journal of Nursing Administration* 11(4):30-33, 1981.

HODGMAN, EC: "Research policy for nursing services: Part 2." *Journal of Nursing Administration* 11(5):33-36, 1981.

INZER, F AND ASPINALL, MJ: "Evaluating patient outcomes." *Nursing Outlook* 29(3):178-181, 1981.

JOINT COMMISSION ON STANDARDS FOR EDUCATIONAL EVALUATION: *Standards for Evaluations of Educational Programs, Projects and Materials.* McGraw-Hill, New York, 1981.

LANG, NM: "A model for quality assurance in nursing." In DAVIDSON, S (ed): *PSRO: Utilization and Audit in Patient Care.* C.V. Mosby, St. Louis, 1976.

MISCHEL, W: "Continuity and change in personality." *American Psychologist* 24:1012-1018, 1969.

MISCHEL, W: "Toward a cognitive social learning reconceptualization of personality." *Psychological Review* 80:252-283, 1973.

NORBECK, JS, LINDSEY, AM, AND CARRIERI, VL: "The development of an instrument to measure social support." *Nursing Research* 30(5):264-269, 1981.

PHANEUF, M: *The Nursing Audit: Self-Regulations in Nursing Practice,* ed. 2. Appleton-Century-Crofts, New York, 1976.

REGAN, GM: "Response to Dr. Aroskar." In LENZ, E, et al (eds): *Ethical Dimensions of Nursing Research.* University of Maryland School of Nursing, Baltimore, MD, 1980, 16-19.

ROYAL COLLEGE OF NURSING OF THE UNITED KINGDOM: *Ethics Related to Research in Nursing.* Royal College of Nursing of the United Kingdom, London, 1977, (Portions are reprinted in BEAUCHAMP, TL, AND WALTERS, L: *Contemporary Issues in Bioethics,* ed. 2. Wadsworth Publishing Company, Belmont, CA, 1982, 513-516).

SCHLENKER, BR AND FORSYTH, DR: "On the ethics of psychological research." *Journal of Experimental Social Psychology* 13:369-396, 1977.

VENTURA, MR, HINSHAW, AS, AND ATWOOD, JR: "Instrumentation: The next step." *Nursing Research* 30(5):257, 1981.

WALTZ, CF AND STRICKLAND, OL: "Measurement of nursing outcomes: State of the art as we enter the eighties." In WE FIELD (ed): *Measuring Outcomes of Nursing Practice, Education, and Administration: Proceedings of the First Annual Southern Council on Collegiate Education for Nursing Research Conference.* Southern Regional Education Board, Atlanta, 1982, pp. 47-62.

WANDELT, MA AND AGER, JW: *Quality Patient Care Scale.* Appleton-Century-Crofts, New York, 1974.

WINTER, WD, FERREIRA, AJ, AND RANSOM, R: "Two measures of anxiety: A validation." *Journal of Consulting Psychology* 27:520-524, 1963.

ZUCKERMAN, M: "The development of an affect adjective checklist for the measurement of anxiety." *Journal of Consulting Psychology* 24:457-462, 1960.

ZUCKERMAN, M AND BIASE, DV: "Replication and further data on the validity of the affect adjective check list measure of anxiety." *Journal of Consulting Psychology* 26:291, 1962.

ZUCKERMAN, M AND LUBIN, B: *Manual for the Multiple Affect Adjective Check List.* Educational and Industrial Testing Service, San Diego, 1965.

ZUCKERMAN, M, LUBIN, B, VOGEL, L, AND VALERIUS, E: "Measurement of experimentally induced affects." *Journal of Consulting Psychology* 28:418-425, 1965.

APPENDIX

NURSING THEORIES, MEASUREMENT RESOURCES, AND METHODS FOR DATA COLLECTION IN NURSING*

This appendix is designed to serve three purposes. It will provide the reader with:

1. a summary of selected nursing theories and their measurement implications;
2. a list of resources useful in selecting tools and devices for measuring nursing variables;
3. and an overview of selected tools and procedures employed in nursing measurement.

The effort to accumulate a body of nursing knowledge through empirical investigation is a relatively new endeavor when compared with other disciplines such as physiology, psychology, or anthropology. In recent years, nursing has made major contributions to a rapidly expanding body of knowledge and has succeeded in delineating the boundaries of the discipline to some extent. These activities have left in their wake numerous and varied conceptual models, methodologies, and devices for the measurement of nursing phenomena. However, repeated testing of models and concepts to establish their validity for nursing practice and repeated use of existing instruments for nursing measurement are minimal, at best, or lacking altogether. Although the development of new theoretical models and the construction and testing of new measurement devices should not be discouraged, neither should existing models and devices be perfunctorily dismissed for their lack of novelty. For it is by replicating efforts that test key concepts and relationships, resulting in validation of some and discon-

---

*Prepared by Joan L. Creasia, Doctoral Student, University of Maryland School of Nursing.

firmation of others, that a scientific body of nursing knowledge to serve as the basis for nursing practice will ultimately be built.

Accordingly, the focus of this appendix is on currently available conceptual frameworks and tools for measurement in nursing. Contained in this appendix is an overview of selected nursing theories in common use and a review of sources that may be useful to identify appropriate instruments for the measurement of nursing phenomena, followed by a somewhat more detailed description of selected tools and procedures developed for or used in nursing.

SELECTED NURSING THEORIES
AND THEIR MEASUREMENT IMPLICATIONS

A number of theories, models, or conceptual frameworks, derived from nursing and related disciplines, are currently available, which can provide the basis upon which to systematically structure education, practice, or research. One of the major considerations in selecting an appropriate framework is the degree of compatibility of the framework with its intended use. For example, when a framework is selected to examine a nursing problem, one that is specific to nursing is usually the most appropriate. But that is not to say that frameworks from related disciplines do not have a place in nursing research. On the contrary, for certain types of studies such as one involving the nurse's autonomy in the practice setting, an organizational framework borrowed from sociology would be a valid approach. However, for research dealing with the effects of nursing action in a particular patient care situation, a nursing framework is probably indicated.

There are several nursing frameworks or theories in common use which offer a variety of perspectives and relationships. These frameworks differ in varying degrees in the assumptions underlying the model, the conceptualization of nursing, health, and illness, and the specific concepts inherent in the models. Some examples have been selected for comparison and are presented in Table A-1.

In constructing the table, the critical considerations were identified and a comparative approach was taken to present the basic assumptions, the definition and goal of nursing, the definitions of health and illness, and the key concepts identified by the theorists. Comparison of the assumptions has been made in terms of how man functions, his relationship with his environment, the cumulative influence of life's experiences on his perceptions or behavior, particular characteristics of man which may affect his reaction to the life process, and specific assumptions unique to a given model. Some of the assumptions have been made explicit by the theorists, while others are more implicit, being derived, for example, from the specified relationships between the concepts. The other elements or concepts inherent in the framework, such as nursing, illness, and health, are presented as explicitly stated by the theorists. By glancing across the table, similarities and differences between the theories become readily apparent.

There are certain implications for measurement when a particular framework is used to measure nursing phenomena. Some of these have also been highlighted in the table in terms of the unit of analysis, the interpretation of scores (the measurement framework), and the appropriate devices and techniques for data collection.

Table A-1 is not intended to be an exhaustive presentation of the various theories. In fact, it should be used only as a preliminary source to assist the potential user to decide whether to investigate the appropriateness of a given theory in greater depth. Most of the theories included are fairly global in scope and by forcing such global models into somewhat restrictive categories, some of the true essence of the relationships may be obscured. Therefore, the primary source which describes the theory in detail should be consulted before attempting to use it as a framework.

It is quite evident that the nursing theories included in Table A-1 offer a wide variety of perspectives. Some are process oriented and dynamic, such as King's theory of goal attainment and Rogers's theory of unitary man, while others are more outcome oriented, such as Roy's adaptation model, Johnson's behavioral system model, and Orem's theory of self-care. Rogers's model focuses on the wholeness of man and conceptualizes nursing as one component of man's life process. King's theory is directed toward the interaction of the nurse and the client, and for the purpose of nursing measurement, they are inseparable. Johnson and Roy conceptualize the nurse as an external regulator whose function is to promote system balance or adaptation. Orem views the nurse as one who assists man with his self-care practices when he is unable to effectively care for himself. Given this variety of perspectives, it is clear that the compatibility of the framework with the intended use is a critical consideration when selecting a model for use in education, practice, or research. The different perspectives also have certain implications for measurement. Based upon the assumptions of the theory and the concepts and relationships proposed by the theorists, there may be variations in the unit of analysis, the measurement framework within which the data are interpreted, and the techniques and devices that are most appropriate to collect the data.

RESOURCES USEFUL IN SELECTING TOOLS AND DEVICES FOR MEASURING NURSING VARIABLES

The lack of reliable and valid instruments for nursing measurement has frequently been cited as a major barrier to effective and efficient data collection in nursing. It is possible, however, that instruments appropriate for a specific purpose or study do exist but their existence is unknown to the researcher, practitioner, or educator, necessitating construction and testing of new tools for each study. Since instrument development and testing is a time consuming and often expensive effort, the use of appropriate existing measures could facilitate the measurement of nursing phenomena.

JOURNALS

How can such instruments be located? The most common method is to engage in an extensive search of journals, in nursing and allied disciplines, that publish research findings. Some of the nursing journals that may publish such studies include Communicating Nursing Research (WICHEN);

TABLE A-1 Summary of selected theories/conceptual frameworks for nursing measurement*

Critical Considerations	Johnson's Behavioral System Model	King's Theory of Goal Attainment	Orem's Theory of Self-Care	Rogers's Theory of Unitary Man	Roy's Adaptation Model
Brief Overview	Views man as a collection of interrelated behavioral subsystems whose response patterns form an organized and integrated whole.	Views man as an open system and as one component of a nurse-client interpersonal system whose interactions lead to the attainment of mutually agreed upon goals.	Views man as a unity whose functioning is linked to the environment and who, with the environment, "form an integrated functional whole or system." (Orem, 1980, p. 41)	Views man as a unified whole in constant interaction with his environment, whose behaviors cannot be predicted by knowledge of the parts.	Views man as a biopsychosocial adaptive system who interacts with the environment and copes with environmental change through the process of adaptation.
Basic Assumptions about Man	The patient as a behavioral system is characterized by organization, interaction, interdependency, and integration of the parts and elements (subsystems).

Man continually strives to maintain behavioral system balance by "more or less automatic adjustments and adaptation to the 'natural' forces impinging on him." (Johnson, 1980, p. 208)

A behavioral system is essential to man in that it is functionally significant and serves a useful purpose.

Behavioral system balance reflects adjustments and adaptation that are | An individual's state of health is determined by his ability to function in social roles. (King, 1981, p. 143)

"Human beings are open systems interacting with the environment." (King, 1981, p. 10)

Perceptions, goals, needs, and values of the nurse and client influence the interaction process. (King, 1981, p. 143)

Individuals are conceptualized as social, sentient, rational, perceiving, controlling, purposeful, action-oriented, and time-oriented beings.

Individuals have a right to knowledge about themselves, to participate in decisions that influence | Man functions "biologically, symbolically, and socially." (Orem, 1980, p. 41)

Man and environment are linked, forming an integrated system.

In response to recurring self-care requisites, self-care is a set of learned behaviors.

"All things being equal, human beings have the potential to develop their intellectual and practical skills and the motivation essential for self care." (Orem, 1980, p. 29) Self-care actions are deliberate choices which are rationally selected.

Self-care is "necessary for life itself, for health, for human development | "Man is a unified whole possessing his own integrity and manifesting characteristics that are more than and different from the sum of his parts." (Rogers, 1970, p. 47)

"Man and environment are continually exchanging matter and energy with one another." (Rogers, 1970, p. 54)

"Life process evolves irreversibly and unidirectionally along the space-time continuum" (Rogers, 1970, p. 59), resulting in changing patterns in both man and environment.

Pattern and organization identify man and reflect his innovative wholeness, are directed toward | "The person consists of biological, psychological and social components." (Roy, 1980, p .180)

"The person is in constant interaction with a changing environment." (Roy, 1980, p .180)

Health and illness are dimensions of the total life experience.

"To respond positively to environmental change, a person must adapt." (Roy, 1980, p. 181) To cope with a changing world, the person uses both innate and acquired biologic, psychologic, or social adaptive mechanisms.

"The person is conceptualized as having four modes of adaptation: physiologic needs, |

	(Johnson)	(King)	(Orem)	(Rogers)	(Roy)
	"successful" in some way or to some degree. Man actively seeks new experiences which may temporarily disturb behavioral system balance and require adaptation or behavioral modification to return to a steady state.	their lives, health and community services, and to accept or reject health care. (King, 1981, p. 143) "Goals of health professionals and goals of recipients of health care may be incongruent." (King, 1981, p. 144)	and for general well-being." (Orem, 1980, p. 29)	increasing complexity rather than achieving equilibrium, and are maintained amidst constant change due to continuous interaction between man and environment. "Man is characterized by the capacity for abstraction and imagery, language and thought, sensation and emotion." (Rogers, 1970, p. 73)	self-concept, role function, interdependence relations." (Roy, 1980, p. 182) The person's adaptation level comprises a zone indicating the range of stimulation that will lead to a positive response and is determined by the combined effect of three classes of stimuli—focal, contextual, and residual. "The person's adaptation is a function of the stimulus he is exposed to and his adaptation level." (Roy, 1980, p. 181)
Definition of Nursing	Nursing is "an external regulatory force which acts to preserve the organization of the patient's behavior on an optimal level under those conditions in which the behavior constitutes a threat to physical or social health, or in which illness is found" (Johnson, 1980, p. 214) by imposing external control mechanisms to fulfill the functional requirements of the subsystem(s).	"Nursing is defined as a process of action, reaction and interaction" (King, 1981, p. 2) whereby the nurse and client "each perceive the other and the situation; and through communication, they set goals, explore means and agree on means to achieve goals." (p. 144) The domain of nursing includes promoting, maintaining, and restoring health, caring for the sick and injured, and caring for the dying. (p. 4)	Nursing involves assisting man with his self-care practices in order to sustain life and health, recover from disease or injury, and cope with their effects. (Orem, 1980, p. 6) Candidates for nursing services are those whose self-care demands exceed their self-care deficit. (p. 25) Nursing has social, interpersonal, and technological aspects and has biologic, behavioral, and social foundations.	Nursing is a science and an art. The science of nursing should be concerned with studying "the nature and direction of unitary human development integral with the environment, evolve descriptive, explanatory, and predictive principles basic to knowledgeable practice in nursing." (Rogers, 1980, p. 330) The art of nursing refers to the use of scientific principles of nursing for human betterment. The uniqueness of nursing is its concern with unitary man as a synergistic phenomenon.	"Nursing acts as an external regulatory force to modify stimuli affecting adaptation" by increasing, decreasing, or maintaining stimuli. (Roy, 1980, p. 186) The uniqueness of nursing is its focus on the person adapting to those stimuli present as a result of his position on the health-illness continuum.

TABLE A-1 Continued

Goal of Nursing	The goal of nursing action is "to restore, maintain or attain behavioral system balance and stability at the highest possible level for the individual." (Johnson, 1980, p. 214)	The goal of nursing is "to help individuals maintain their health so they can function in their roles." (King, 1981, p. 3 and 4)	Nursing agency is aimed at moving a patient toward responsible self-care (Orem, 1980, p. 58) or at meeting the existing health-care requisites of others in the event of health-derived or health-related self-care deficits. (p. 92)	Nursing "seeks to promote symphonic interactions between humans and environments, to strengthen the coherence and integrity of the human field and to direct and re-direct patterning of the human and environmental fields for the realization of maximum health potential." (Rogers, 1970, p. 122) The goal of nursing is the attainment of the best possible state of health for man who is continually evolving.	Nursing activity is aimed at promoting the person's adaptation in the four adaptive modes.
Health and Illness	It may be inferred that health is a state in which "the subsystems and the system as a whole are self-maintaining and self-perpetuating due to orderly conditions in the internal and external environment, the resources necessary to their functional requirements are met and the interrelationships among the subsystems are harmonious. If these conditions are not met, malfunction becomes apparent in behavior that is in part disorganized, erratic, and dysfunctional. Illness or other sudden internal or external	Health is "the dynamic life experiences of a human being, which implies continuous adjustment to stressors in the internal and external environment through optimum use of one's resources to achieve maximum potential for daily living" (King, 1981, p. 5) and the ability to function in social roles. Illness is "a deviation from normal, that is, an imbalance in a person's biological structure or in his psychological make-up, or a conflict in a person's social relationships." (p. 5)	Health, which has physical, psychological, interpersonal, and social aspects (Orem, 1980, p. 119), is a state in which human beings are "structurally and functionally whole or sound." (p. 118) Illness occurs when a person has health-related limitations which affect specific structures, physiological or psychological mechanisms or integrated human functioning that render him incapable of maintaining self-care.	Health and illness are part of the same continuum, are not dichotomous notions, are value laden, arbitrarily defined, and culturally infused. Health seems to occur when patterns of living are coordinate with environmental change, while illness occurs when patterns of living are in conflict with environmental change and are deemed unacceptable.	Both health and illness are aspects of the total life experience and are viewed as a continuum.

Key Concepts				
environmental change is most frequently responsible for such malfunctions." (Johnson, 1980, p. 212) Behavioral system—composed of "all the patterned, repetitive and purposeful ways of behaving that characterize each man's life." (Johnson, 1980, p. 209) Behavioral subsystem—"a formed set of behavioral responses, responsive tendencies or action systems that seem to share a common drive or goal" which are modified over time through maturation, or learning. (Johnson, 1980, p. 209 and 210) Each subsystem has a specific structure and function and its action pattern is observable. 7 subsystems: Affiliative—serves the function of security and has "the consequences of social inclusion, intimacy and the formation and maintenance of a strong social bond." (Johnson, 1980, p. 212)	Personal system—an individual Interpersonal system—two or more interacting individuals. Social system—organizations formed by groups with special interests and needs which make up communities and societies. (King, 1981, p. 141) Concepts of goal attainment theory as derived from interpersonal systems framework: Interaction—"a process of perception and communication between person and environment and between person and person, represented by verbal and nonverbal behaviors that are goal-directed." (King, 1981, p. 146) Perception—"each person's representation of reality." (King, 1981, p. 146) Communication—"a process whereby	Self-care—a set of learned behaviors which purposely "regulates structural integrity, human functioning and human development." (Orem, 1980, p. 26) Self-care requisites—three categories of purposes to be attained through self-care actions: Universal—common to all human beings, "they are associated with life processes and with the maintenance of the integrity of human structure and functioning." (Orem, 1980, p. 41) Developmental—associated with human developmental processes, with conditions and events occurring at various stages of the life cycle, and with events that can adversely affect development. (Orem, 1980, p. 41) Health-deviation—"associated with	Energy fields—dynamic fields having no real boundaries; the fundamental level of unitary man and the environment. Two types: Human energy field—more than the biological, psychological, and sociological fields, taken separately or together. Man possesses integrity and cannot be generalized from parts to whole. Environmental energy field—all that which is outside a given human field. Openness—as energy fields, man and environment are continuously open and extending to infinity. Pattern and organization—characterize human and environmental fields and are continuously changing. "The nature of the pattern and organization is always novel, always emerging,	Adaptation—man's ability to cope with the constantly changing environment. Adaptive modes—ways a person adapts. Four adaptive modes: Physiologic—determined by physiologic needs. Self-concept—determined by interactions with others. Role function—the performance of duties based on given positions within society. Interdependence—involves ways of seeking help, affection, and attention. Adaptive level—determined by the combined effect of stimuli: Focal stimuli—stimuli immediately confronting the person. Contextual stimuli—all other stimuli present. Residual stimuli—beliefs, attitudes, or traits that have an indeterminate effect on the present situation.

347

Dependency—succoring behavior that calls for the response of nurturing and has as its consequence approval, attention, or physical assistance.

Ingestive—serves the broad function of appetitive satisfaction but is governed by social and psychological considerations.

Eliminative—functions difficult to differentiate from the biologic system; based on the notion that humans learn expected behavior in the excretion of wastes which strongly influence purely biological eliminative acts.

Sexual—with its dual functions of procreation, the response originates with gender role identity and covers the broad range of behaviors dependent on one's biologic sex.

Achievement—function is mastery or control over some aspect of the self or environment as measured against some standard of excellence and includes intelligence, physical, creative, mechanical, and social skills.

information is given from one person to another either directly," or indirectly. (King, 1981, p. 146)

Transaction—"observable behavior of human beings interacting with their environment." (King, 1981, p. 147)

Role—"a set of behaviors expected of persons occupying a position in a social system; rules that define rights and obligations in a position; a relationship with one or more individuals interacting in a position; a relationship with one or more individuals interacting in specific situations for a purpose." (King, 1981, p. 147)

Stress—"a dynamic state whereby a human being interacts with the environment to maintain balance for growth, development, and performance." (King, 1981, p. 147)

Growth and Development—"continuous changes in individuals at the cellular, molecular, and behavioral levels of

genetic and constitutional defects and structural and functional deviations," (Orem, 1980, p. 41) which impair the individual's power of self-care agency.

Therapeutic self-care demands—"The totality of self-care actions to be performed for some duration in order to meet known self-care requisites." (Orem, 1980, p. 39) The self-care agent may be the nurse or self.

Self-care deficits—occur when a person is incapable of continuous self-care or has health related limitations that render him incapable of effective or complete care to meet his self-care demands. (Orem, 1980, p. 27)

Nursing Systems—"are formed when nurses use their abilities to prescribe, design and provide nursing for legitimate patients" for the purpose of regulating the individual's capabilities to engage in self-care and meet his self-care requisites. (Orem, 1980, p. 29) Three types:

always more diverse." (Rogers, 1980, p. 331)

Four dimensionality —thought to characterize human and environmental fields beyond the traditional time-space dimensions

Principles of Nursing Science—(homeodynamics)— postulate the nature and direction of unitary human development:

Helicy—"The nature and direction of human and environmental change is continuously innovative, probabilistic, and characterized by increasing diversity of human field and environmental field pattern and organization emerging out of the continuous, mutual, simultaneous interaction between the human and environmental fields and manifesting nonrepeating rhythmicities." (Rogers, 1980, p. 333)

Resonancy—"The human field and the environmental field are identified by wave pattern and

Aggressive—functions to preserve and protect self (and thus, society) within the limits imposed by society.

activities." (King, 1981, p. 148)

Time—"a sequence of events moving onward to the future," . . . "a duration between one event and another uniquely experienced by each human being." (King, 1981, p. 148)

Space—"a physical area called territory, and is defined by the behavior of individuals occupying space, such as gestures, postures, and visible boundaries erected to mark off personal space." (King, 1981, p. 148)

Wholly compensatory—the nurse compensates for the patient's total inability to engage in self-care activities.

Partly compensatory—the nurse compensates for the patient's partial inability to perform self-care actions (i.e., can perform some but not all).

Supportive-educative (developmental)—the nurse assists the patient in decision-making, behavior control, acquisition of knowledge and skill. The patient is able to perform all self-care activities.

Each nursing system has three subsystems:

Social—the complementary role of the nurse and the client and the contractual relationship between them.

Interpersonal—the nurse-client interaction.

Technological—the use of regulatory, social, and interpersonal mechanisms to effect self-care. (Orem, 1980, p. 90)

organization manifesting continuous change from lower-frequency, longer wave patterns to higher-frequency, shorter wave patterns." (Rogers, 1980, p. 333)

Complementarity—"The interaction between human and environmental fields is continuous, mutual, simultaneous." (Rogers, 1980, p. 333)

TABLE A-1 Continued

Major Implications for Measurement

Unit of Analysis	The individual as a behavioral system is the unit of analysis. The state of each component subsystem is assessed separately and in relationship to other subsystems.	The nurse-client interaction is the unit of analysis. Since the interpersonal system includes interaction between dyads, triads, and small groups, analysis of nurse-individual or nurse-family interactions would be appropriate.	The individual, as a self-care agent or care recipient, is the unit of analysis. Since the term 'agent' is defined as the "person taking action" (Orem, 1980, p. 35), the agent could be the patient self-care agent, a parent or other dependent care agent, or the nurse-agent. The patient as care-recipient might be the unit of analysis in the situation in which a person's health state necessitates total or almost total care.	The theory of unitary man as a human energy field implies that the individual is the unit of analysis. Since the model depicts man as being inseparable from his environment, the units of analysis may also include man-family, man-society, man-physical environment, etc.	"The system of the person and his interaction with the environment are the units of analysis of nursing assessment." (Roy, 1980, p. 179). Thus, the individual as a biopsychosocial adaptive system, the family as an adaptive system, and/or individual-environmental or family-environmental interactions could be the unit of analysis.
Framework for Measurement	The framework for subsystem measurement provides for either a norm-referenced or criterion-referenced approach, depending upon conceptualization and operationalization. Achievement, for example, as mastery of the self or environment, implies a criterion-referenced frame while affiliative subsystem concepts such as security or intimacy favor a norm-referenced approach.	Interaction implies a norm-referenced framework for measurement since the concepts are defined as dynamic, continuous processes. However, goal attainment suggests an end-point in the nurse-patient interaction and goals arising out of the interaction process could be appropriately measured within a criterion-referenced framework.	The definitions of health and self-care suggest that there is a point at which a person is structurally sound or whole and has mastered the necessary self-care behaviors to remain so. These interpretations imply a criterion-referenced approach. If, however, concepts such as developmental or health-deviation are conceptualized as a continuum, then a norm-referenced measurement framework may be employed.	Since the model represents man as a dynamic human energy field in constant interaction with a dynamic environmental energy field, a norm-referenced approach to the measurement of the concepts is indicated.	It is suggested that the criterion for judging when the goal of adaptation has been reached is "any positive response made by the recipient to the stimuli present and frees energy for responses to other stimuli. The criterion must be applied to each specific instance of nursing intervention for which a specific goal of adaptation has been set." (Roy, 1980, p. 183) Operationalization of adaptation in this way implies a criterion-referenced approach to measurement. Norm-referenced measures may be useful in operationalizing other key concepts such as self-concept and/or

Measurement Devices and Techniques	For subsystem assessment, psychological, social, cognitive, or behavioral measures may be used. Cognitive measures might be employed to assess the achievement subsystem, while attitude scales, developmental measures, or other behavioral devices may be useful for the assessment of the other subsystems. Although some of the subsystems have strong physiological connotations (e.g., ingestive, eliminative, sexual), the model focuses primarily on behavioral responses rather than biologic functioning. (Johnson, 1980, p. 213)	The definitions of the concepts suggest the use of psychological, behavioral, developmental, and/or social measures for their operationalization. Such techniques as attitude scales, affective measures, and developmental scales may be useful for operationalizing perception, role, stress, growth, and development. Participant or nonparticipant observation would be particularly useful for data collection related to the processes of interaction, transaction, and communication. While none of the concepts are defined from a physiological perspective, growth and development include cellular, molecular, and behavioral levels of activities which imply biobehavioral or physiological measurement.	Since health has physical, psychological, interpersonal, and social aspects (p. 119), physiological, psychological, behavioral, and cognitive tools and techniques may be used to assess the level of self-care. Possible devices include self-report inventories, behavioral and cognitive measures, developmental scales, and physiological instrumentation as well as interview and observation.	Psychological, physiological, behavioral, social, or cognitive tools could be appropriate measurement devices, depending on the concept chosen. Possible measurement techniques are physiological instrumentation, developmental scales, affective or cognitive measures, interview, or observation.	The use of physiological, psychological, social, cognitive, or behavioral tools are appropriate, depending on the adaptive mode being assessed. For the physiologic mode, physiological instrumentation or observation may be employed. For the self-concept, role mastery and interdependence modes, affective measures such as self-report inventories, scales, cognitive measures, and observation would be appropriate.
Examples of Use in Education, Practice, and Research	Broncatello, Karen R.: "Auger in Action—Application of the Model." *Advances in Nursing Science*, 2:1, January, 1980, pp. 13–23.	Daubenmire, M. Jean and Imogene M. King: "Nursing Process Models: A Systems Approach." *Nursing Outlook*, 21:8, August, 1973, pp. 512–515.	Bromley, Barbara: "Applying Orem's Self-Care Theory in Enterostomal Therapy." *American Journal of Nursing*, 17:2, February, 1980, pp. 245–249.	Gill, Barbara and Jan Atwood: "Reciprocity and Helicy Used to Relate mEGF and Wound Healing." *Nursing Research*, 30:2, March-April, 1981, pp. 68–72.	Laros, Jaydene: "Deriving Outcome Criteria from a Conceptual Model." *Nursing Outlook*, 25:5, May, 1977, pp. 333–336. Roy, Sister Callista: "Relating Nursing Theory to Education:

TABLE A-1 Continued

Bruce, Glenda, et al: "Implementation of ANA's Quality Assurance Program for Clients with End Stage Renal Disease." *Advances in Nursing Science*, 2:2, January, 1980, pp. 79–91.

Damus, Karla: "An Application of the Johnson Behavioral System Model for Nursing Practice." In Joan P. Reihl and Sister Callista Roy: *Conceptual Models for Nursing Practice*, 2nd Ed. New York: Appleton-Century-Crofts, 1980, pp. 274–289.

Glennin, Claire G.: "Formulation of Standards of Nursing Practice Using a Nursing Model." In Joan P. Reihl and Sister Callista Roy: *Conceptual Models for Nursing Practice*, 2nd Ed. New York: Appleton-Century-Crofts, 1980, pp. 274–89.

Daubenmire, M. Jean: "Nurse-Patient-Physician Interaction Process." In Harriet Werley et al, Eds.: *Health Research: The Systems Approach*. New York: Springer Publishing Co., Inc., 1976, pp. 139–153.

King, Imogene: *A Theory for Nursing: Systems, Concepts, Process*. New York: John Wiley and Sons, 1981, pp. 150–157 and 163–177.

Facteau, Lorna M.: "Self-Care Concepts and the Care of the Hospitalized Child." *Nursing Clinics of North America*, 15:1, March, 1980, pp. 145–154.

Fenner, Kathleen: "Developing a Conceptual Framework." *Nursing Outlook*, 27:2, February, 1979, pp. 122–126.

Mullin, Virginia I.: "Implementing the Self-Care Concept in the Acute Care Setting." *Nursing Clinics of North America*, 15:1, March, 1980, pp. 177–190.

Porter, Luz: "Impact of Physical-Physiological Activity on Infants' Growth and Development." *Nursing Research*, 21:3, May-June, 1972, pp. 210–219.

Swanson, Ardis R.: "Fearlessness of Children in Relation to Maternal Anxiety, Self-Differentiation and Accuracy of Perception." In Florence Downs and Margaret Newman, Eds.: *A Sourcebook for Nursing Research*. Philadelphia: F.A. Davis, 1977, pp. 178–186.

Whelton, Beverly: "An Operationalization of Martha Rogers' Theory Throughout the Nursing Process." *International Journal of Nursing Studies*, Vol. 16, 1979, pp. 7–20.

A New Era." *Nurse Educator*, March-April, 1979. pp. 16–21.

Schmitz, Marh: "The Roy Adaptation Model: Application in a Community Setting." In Joan P. Reihl and Sister Callista Roy: *Conceptual Models for Nursing Practice*, 2nd Ed. New York: Appleton-Century-Crofts, 1980, pp. 274–289.

Starr, Suzan L.: "Adaptation Applied to the Dying Client." In Joan P. Reihl and Sister Callista Roy: *Conceptual Models for Nursing Practice*, 2nd Ed. New York: Appleton-Century-Crofts, 1980, pp. 189–192.

* Adapted in part from Newman, Margaret: *Theory Development in Nursing*. Philadelphia: F.A. Davis, 1979, with permission.

Heart and Lung; Image; Journal of Nursing Administration; Journal of Nursing Education; MCN: American Journal of Maternal Child Nursing; Nurse Educator; Nursing Research; Research in Nursing and Health; and Western Journal of Nursing Research.

There are numerous journals in related disciplines that may also be useful. A small sample of the available resources includes Administrative Science Quarterly; Advances in Psychological Assessment; American Journal of Psychology; American Journal of Public Health; American Journal of Sociology; American Pharmacy; Annals of Clinical Research; Annals of Internal Medicine; Child Development; Developmental Psychology; Educational and Psychological Measurement; Evaluation and the Health Professions; Health Care Management Review; Hospital Administration; Journal of the American Medical Association; Journal of Educational Psychology; Journal of Educational Research; Journal of Marriage and the Family; Medical Care; New England Journal of Medicine; and Pediatrics.

Undertaking an extensive search of the literature is a laborious and often inefficient approach to locate appropriate measuring devices. Once a relevant study has been located, it is not surprising to find relatively little information about the instruments used for data collection. Often, however, the journal article will contain a description of the conceptual basis for measurement which can assist the researcher to decide whether further investigation of the tool is warranted.

INSTRUMENT COMPENDIA/RESOURCE BOOKS

An alternative approach is to use compendia of instruments. There are several available compilations of tools which are potentially useful to identify instruments appropriate for nursing measurement. These volumes contain varying types and amounts of information. Some provide only the bibliographical source in which the tools have been used or described. Others present a critical review of the tools and include such valuable information as the conceptual basis, a description of the variables, procedures for administration and scoring, and the instruments' psychometric properties. Still others include a copy of the tool.

The following section contains descriptions of compendia of instruments that may have utility for identifying measurement devices that are relevant to nursing education, practice, or research. Although only two sources contain tools designed specifically for nursing, it is likely that many instruments designed for use in related disciplines might also be appropriate for certain types of nursing studies. Therefore, volumes compiled by other disciplines that may be useful for nursing measurement have also been included.

The sources specific to nursing are presented first. The remaining compendia are grouped according to the kind of measures included (attitudinal, behavioral, health-related, mental, physiologic, and sociologic-occupational), the specific populations addressed (women, children, families), or the specific attributes being measured (intelligence, personality). The classification scheme is an arbitrary one, since there is a great deal of overlap among the contents of the compilations. However, the sources have been clustered as described for the convenience of the reader on the basis of the stated purpose of the compendium.

Each review is headed by the bibliographical citation and contains a general overview of the contents such as the approximate number of measures described, the particular topics addressed, major variables or concepts included, a description of the format for presentation, and the identification of special features such as tables, indices, and so forth. Following this, reliability and validity of the instruments included in the compilation are briefly described in terms of the predominant types and the availability. Unless it is specifically noted to the contrary, it may be assumed that reproductions of instruments are *not* included in the compendium.

INSTRUMENTS SPECIFIC TO NURSING

Ward, Mary Jane and Mark E. Felter: *Instruments for Use in Nursing Education Research*. Boulder, Colorado: Western Interstate Commission for Higher Education, 1979.

Descriptions and reproductions of 78 instruments for use in nursing education research as well as descriptions and bibliographical information for 39 others are included in this compendium. Specific descriptions for each instrument include author, title, key concepts, variables, general description, development, reliability and validity, uses in nursing education research, and comments. The general description contains information relative to the nature and content of the tool and administration and scoring procedures. An overview of the rationale for development, the source of the items, and the procedure for development is also presented. The utility of each instrument in nursing education research is discussed, followed by a brief critique and overview of the measure.

The instruments are indexed according to the key concepts embedded in the framework as well as by author and title. The wide variety of key concepts is also highlighted in the heading of the descriptive information, and the variables each instrument seeks to measure are identified.

Descriptions of the psychometric properties of the tools are presented based on available information. Methods for estimating reliability and validity are briefly described and statistical data are furnished when available. For slightly less than half of the instruments, no reliability or validity information was provided by the developer or researcher.

Ward, Mary Jane and Carol Lindeman, Eds.: *Instruments for Measuring Nursing Practice and Other Health Care Variables*. Hyattsville, Md.: DHEW Publication No. HRA 78-53 (Volume 1) and HRA 78-54 (Volume 2), 1979.

This compilation is limited to instruments judged to relate directly to nursing practice. Descriptions of 138 psychosocial instruments and 19 instruments to measure physiologic variables are presented and copies of 133 psychosocial instruments are included.

The psychosocial measures are organized according to the following scheme: health-care provider, provider-client interaction, client-significant others interaction, and significant others. For each instrument, the title, author, description of variables, development, and uses in research are provided. The description of the tool includes information about its nature and content and the methods of scoring and administration. Under the heading of development, the conceptual or theoretical framework is described, as are the source of the items and the psychometric properties of the tool. Some reliability or validity information is available for approximately 75 percent of the instruments, with validity estimates being reported more frequently than reliability. A commentary at the end of each description summarizes the apparent strengths and weaknesses of the instrument. References and copyright information are provided. The psychosocial measures are indexed by author, title, and key concepts.

The physiologic instruments described are those judged to be suitable for nursing research in patient care settings. They are organized according to body systems. Information provided includes the name of the instrument, a discussion of the variable, the parameters (including background information and uses), research application, description of its operation, and a commentary. The fetal heart monitor, electrocardiograph, and spirometer are among those included.

ATTITUDINAL MEASURES

Robinson, John P. and Philip R. Shaver: *Measures of Social Psychological Attitudes*. Ann Arbor, Michigan: Institute for Social Research, University of Michigan, 1973.

The attitudinal measures presented in this volume are organized under the general headings of self-esteem and related constructs, locus of control, alienation, authoritarianism, sociopolitical attitudes, values, attitudes toward people, religious attitudes, and social desirability scales. In all, 126 instruments are reviewed and evaluated, most of which are reproduced in the compendium. Bibliographical information is provided for 30 additional self-concept measures, and there is a review and discussion of previous attempts to measure the constructs of happiness and life satisfaction.

Each section begins with a broad definition or description of the construct of interest, followed by the presentation of various measurement issues and a general overview of the measuring devices included. Individual instruments are then reviewed and critiques are also provided. Information provided for each tool includes a description of the variables, the format of the tool, the samples to which it has been administered, reliability, validity, the bibliographical sources in which it was described or used, and the method of administration. An evaluative commentary follows.

Estimates of reliability or validity are available for 75 to 80 percent of the instruments. Validity is often discussed quite extensively, with particular attention given to convergent and discriminant validity for the constructs of self-esteem and locus of control.

Shaw, Marvin E. and Jack M. Wright: *Scales for the Measurement of Attitudes*. New York: McGraw-Hill, 1967.

Following a discussion of the nature of attitudes and the methods of attitudinal scale construction, descriptions and exhibits (reproductions) of 176 attitude scales are presented. The scales fall into the general categories of social practices, social issues and problems, international issues, abstract concepts, political and religious attitudes, ethnic and national groups, significant others, and social institutions. There are several subheadings under each category. Accompanying each scale is a general description of the tool and the subjects (samples) used for testing, as well as relevant measurement properties such as response mode, scoring, reliability, and validity. Evaluative comments are made by the authors regarding each scale's strengths and weaknesses.

Some reliability or validity information is provided for nearly all of the scales. The most common form of reliability is the split-half method to estimate internal consistency, a technique used for approximately 54 percent of the instruments. Test-retest stability is reported for nearly 30 percent of the scales and parallel forms reliability for approximately 18 percent (p. 562).

The content and method of item generation are most often cited as evidence for validity, followed by reports of concurrent validity using known groups. The infrequent estimations of predictive and construct validity may be partially accounted for by the fact that many of the scales were developed before such methodologies were widely used. The scales span a time period from 1925 to 1964.

BEHAVIORAL MEASURES

Andrulis, Richard: *A Source Book of Tests and Measures of Human Behavior.* Springfield, Ill.: Charles C Thomas, Publisher, 1977.

Compiled in this volume are descriptions of 155 commercially available tests to assess adult behavior. Appropriate for subjects aged 16 or over, the devices are categorized according to 10 dimensions of human behavior: intelligence and aptitude; achievement; cognitive style; general measures of personality; specific measures of personality; personality adjustment; vocational and interest inventories; attitude devices; personal performance and history measures; and managerial and creativity devices.

The first three chapters deal with such measurement issues as functions and styles of testing, considerations in choosing tests and measures, and a discussion of reliability and validity. Instrument descriptions follow and include the title, author, the variables measured, the type of measure, where to obtain it, psychometric properties, and a general description. The purpose of the tool, the number of items, the scoring application, and the groups on which it has been normed are included in the general description. Some reliability and validity data are available for approximately 90 percent of the tools, although the amount of information about the psychometric properties of a given tool varies.

Ciminero, Anthony R., Karen S. Calhoun, and Henry E. Adams, Eds.: *Handbook of Behavioral Assessment.* New York: John Wiley and Sons, Inc., 1977.

This handbook provides a comprehensive review of general and critical issues in behavioral assessment, as well as specific approaches used to measure behavior. The book is divided into three parts. Part one consists of a general overview, a discussion of basic issues in behavioral assessment, a system to classify psychological responses that may be used as a framework for research, and instrumentation. The instrumentation chapter deals with physiologic instrumentation and is based on the premise that psychological measures have a physical referent. A table of selected behavioral systems and methodologies and a table of descriptions of commercial instruments with application to behavioral assessment provide some sense of the wide range of tools and methods available for physical measurement of behavior.

Part two deals with general approaches to behavioral assessment. Included are chapters on interviews, self-report schedules and inventories, self-monitoring procedures, direct observation in both analogue and naturalistic settings, and psychophysiologic techniques. Issues involving these approaches are discussed and examples of their use are cited.

Part three describes how these measurement approaches are used to assess anxiety, addiction, sexual behavior, social skills, marital conflict and accord, child behavior problems, and psychotic behavior. A number of sources are identified in which relevant instruments may be found. Occasionally instruments are described in some depth in the text, providing such information as the purpose, number of items, source of the items, target population, scoring, reliability, and validity.

Lake, Dale G., Matthew B. Miles, and Ralph B. Earle, Jr.: *Measuring Behavior*. New York: Teachers College Press, 1973.

A description and critique is provided for each of 84 behavioral instruments oriented toward personal, interpersonal, group, or organizational variables. Information for each tool is presented in the following format: title, author, variables, description, administration and scoring, development, critique (including psychometric properties and possible measurement difficulties), and comments evaluating its usefulness. Bibliographical information is provided for work referred to in the body of the review. Uniterms or key concepts are identified for each instrument and are cross-referenced in the index.

A variety of approaches have been used to estimate the psychometric properties of these behavioral instruments and they are extensively discussed. Particularly emphasized are methods employed, results obtained, the adequacy of the norms, and the potential degree of item transparency. Virtually all of the instruments have been tested for reliability and validity using one or more techniques.

Lyerly, Samuel: *Handbook of Psychiatric Rating Scales*, 2nd Ed. Rockville, Maryland: National Institute of Mental Health, 1973.

Descriptions of 61 rating scales that are being used or have frequently been used in psychiatric settings are included in this compilation. Detailed descriptions of 11 scales for rating the behavior and symptomatology of children and 27 scales for rating the behavior and symptomatology of adults are provided, as are very brief reports of 23 additional scales. A table of relevant scale characteristics has been constructed which allows the researcher to obtain information at a glance on the relevant population, the type of rater, the source of data, and the reliability and validity of the 38 scales, which are described in detail.

The detailed descriptions include the title, original source or commercial publisher, a general description, the type of subject for whom appropriate, the type of rater (i.e., nurse, teacher, psychiatrist), the basis for rating, the source of the items, sample items, norms, reliability, validity, and related references. Reliability statistics are provided for over 90 percent of the scales. Although validity information is available for approximately 80 percent of the scales, statistics are rarely provided. Rather, studies giving evidence of validity are described.

HEALTH-RELATED MEASURES

Comrey, Andrew L., Thomas E. Backer, and Edward M. Glaser: *A Sourcebook for Mental Health Measures.* Los Angeles: Human Interaction Research Institute, 1973.

Contained in this volume are abstracts of approximately 1100 psychological and mental health–related measures, with major well-known tools purposely excluded. Among the 45 clusters or categories of instruments are such topics of interest to nurses as alcoholism, drugs, family interaction, geriatrics, mental retardation, and evaluation of professional service delivery.

Each abstract is headed by the title of the instrument, its source, and the author's name and address. Presented in the abstract is information related to the purpose of the tool, a description which may include the number of items, sample items, and administration time, the method of development, the psychometric properties, major applications in research, and where it may be obtained. Since the information in the abstract has usually been supplied by the developer of the instrument, the amount and type of information varies.

Although occasionally reliability and validity statistics are provided, more often the abstract indicates whether such information is available and where it may be obtained. The psychometric properties of many instruments included in this compendium are unknown.

Reeder, Leo G., Linda Ramacher, and Sally Gorelnik: *Handbook of Scales and Indices of Health Behavior.* Pacific Palisades, Calif.: Goodyear Publishing Co., Inc., 1976.

Seventy-eight studies focusing on a defined segment of health services behavior research were selected for inclusion in this volume. They are grouped according to preventive health behavior, health status, health orientation, illness behavior, and use of health services.

In an effort to link theory with research, information from each study has been abstracted in the following format: major health concept investigated; research design (method of data collection); theoretical framework; research hypothesis and research questions; conceptual model (graphically presented); major variables (identified as independent, dependent, or intervening variables); operationalization of major variables; description of the sampling frame (unit of analysis, population, sampling design, and sample size); and major findings and interpretation.

Approximately 85 percent of the studies employed the survey method of data collection. For approximately one fourth of the studies, the instrument or sample items are included in the compendium. For several others, the content of the instrument may be discerned from the tables included in the presentation of the findings. Information describing the psychometric properties of the tools is provided for a small number of studies.

MISCELLANEOUS MENTAL MEASURES

Buros, Oscar K., Ed.: *Tests in Print II.* Highland Park, N.J.: Gryphon Press, 1974.

A guide to the tests of mental measurement in print as of early 1974 and a cumulative index to the first seven *Mental Measurements Yearbooks,* this volume contains 2467 test entries. Included are bibliographical sources that refer to the construction, use, and validity of specific tests through 1971, a cumulative index of all tests with references, a directory of publishers, an author index, a title index of tests in and out of print, a list of tests out of print since the 1961 edition of this compendium, and a scanning index giving populations for which each test is intended. According to the editor, it is necessary to combine the use of this volume with *The Eighth Mental Measurements Yearbook* for a complete index to all tests, reviews, excerpts, and references for mental measurements.

Buros, Oscar K., Ed.: *The Eighth Mental Measurements Yearbook.* Highland Park, N.J.: Gryphon Press, 1978.

This compendium has three major sections. The first section, tests and reviews, contains a listing of 1184 tests of mental measurements, 898 of which are critically reviewed by a variety of reviewers. An additional 140 reviews were excerpted from journals, thereby providing reviews for nearly all of the tests listed. The second section, books and reviews, lists 576 books on testing, most of which were published between 1970 and 1977. Reviews of 229 books are included. The final section is composed of 6 indices: author, test title, book title, publishers directory, periodical index, and scanning index. Included in the introduction is a list of test titles, each of which has been referenced 100 or more times.

The tests are organized according to 14 categories: achievement batteries, English, fine arts, foreign language, intelligence, mathematics, miscellaneous, reading, science, sensory and motor, social studies, speech and hearing, and vocations. Among the entries for each test are title, population for which use is intended, variables (listed as partial scores), available forms, and copyright information. References to the psychometric properties are contained either in the test information or in the critical review and sometimes in both. A list of all known references to the test follows the descriptive information. This volume and its companion, *Tests in Print II,* provide a complete index to all tests of mental measurements.

Tests of personality, intelligence, reading, and vocational skills have been separated into individual volumes. The monographs, referenced below, cover the time period between 1938 to the time of publication and contain all reviews from the earlier editions of *Mental Measurements Yearbooks* as well as some new information.

Buros, Oscar K., Ed.: *Intelligence Tests and Reviews.* Highland Park, N.J.: Gryphon Press, 1975.

Buros, Oscar K., Ed.: *Reading Tests and Reviews.* Highland Park, N.J.: Gryphon Press, Vol. I, 1968 and Vol. II, 1975.

Buros, Oscar K., Ed.: *Personality Tests and Reviews.* Highland Park, N.J.: Gryphon Press, Vol. I, 1970 and Vol. II, 1975.

Buros, Oscar K., Ed.: *Vocational Tests and Reviews.* Highland Park, N.J.: Gryphon Press, 1975.

Chun, Ki-Taek, Sidney Cobb, and John R. French, Jr.: *Measures for Psychological Assessment: A Guide to 3,000 Original Sources and Their Applications.* Ann Arbor, Michigan: Institute for Social Research, University of Michigan, 1975.

A search of 26 psychological and sociological journals and publications between 1960 and 1970 resulted in this compilation of annotated references to measures of mental health and related concepts, and the uses of these measures. The two major sections of the book are designed to lead the user from the primary source that originally described the measure to additional sources describing its application.

More specifically, the Primary Reference section lists approximately 3000 references to publications in which the measure of interest was initially described. For each listing, key words that describe the content of the instrument are identified. The user is then referred to the second or Application section of the book if the measure has been used in additional studies or work. Contained in this section is a bibliographical listing of the source of the application and a notation indicating the type of information available in the article such as reliability, validity, normative data, and sample description. Also included is a descriptive index—an alphabetical listing of key words or concepts contained in this volume which cross-references the Primary Reference section.

Goldman, Bert A. and John L. Saunders: *Directory of Unpublished Experimental Measures.* New York: Behavioral Publications, Vol. 1, 1974 and Vol. 2, 1978.

In combination these volumes contain information on a total of 1034 mental measures. These were identified by reviewing 43 psychology, sociology, and educational journals for 1970, 1971, and 1972. The measures are organized under 23 headings, among which are adjustment, behavior, development, motivation, and perception. An effort was made by the authors to exclude tests that are commercially sold and to include those deemed to be of value to researchers.

Information for each test includes the name, purpose, description (number of items, time required for administration, and format), reliability, validity, bibliographical source of the tool, and related research references. Since the inclusion of this information was subject to availability, not all test entries have a complete set of descriptors.

When psychometric data are reported, the types of reliability and validity and the statistics are provided. In general, reliability is reported more frequently than is validity, but often no psychometric data are available.

PHYSIOLOGIC MEASURES

Many laboratory manuals and reference books provide useful information about methods and devices to measure physiologic phenomena. Of particular interest are instruments and procedures used in the clinical laboratory as well as devices employed in direct patient monitoring. The following selections are a sample of the variety of available resources in this area. Some of these volumes have undergone extensive revisions, as major technological innovations such as automated chemical analyzers and computerized axial tomography have made less sophisticated equipment obsolete. Since such resources become quickly outdated as technology continues to expand, the use of recent editions is advised.

Bauer, John D., Philip G. Ackerman, and Gelson Toro: *Clinical Laboratory Methods*, 8th Edition. St. Louis: C.V. Mosby Co., 1974.

Laboratory methods in urinalysis, hematology, clinical chemistry, enzymology, stool analysis, parasitology, toxicology, and tissue examination are among the topics included in this compendium. Descriptions of specific tests and procedures may include such information as general principles, necessary equipment, methodology, physiologic variations, calculations, normal values, and interpretation.

A chapter on quality control in the laboratory addresses sources of potential measurement error and offers suggestions for maintaining or improving the precision and accuracy of various instruments and procedures. In addition, quality control methods pertaining to specific tests are identified and discussed within the test description.

Cromwell, Leslie, Fred J. Weibell, and Erich A. Pfeiffer: *Biomedical Instrumentation and Measurements*, 2nd Edition. Englewood Cliffs, New Jersey: Prentice-Hall, 1980.

After a general overview of biomedical instrumentation and bioelectric potentials, specific classes of instruments such as transducers, electrodes, ultrasonic devices, biotelemetry, and x-ray and radioisotopes are described in some depth. For each of the major body systems, the basic physiology is presented, variables to be measured are identified, and principles of instrumentation are discussed. Typical medical, behavioral, and biologic applications of various instruments are also described. Chapters on intensive-care monitoring and biomedical computer applications illustrate some of the recent advances in physiologic measurement. Several appendices, including a glossary of terms and a summary of physiologic measurements, are provided.

Ferris, Clifford: *A Guide to Medical Laboratory Instruments*. Boston: Little, Brown and Company, 1980.

This volume is designed to provide a basic understanding of the operating principles of various classes of electronic instruments used in the clinical laboratory. Following an overview of the basic principles of electricity, instrumentation systems, and optical devices, chapters describing the design and use of special classes of instruments are presented. Instruments that employ exciter lamps (e.g., spectrophotometers) and flame excitation (e.g., flame photometers), as well as selected instruments to measure electrolyte and water balance (e.g. osmometers) are described. Additional classes of instruments include ion selective electrodes, particle counters, nuclear counters, automated chemistry analyzers, chromotography, and electrophoresis. Principles of laboratory safety and instrument trouble-shooting are discussed, and methods to promote accuracy in measurements, such as instrument calibration and the use of standard reagents and solutions, are presented.

Geddes, Leslie A. and L.E. Baker: *Principles of Applied Biomedical Instrumentation.* New York: John Wiley and Sons, 1975.

The first eight chapters of this volume concern the principles of transduction and descriptions and applications of various classes of transducers. Electrodes for transduction of bioelectric events, detection of physiologic events by impedance, bioelectric events and related bio-instrumentation, and semi-conductor transducers are the topics of the remaining chapters. Finally, a somewhat technical discussion of the criteria necessary for the faithful reproduction of a bioelectric event is presented.

Weiss, Marvin: *Biomedical Instrumentation.* Philadelphia: Chilton Book Co., 1973.

After several chapters to acquaint the reader with the terminology, the principles of physiology and electronics, and the techniques necessary for a basic understanding of biomedical instrumentation, some of the prevalent applications to patient monitoring and diagnosis are discussed. Descriptions of monitoring devices such as sensors, electrocardiographs, bedside monitors, and telemetry are provided. Also included are descriptions of diagnostic equipment such as electroencephalography, phonocardiography, ultrasound, and instruments to measure cardiac output and respiratory function. The uses of analog and digital computer systems to handle and manipulate the data produced by biomedical instruments are discussed. A glossary of physiologic and electronic terms is also provided.

SOCIOLOGIC/OCCUPATIONAL MEASURES

Bonjean, Charles M., Richard J. Hill, and S. Dale McLemore: *Sociological Measurement: An Inventory of Scales and Indices.* San Francisco: Chandler Publishing Co., 1967.

This volume contains bibliographical information for 2080 sociologic scales and indices that were identified by analyzing the content of four sociologic journals published during the years 1954 to 1965. Authoritarianism, family cohesion, and attitudes toward medicine and health are examples of the 78 conceptual categories used to classify the instruments. The 47 most frequently used and cited measures are displayed in a table, and these measures are subsequently discussed as they appear in the text.

The extent of each discussion varies, with approximately half containing some information about the scale's psychometric properties. The discussion of a particular scale generally includes such topics as its development, use, administration, scoring, and a description of the sample with whom it was used. Occasional examples of items are provided and copies of a few instruments are included. The tools are indexed by author and topic.

Miller, Delbert C.: *Handbook of Research Design and Social Measurement,* 3rd Edition. New York: David McKay Co., 1977.

As its title implies, this book is concerned with all phases of the research process including design, sampling, data collection, statistical analysis, reporting, and funding. Forty-eight sociologic scales and indices covering a wide range of topics are briefly reviewed and reproductions of most of them are provided. The scales fall under the general headings of social status, group structure and dynamics, social indicators, measures of organizational structure, evaluation research and organizational effectiveness, community, social participation, leadership in the work organization, morale and job satisfaction, and scales of attitudes, norms, and values.

Descriptive information provided for most scales includes the variable measured, description, reliability, validity, location, and bibliographical sources which describe its application in research. Reliability and validity data, when available, are difficult to evaluate, primarily because of the lack of a detailed description of the methodologies employed in psychometric testing. For some instruments, bibliographical notations indicating where this information can be obtained are provided. The tools contained in this volume are indexed by author and title.

An inventory of all instruments used in the *American Sociological Review* between 1965 and 1974 is also included. The list is organized according to the same categories as are the scales in this handbook, and bibliographical information is provided for each of these measures.

Pfeiffer, William J., Richard Heslen, and John E. Jones: *Instrumentation in Human Relations Training*, 2nd Ed. La Jolla, Calif.: University Associates, Inc., 1976.

Part one of this book deals with such instrumentation issues as administration, validity, reliability, instrument development, and problems of instrumentation in research. Part two consists of a guide to 92 instruments appropriate for use in the behavioral sciences. The tools are categorized according to their particular focus: personal, interpersonal (i.e., group dynamics, marriage, family), and organizational (i.e., organizational climate, management/leadership style, superior-subordinate relations).

Information provided for each tool varies. The length of the test, length of time to administer, a description of the scales and subscales, and purchase information are provided for all measuring devices. Occasionally, sample items are included. For some tools, uses, positive features, and concerns are identified. Administration, scoring, or interpretation issues may also be included. When reliability or validity are mentioned, it is within the discussion of positive features or concerns, and little information is provided.

Price, James L.: *Handbook of Organizational Measurement*. Lexington, Mass.: D.C. Heath Co., 1972.

Twenty-two organizational concepts provide the framework for this handbook, among which are absenteeism, autonomy, centralization, communication, effectiveness, satisfaction, and span of control. Each chapter begins with a general discussion and definition of the concept, followed by a presentation of issues pertaining to its measurement and descriptions of from one to three relevant instruments. According to the author, these instruments use the organization as the unit of analysis and the data are mainly ordinal or nominal in nature.

Specific descriptors for each measuring device include a general description, operational definition of the concept, data collection information, computation methods, reliability, validity, evaluative comments, and bibliographical source. Within the data collection description, the source of the data is identified (data bank, archives, sample description,) and sample items are often provided. In a few instances, the entire instrument is included.

For slightly more than half of the instruments, no reliability data are available. Evidence of validity is often presented as the findings of a study in which the tool was used. Less often, developers of the tool made an effort to do their own validity studies.

Robinson, John P., Robert Athanasiou, and Kendra B. Head: *Measures of Occupational Attitudes and Occupational Characteristics.* Ann Arbor, Michigan: Institute for Social Research, University of Michigan, 1969.

Copies and reviews of 77 scales used to measure occupational-related variables are included in this volume. The scales are classified under ten general headings: job attitudes, general job satisfaction, job satisfaction for particular occupations, satisfaction with specific job features, concepts related to job satisfaction, occupational values, leadership styles, other work-related attitudes, vocational interest, and occupational status. With the exception of the occupational status indices, information provided for each scale includes variable, description, sample, reliability/homogeneity, validity, location, and results and comments. A less structured approach is used to describe the occupational status scales.

Some reliability or validity data are provided for over one half of the instruments. Perhaps because the earliest scale included in this compendium was developed in 1935 and the latest in 1968, there is wide variability in the type and extent of reliability and validity studies reported. The comments highlight the strengths and weaknesses of each scale in terms of its psychometric properties and evaluate the scale in terms of the degree of response set, item content, wording, and analysis.

In addition to the tool descriptions, several chapters are devoted to such topics as status inconsistency, occupational similarity, and social mobility. An overview of research and a summary of the literature related to job attitudes and job performance are also included.

MEASURES FOR SPECIFIC POPULATIONS

Beere, Carole A.: *Women and Women's Issues: A Handbook of Tests and Measurements.* San Francisco: Jossey-Bass Publishing Co., 1979.

The literature was searched through 1977 to identify instruments that measure variables pertinent to women and women's issues. The 235 instruments are divided into 11 categories including sex roles, sex stereotypes, sex role prescriptions, children's sex roles, gender knowledge, marital and parental roles, employee roles, multiple roles, attitudes toward women's issues, somatic and sexual issues, and unclassified. The sections on sex roles and attitudes toward women's issues contain the greatest number of instruments.

Each of the 11 categories constitutes a chapter, each beginning with an overview of the concept or category involved. Two-hundred and twenty of the instruments are presented in the following format: title, author(s), date mentioned in the literature, variables, type of instrument (22 different types are included in this compendium), description of the item content, length of the tool and response options, the group or individual for whom the tool is appropriate, at least two sample items, the method of scoring, the theoretical basis for development, reliability, validity, notes and comments (i.e., factor analysis as it relates to reliability and validity, information relative to modification, evaluative comments, subscores), the source, and bibliographical information. Descriptions of the remaining instruments are abbreviated, referring the researcher to other sources (e.g., Personality Tests in Review). The instruments are indexed by variable, author, and title.

Both reliability and validity information is available for approximately 75 percent of the instruments, with validity being reported more frequently than reliability. According to the author, content validity may be inferred from the method of development of the instrument. Therefore, discussion of a tool's validity is focused on evidence of construct or criterion-related validity.

Johnson, Orval G. and James W. Commarito: *Tests and Measurements in Child Development: Handbook I.* San Francisco: Jossey-Bass Publishing Co., 1971.

This compendium contains descriptive information for more than 300 unpublished (not commercially sold) instruments through 1965 which are suitable for research involving children from birth to 12 years. The instruments are grouped into 10 major categories: cognition, personality and emotional characteristics, perceptions of environment, self-concept, environment, motor skills, brain injury and sensory perception, physical attributes, miscellaneous attitudes and interests, social behavior, and unclassified. Descriptive information includes title, author, age for which appropriate, variables, format of the instrument, availability, description, reliability and validity, and bibliographical information. The tests are indexed by author, title, and subject.

According to the authors, data on reliability and validity were not usually supplied by the developers of the instrument. Rather, they were extracted from research reports in which the tool was used, interpreted by the authors, and summarized. Construct validity was often inferred from the results of a study designed to test a hypothesis. By using this approach, some reliability and validity estimates are available for a large majority of the instruments.

Johnson, Orval G.: *Tests and Measurements in Child Development: Handbook II.* Volumes 1 and 2, San Francisco: Jossey-Bass Publishing Co., 1976.

These volumes represent an extension of *Handbook I*, containing descriptions of approximately 900 additional tools and covering the literature from 1965 through 1974. The categories are essentially the same as those in the earlier work, but a vocational category has been added. The upper age limit has been increased from 12 to 18 years.

Data to estimate reliability and validity have typically been collected by the developers of the instrument, and descriptions of these studies are frequently provided in the review. For a few instruments, the potential user is referred to a bibliographical source to obtain information on the psychometric properties. For a small percentage of tools, no reliability or validity data are reported.

Strauss, Murray A. and Bruce W. Brown: *Family Measurement Techniques—Abstracts of Published Instruments, 1935–1974*. Revised Edition, Minneapolis: University of Minnesota Press, 1978.

This compilation includes abstracts of 813 instruments to measure the properties of the family or the behavior of people in family roles. The instruments are classified into four broad categories, each of which is further divided into several subcategories. The major categories are husband-wife relationship measures, parent-child and sibling-to-sibling relationship measures, measures covering husband-wife and parent-child variables, and sex and premarital relationships. The instruments are indexed according to author, test title, and subject of the test.

The format of the abstract is as follows: author, test name, variables measured, test description, sample item (including scoring method), length, availability, and references. In contrast to the earlier edition, the psychometric properties of the instruments are not included, because this information is usually not provided by the author but must be inferred by the abstractor. Thus, the accuracy of the information is compromised, according to the authors (p. 14). Some of the instruments presented in this volume were also presented in the earlier edition.

Walker, Deborah K.: *Socioemotional Measures for Pre-School and Kindergarten Children*. San Francisco: Jossey-Bass Publishing Co., 1973.

By consulting a number of sources, 143 instruments to assess the affective growth in children from 3 to 6 years were located. The tools are organized according to attitudes, general personality and emotional adjustment, interests or preferences, personality or behavior traits, self-concept, and social skills or competency. Following an overview of socioemotional measurement technology for young children, a description of each measure is presented.

Specific descriptors include author, appropriate age range, measurement technique, bibliographical source, address where the tool can be obtained, description (variables, administration, scoring, item examples, and special considerations), norms, reliability, and validity. For approximately 33 percent of the measures, no reliability data are available. In a fewer number of instances, the scale's validity is unknown.

MEASURES OF SPECIAL ATTRIBUTES

Anastasi, Anne: *Psychological Testing*, 4th Ed. New York: Macmillan Publishing Co., Inc., 1976.

With the primary goal of this volume being to contribute toward the proper evaluation of psychological tests and the correct interpretation of test results, a great deal of space is devoted to the content and principles of psychological testing. Following this, tests of general intelligence level, tests of separate abilities, and personality tests are discussed. The content and format of these sections vary. For example, intelligence tests

are presented in the context of individual tests, tests for special populations, and group testing. In some instances, specific tests are described
in great detail including the development, administration and scoring,
normative interpretation, reliability, and validity. In others, only a short
description of the test is provided.

An appendix lists over 250 tests, most of which are discussed in the
text. The appendix is categorized according to intelligence tests and developmental scales, multiple aptitude batteries, tests of creativity and
reasoning, educational tests, occupational tests, clinical tests for cognitive dysfunction and learning disabilities, self-report personality inventories, tests of interests, attitudes and values, projective techniques, miscellaneous personality tests, and measures of environment. The
publisher of each test is listed as is the entry number in the *Mental Measurements Yearbook* or the date of the revised edition of the test.

Cattell, Raymond B. and Frank Warburton: *Objective Personality and Motivation Tests: A Theoretical Introduction and Practical Compendium.* Ur-
bana: University of Illinois Press, 1967.

Following a 186-page theoretical introduction describing the state of
the art of objective personality tests is a compendium of 412 tests. Each
test has two titles: that used by the psychologist (determined by the psychological purpose) and that given to the subject (determined by surface
content). Descriptive information includes the age range, length of the
test, the test structure (which contains 12 categories such as ability, perceptual, questionnaire), variables, theory, rationale, design, sample
items, administration, and scoring. The authors' names and location of
the tests are not provided.

Twenty-one bipolar personality factors provide the basis for categorizing tests for one of the 6 indices. Tests are also indexed according to
psychologist's test title, variable title in alphabetical order, apparent
content, published research in which tests have been used, and variables
grouped according to personality factors. The factor loadings provided
in Index VI and the occasional mention of them in the test description
constitute the only references to the psychometric properties of the tests.

The foregoing reviews provide some sense of the wide variety of existing tools that may be relevant for nursing measurement. Many of these
compendia can be found in the reference sections of major libraries.
Those that are specific to a particular discipline, such as nursing, may be
located in the libraries of universities that offer courses in that discipline.

SELECTED TOOLS AND PROCEDURES
EMPLOYED IN NURSING MEASUREMENT

There are a number of tools and procedures that have gained special recognition in nursing on the basis of their continued use over the years or their

potential utility for nursing measurement. Several of these instruments were developed for quality of care evaluation, either to measure the quality of care received by the patient (Nursing Audit, QualPacs, Rush Medicus Methodology) or the competencies displayed by the nurse (Slater Scale). Others, such as the Nursing Child Assessment Series (NCAST), were developed for use in direct patient care. A recently developed tool, the Nurse Practitioner Rating Form (NPRF) was designed to assess the dimensions of the nurse's role during the process of care delivery. These instruments will be described in some detail.

The format for presentation includes the title, source, and authors, followed by the variable the tool seeks to measure and a general description of the contents including the type of tool, the number of items, and the existence of subscales. In describing the development of the tool, particular attention is given to the conceptual basis and the source of the items. A brief description of the format of the items or the tool as a whole, the population for which it is intended, administration and scoring techniques, and the measurement framework within which the scores are interpreted are provided. The psychometric properties are discussed, highlighting published reports of reliability and validity as well as recommended methods. Finally, past and potential uses of the devices are noted and issues that merit careful consideration are raised. Additional references and instrument copyright information are provided.

SELECTED INSTRUMENTS FOR DATA COLLECTION IN NURSING

THE NURSING AUDIT.
Source: *The Nursing Audit: Self-regulation of Nursing Practice.* New York: Appleton-Century-Crofts, 1976.
Author: Maria C. Phaneuf
Variable: The *quality of nursing care received by a patient* in any setting, as reflected in the patient care record, after the cycle of care has been completed.
Description: This 50-item instrument, designed to be completed by a rater, consists of one dependent and six independent functions of professional nursing practice:

I.   Application and execution of physician's legal orders—6 items.
II. Observation of signs and symptoms and reactions—6 items.
III. Supervision of the patient—7 items.
IV. Supervision of those participating in care (except the physician)—4 items.
V.   Reporting and recording—5 items.
VI. Application and execution of nursing procedures and techniques—16 items.
VII. Promotion of physical and emotional health by direction and teaching—6 items.

Development: The conceptual basis for the Nursing Audit is the seven functions of professional nursing (Lesnik and Anderson, 1955) which recognizes the social and legal expectations of nursing practice. For each of the major components, subcomponents were developed. Each subcomponent is a question to be answered by the auditor. Key subcomponents included in the audit are those considered essential to the major component or function.

After a trial use of the audit, technical assistance was obtained for scoring (weighting) the subcomponents. This led to the development of subscale scores. Finally, five numerical ranges were established in which the final quality score for each case might be ranked.

Format: One of three responses (yes, no, or uncertain) is checked by the rater for each item in components I through V. For components VI and VII, an additional response is available when the item does not apply.

Application: The audit is intended to be used by a committee of nurses to evaluate the quality of care received by patients, after the cycle of care has been completed, through retrospective review of the patient care record.

Administration: Records are randomly selected for chart review. It is recommended that 10 percent of the monthly discharges be audited if the number per month exceeds 50. If the number of monthly discharges is 50 or less, it is recommended that all records be reviewed. Thirty-five to 40 hours of orientation are required to train a committee of raters. The length of time of administration varies with the patient's length of stay (i.e., size of the record). However, after audit skills are well developed, approximately 15 minutes per case is required for patients whose length of stay is 3 months or less.

Scoring: The items of each major component are weighted. The weights for yes responses range from 2 to 7, and for uncertain responses the range is from 0.5 to 3. All no responses receive a score of 0. The does not apply weights range from 2 to 3.

When the chart review has been completed and the appropriate responses checked, the subcomponent scores (excluding does not apply scores) are summed to provide a component score. Similarly, the component scores are summed to provide a total score. In order to compute the final score, it is necessary to correct for the does not apply scores by summing these scores and consulting a guide to obtain a correction value. The total score is multiplied by the correction value to obtain a final score. The final score falls into one of five ranges:

Excellent	161–200
Good	121–160
Incomplete	81–120
Poor	41–80
Unsafe	0–40

Interpretation: The provision of numerical ranges denoting levels of quality imply a criterion-referenced interpretation of scores.

Reliability and Validity: It is recommended that interrater reliability be established during the committee's period of orientation. "Interrater reliability has been established when any given patient care record privately reviewed by each committee member yields a common *overall* judgment of quality" (p. 72). The instrument's validity is not addressed by the author.

In a study to assess the reliability and validity of the Nursing Audit (Stanhope and Murdock, 1982), the charts of 358 patients who were discharged from a home health care agency were reviewed. Cronbach's alpha, used to assess the internal consistency of the tool, yielded an overall alpha of 0.95. The alphas of the major components ranged from 0.227 for component V to 0.912 for component VI. Intrarater reliability yielded a correlation coefficient of 0.80. Stepwise discriminant analysis indicated that the cases fell into the correct quality range 97.5 percent of the time, providing some evidence for discriminant validity.

Uses: The Nursing Audit has been used in nursing homes, public health agencies, and hospitals as the measuring device for nursing quality assurance programs. In the examples provided (pp. 111–124), quality of care improved six months after the implementation of the Nursing Audit in each of these sites. More detailed descriptions of its use are provided by Husung, Ruth J.: University Hospital: "Nursing Audit Experience" in Maria Phaneuf: *The Nursing Audit: Self-Regulation in Nursing Practice,* 2nd Ed. New York: Appleton-Century-Crofts, 1976, pp. 125–138; Peabody, Sylvia R.: "Visiting Nurse Agency: Nursing Audit Experience" in Maria Phaneuf: *The Nursing Audit: Self-Regulation in Nursing Practice,* 2nd Ed. New York: Appleton-Century-Crofts, 1976, pp. 139–143.

Comments: An audit committee of at least five nurses is recommended. In larger settings, more members may be required so that one member does not review more than 10 cases per month.

Additional References: In addition to the major source cited at the beginning of this section, material was also gained from the following:

Lesnik, M.J. and B.E. Anderson: *Nursing Practice and the Law,* 2nd Ed. Philadelphia: J.B. Lippincott Co., 1955, p. 247–293.

Phaneuf, Maria C.: *The Nursing Audit: Profile for Excellence.* New York: Appleton-Century-Crofts, 1972.

Stanhope, Marsha and Marianne Murdock: "Psychometric Evaluation of a Retrospective Nursing Audit." In *Proceedings of the Fifth Biennial Eastern Conference on Nursing Research,* University of Maryland School of Nursing, Baltimore, Md., April 15–17, 1982, pp. 48–51.

Copyright: Appleton-Century-Crofts
292 Madison Avenue
New York, New York 10017

SLATER NURSING COMPETENCIES RATING SCALE.

Source: *Slater Nursing Competencies Rating Scale.* New York: Appleton-Century-Crofts, 1975.

Authors: Mabel A. Wandelt and Doris Slater Stewart

Variable: The *competencies displayed by the nurse* while caring for the patient.

Description: This 84-item observation scale is subdivided into 6 categories:

1. Psychosocial: Individual—18 items
2. Psychosocial: Group—13 items
3. Physical—13 items
4. General—16 items
5. Communication—7 items
6. Professional Implications—17 items

Each category is defined and the tool is accompanied by a 20-page cue sheet listing several examples of activities or behaviors illustrative of each item.

Development: The items were derived from a review of the literature and the personal experience of the developers, in consultation with colleagues and peers. The scale was developed with the view of enhancing objectivity in the ratings of nurse performance in the clinical setting. No standard of measurement is defined, but the assumption is made that there is a common conception of the level of skill expected of first-level staff nurse performance. Thus, each rater uses his or her own frame of reference to define first-level staff nurse performance, which is the basis for measurement.

Format: A 5-point rating scale is used to rate each item using the categories best nurse, between, average nurse, between, and poorest nurse. There are also spaces to check not applicable or not observed.

Application: The scale is intended to be used by an observer-rater to rate the performance of a nurse as she provides patient care. However, it may also be used as a retrospective evaluation tool to evaluate nursing or student performance.

Administration: Before attempting to rate nursing performance, the rater must establish his or her frame of reference for the first-level staff nurse against which the ratings can be made. Practice with retrospective evaluation is recommended before attempting to do real ratings. Thirty to 40 minutes is required to complete a retrospective evaluation after four practice opportunities.

Since ratings of at least 60 items are necessary to provide a reliable and valid score (p. 41), the time required for live administration varies. Early testing has indicated that $2\frac{1}{2}$ to 3 hours is sufficient to observe 60 or more behaviors. Raters usually rate 5 to 6 items per episode before moving on to the next episode.

Scoring: Each item is scored according to the following scale: 5 = best nurse, 4 = between best and average nurse, 3 = average nurse, 2 = between average and poorest nurse, 1 = poorest nurse. No score is given for not observed or not applicable. If an item has been scored more than once, an average item score is obtained. The mean item scores are then summed for a total competency score.

Interpretation: Since a nurse is being rated with reference to others in a well-defined norming group (i.e., first-level nurses), a norm-referenced interpretation is required.

Reliability and Validity: To estimate interrater reliability, three groups of students (N = 74) were rated retrospectively by pairs of raters from educational and practice settings. One to seven students were rated by a given pair of raters. Interclass correlations for the three groups were 0.78, 0.75, and 0.72; and for the total group, the interclass correlation was 0.77.

Internal consistency was assessed using Cronbach's alpha (0.74) and odd-even split-half correlation (0.98). The stability of the scale was tested by rating 103 staff nurses initially and again six months later, obtaining a correlation of 0.60 between the two administrations.

The scale has undergone extensive content validation over the years by nurse educators and nurse practitioners from all major clinical areas. Construct validity was assessed using factor analysis. By this method, a large general factor was obtained, accounting for 55 percent of the variance. Twelve factors had eigenvalues of 1 or more.

The extent of the tool's predictive validity was estimated by correlating the scores with other measures of nursing knowledge and practice. The correlations ranged from 0.54 (with NLN Achievement Test scores) to 0.72 (with instructor practice grades).

Uses: The scale has been widely used to evaluate the clinical nursing performance of practicing nurses and students. One such example is Shulka, Ramesh K.: "Structure vs. People in Primary Nursing: An Inquiry." Nursing Research, 30:4, July-August, 1981, pp. 236–41.

Comments: The authors acknowledge the potential difficulties arising out of the absence of defined standards of measurement. Additionally, a first-level nurse may be one with a baccalaureate degree, an associate degree, or a diploma, and the expectation of different levels of care from nurses with different educational backgrounds may complicate the notion that all nurses hold a common view of the level of performance expected of a first-level nurse. However, the authors warn against a flexible standard of measurement, asserting that if the standard is held constant across time, differences in performance will be readily visible.

Copyright: Appleton-Century-Crofts
              292 Madison Avenue
              New York, New York 10017

QUALITY PATIENT CARE SCALE (QualPaCS).

Source: Quality Patient Care Scale. New York: Appleton-Century-Crofts, 1975.

Authors: Mabel A. Wandelt and Joel Ager

Variable: The quality of nursing care received by the patient in any setting where nurse-patient interactions occur.

Description: QualPaCS is a 68-item observation scale, subdivided into 6 categories:

1. Psychosocial: Individual—15 items
2. Psychosocial: Group—8 items
3. Physical—15 items
4. General—15 items
5. Communication—8 items
6. Professional Implications—7 items

Each category is defined and the instrument is accompanied by a 20-page cue sheet listing concrete examples of activities illustrative of each item. The cues are relevant to a variety of settings and patient populations.

Development: QualPaCS draws heavily from the Slater Nursing Competencies Rating Scale, but the focus of measurement is the care received by a patient rather than the competencies displayed by a nurse. As with the Slater Scale, the standard of measurement is the quality of care provided by a first-level staff nurse, and the user is expected to establish his or her own frame of reference to define this standard.

Format: A 5-point rating scale is used to rate each item using the categories best care, between, average care, between, and poorest care. Two additional categories may also be used when a particular item is either not observed or not applicable. Each item is followed by a code to signify the type of rater activity required: #D = direct observation, *I = indirect observation, #D/*I = direct or indirect observation.

Application: The scale may be used by one observer-rater to rate the quality of care received by up to three patients during a two-hour observation period.

Administration: Two hours of direct observation are required by an uninvolved observer in the patient care setting. Prior to observation, the rater should learn about the patients and develop a nursing assessment and skeletal care plan for the patients whose care will be evaluated.

Scoring: Each item is scored according to the following scale: 5 = best care given, 4 = between best care and average, 3 = average care given, 2 = between average care and poorest, 1 = poorest care given. No score is given for not observed or not applicable. If a particular item has been scored more than once, a mean score for the item is obtained. The individual mean scores are summed and a mean score for the entire scale is obtained. Thus, the totalled mean score is the indicator of the quality of nursing care received by the patient. Single category mean scores may also be calculated.

Interpretation: The scoring system and the lack of a definition of the standard of measurement imply a norm-referenced interpretation.

Reliability and Validity: Interrater reliability is described as being the most critical reliability requirement. Three separate studies produced interrater reliability coefficients of 0.74, 0.91, and 0.64, respectively. The Kuder-Richardson technique to estimate internal consistency was used in another study and yielded a reliability coefficient of 0.96. To estimate stability, one rater rated five patients during a two-hour observation period on two consecutive days, obtaining a stability coefficient of 0.98.

A concurrent validity study using the Spearman-Brown formula corrected for attenuation resulted in a 0.52 correlation between the ranking of quality of care on 21 wards by 8 supervisors and QualPaCS.

Uses: QualPaCS has been widely used in quality assurance studies as well as in experimental and descriptive research designs. Among several references illustrating its use are Eichhorn, Marsha and Elaine Frevert in: "Evaluation of a Primary Nursing System Using the Quality Patient Care Scale." *Journal of Nursing Administration*, October, 1979, pp. 11–15; Passos, Joyce: "Systems Approach to Evaluation of Quality of Care in an Urban Hospital." In Harriet Werley, et al: *Health Research: The Systems Approach*. New York: Springer Publishing Co., 1976, pp. 193–200.

Comments: It is acknowledged by the authors that the lack of an explicit definition of the standard of measurement (i.e., quality of care provided by a first-level nurse) may be problematic, but the tool is based on the assumption that nurses have a common notion of the level of care a first-level nurse can be expected to provide.

Copyright: Wayne State University
         School of Nursing
         Detroit, Michigan 14828

THE RUSH-MEDICUS QUALITY-MONITORING METHODOLOGY.

Source: *Monitoring Quality of Nursing Care, Part II—Assessment and Study of Correlates*. DHEW Publication No. HRA 76-7, Washington, D.C.: U.S. Government Printing Office, 1976.

Authors: R.K. Dieter Haussmann, Sue T. Hegyvary, John F. Newman.

Variable: *The quality of nursing care* in the hospital setting.
Description: This instrument to evaluate the quality of nursing care consists of 6 major objectives and 28 subobjectives:

1.0 The plan of nursing care is formulated.
   1.1 The condition of the patient is assessed on admission.
   1.2 Data relevant to hospital care are ascertained on admission.
   1.3 The current condition of the patient is assessed.
   1.4 The written plan of nursing care is formulated.
   1.5 The plan of nursing care is coordinated with the medical plan of care.
2.0 The physical needs of the patient are attended.
   2.1 The patient is protected from accident and injury.
   2.2 The need for physical comfort and rest is attended.
   2.3 The need for physical hygiene is attended.
   2.4 The need for a supply of oxygen is attended.
   2.5 The need for activity is attended.
   2.6 The need for nutrition and fluid balance is attended.
   2.7 The need for elimination is attended.
   2.8 The need for skin care is attended.
   2.9 The patient is protected from infection.
3.0 The nonphysical (psychological, emotional, mental, and social) needs of the patient are attended.
   3.1 The patient is oriented to hospital facilities on admission.
   3.2 The patient is extended social courtesy by the nursing staff.
   3.3 The patient's privacy and civil rights are honored.
   3.4 The need for psychological-emotional well-being is attended.
   3.5 The patient is taught measures of health maintenance and illness prevention.
   3.6 The patient's family is included in the nursing care process.
4.0 Achievement of nursing care objectives is evaluated.
   4.1 Records document the care provided for the patient.
   4.2 The patient's response to therapy is evaluated.
5.0 Unit procedures are followed for the protection of all patients.
5.1 Isolation and decontamination procedures are followed.
5.2 The unit is prepared for emergency situations.
6.0 The delivery of nursing care is facilitated by administrative and managerial services.
   6.1 Nursing reporting follows prescribed standards.
   6.2 Nursing management is provided.
   6.3 Clerical services are provided.
   6.4 Environmental and support services are provided (p. 7).

Within each of the 28 subobjectives are numerous criteria for measuring the quality of care. In all, over 300 criteria have been included in the master list. The criteria are coded in terms of their applicability to patient type (operationalized as intensity of nursing care required) and the nursing unit in general, as well as the source of information (i.e., observation, the patient, the record). The criteria are stated in measureable terms which do not promote subjective interpretation, with most requiring a dichotomous yes or no answer.
Development: After an extensive review of the literature, a patient-centered approach to monitor the quality of nursing care was selected. A framework incorporating patient needs with the nursing process model provided the

basis for the organization of criteria relating to assessment, planning, implementation, and evaluation of patient care. It was recognized that provision of direct patient care is dependent on certain indirect components; therefore, relevant unit criteria are included for simultaneous consideration during direct patient care evaluation. Thus, the methodology consists of patient-specific and unit-specific criteria.

Weights, reflecting the subjective level of importance to quality of care, were assigned to the major divisions of objectives, the major objectives and the subobjectives, by two hospital-based advisory committees and one national advisory committee. The master list of criteria was developed by incorporating appropriate criteria from existing methodologies or writing new criteria. These procedures, as well as testing and statistical analysis of the methodology, resulted in the revised objective and subobjective structure (as shown above) and the master list of criteria.

Format: The methodology employs randomly computer-generated observation worksheets which are grouped subsets of criteria specific for type of patient and type of unit. Once selected by the computer, the criteria are organized and coded according to the source of the information, for the observer's convenience. The number of items per worksheet range from 8 to 64. Most of the responses are dichotomous options (yes, no, not applicable), but a few criteria have additional response options (sometimes, always, information not available). The nurse-observer checks the appropriate response for each criterion.

Application: A trained nurse-observer assesses the quality of care received by individual patients using the procedure described above. When the methodology is used in quality assurance programs, it is recommended that 10 percent of the monthly patient census per unit be randomly selected to provide an overall quality index for the unit for each month.

Administration: After a two- or three-day period of orientation, a nurse-observer is usually prepared to use the methodology. Patients are randomly selected from the nursing unit census and classified according to level of care required, and the appropriate worksheets are obtained. The nurse-observer gathers data from several sources: the patient record, patient observation, patient interview, nursing personnel interview, nursing personnel observation, patient environment observation, observer inference, and unit management observation. The time required for administration varies.

Scoring: All of the worksheets for the month are scored by computer and the data are aggregated to produce quality indices for each of the 28 subobjectives. To obtain each index, the subobjective criterion scores are averaged. Each criterion score is the ratio of positive responses to the total number of valid observations for that criterion. Indices for objectives are obtained by averaging the subobjective scores.

Interpretation: By eliminating items that exhibited little variance in the developmental phase, the present methodology is one that promotes wide variability. This, combined with the lack of a cut score to indicate achievement of quality, suggests a norm-referenced interpretation.

Reliability and Validity: Early testing, conducted during the developmental phase, resulted in significant revisions of the structure of the subobjectives and the criteria. Tests during this phase included frequency marginal distributions to assess the discriminatory ability of the criteria, inter-item correlations to determine whether criteria were correlated with subobjectives, correlational analysis to identify redundant criteria, and cluster analysis to test the statistical cohesiveness of the subobjectives. Revisions were made after each test and were incorporated into the next step of the testing sequence. As a result of these procedures, a methodology which seems to be internally consistent and reliable was developed.

The methodology was subjected to further testing using a sample of 19 hospitals across the United States. Observers at each hospital participated in a 2- or 3-day orientation period, following which interrater reliability was assessed. Most observers achieved 90 percent agreement at this time.

Several examples of system validity were presented by the authors. Content validity was demonstrated by the method of tool development and early testing. Using the data obtained from the 19 hospitals in the study group, the findings revealed a number of systematic variations across subobjectives. The fact that nursing administrators and advisory committee members believed that these variations represented the state of the art in quality of care supported, in part, a claim for construct validity. In addition, current trends in nursing education (emphasis on assessment and planning) and nursing practice (interaction between nursing and support services) led to the hypothesis that several parts of the nursing process should be highly correlated in terms of quality. Several intercorrelations significant at 0.001 supported this hypothesis and provided further evidence of construct validity.

Assessment of the methodology's concurrent validity was problematic due to the lack of existing comparable approaches to the measurement of quality. There was, however, high agreement between quality scores and subjective assessments of quality by key nursing administration personnel, leading to the conclusion that the methodology probably has concurrent validity.

There are limited data to support predictive validity, but a few situations occurred in the 19 study hospitals which would be expected to affect the level of quality of care (e.g., prolonged illness of the head nurse, inservice education programs on care planning, organizational and staffing changes). Quality scores were in the direction predicted in each instance. Uses: In addition to its utility in ongoing quality assurance programs, the methodology has also been employed in research designs, as illustrated in the study by Betz, Michael, Thelma Dickerson, and Douglas Wyatt: "Cost and Quality: Primary and Team Nursing Compared." *Nursing and Health Care.* 1:3, 1980, pp. 150–157.

Comments: In order to establish a link between nursing process and patient outcomes, outcome screening criteria have been developed for specific patient populations such as myocardial infarction, abdominal hysterectomy, cholecystectomy and transurethral resection and have been correlated with process criteria. The correlations were inconsistent, although some part of the nursing process was significantly correlated with every type of outcome (Haussmann and Hegyvary, 1977).

This methodology has been extensively tested and refined numerous times on the basis of that testing. A major barrier to the use of the methodology may be the cost involved or the lack of computer facilities to handle the data. Sets of computer-generated criteria may be purchased, thus eliminat-

ing the generation of criteria on site. However, the feasibility of running the required scoring routines on the available computer facilities should be carefully investigated before adopting this approach to quality monitoring.
Additional References: In addition to the major source cited at the beginning of this section, material was also gained from the following:

Haussmann, R.K. Dieter and Sue T. Hegyvary: "Correlates of the Quality of Nursing Care." *Journal of Nursing Administration.* 6:11, November, 1976, pp. 22–27.

Haussmann, R.K. Dieter and Sue T. Hegyvary: *Monitoring Quality of Nursing Care, Part III.* DHEW Publication No. HRA 77-70, Washington, D.C.: U.S. Government Printing Office, 1977.

Jelinek, Richard, R.K. Dieter Haussmann, Sue T. Hegyvary, and John Newman: *A Methodology for Monitoring Quality of Nursing Care.* DHEW Publication No. HRA 74-25, Washington, D.C.: U.S. Government Printing Office, 1974.

Copyright: None.

NURSING CHILD ASSESSMENT SATELLITE SERIES (NCAST).

Source: *Nursing Child Assessment Satellite Training Project Manuals,* University of Washington School of Nursing, Seattle, Washington.
Authors: Kathryn Barnard and Project Staff
Variables: The multiple variables related to *parent-child-environment interaction.*
Description: This series consists of four tools for the assessment of the child-parent-environment interactions, beginning at birth:

1. Home Observation for Measurement of the Environment—45 items
2. Nursing Child Assessment Teaching Scales—73 items
3. Nursing Child Assessment Feeding Scales—76 items
4. Nursing Child Assessment Sleep/Activity Record—a 7-day diary.

The teaching and feeding scales contain 6 subscales specific to parent-child interactions: sensitivity to cues, response to distress, social-emotional growth fostering, cognitive growth fostering, clarity of cues, and responsiveness to parent. The six subscales of the home environment measure are emotional and verbal responsivity of the mother, avoidance of restriction and punishment, organization of environment, provision of appropriate play material, maternal involvement with child, and opportunities for variety in daily stimulation. Recordings on the sleep/activity scale may include feeding, sleeping, crying episodes, parent-child activities, and so forth.
Development: Based on previous research to determine early predictors of child health and developmental problems (Child Health Assessment, 1979), a pattern of the parent and child as an interactive system emerged and provided the conceptual basis for this set of tools. The items are derived from the literature as well as personal observation and experience.
Format: The items on the environment, teaching, and feeding scales are statements that require a binary (yes or no) response from the observer. The sleep-activity record is in graph form with spaces provided for hourly recording of significant activities over a 7-day period.
Application: The scales are intended to be used by an observer to assess the parent-child-environment interaction from birth to 3 years for the teaching and home environment scales and from birth to 1 year for the feeding

scales. The sleep/activity record is appropriate for newborns through an indefinite period of time for the purpose of discerning patterns of behavior. Administration: The sleep/activity scale is administered by the caregiver (parent or other). The remaining scales are administered by an observer in the child's home environment. Although primarily observational measures, some interviewing is required to complete the scales.

Scoring: For the home environment, feeding and teaching scales, the number of yes responses are totalled to obtain subscale scores, which are in turn summed to obtain final scores. The sleep/activity record requires totalling the daily frequencies of specific activities. These are averaged at the end of each 7-day period to obtain a mean daily occurrence for a given activity. Other scores such as length and regularity of activity may also be calculated.

Interpretation: The scales have been used both as norm-referenced and criterion-referenced tools. The parent-child-environment as a dynamic interactive system suggests a norm-referenced interpretation of scores. If data are analyzed at the item level, a criterion-referenced interpretation is indicated.

Reliability and Validity: For the teaching, feeding and home environment scales, the training manual suggests that two raters view and rate taped parent-child interactions with the goal of obtaining 65 percent agreement at least once before attempting to do live assessments. Eighty-five percent interrater agreement is recommended for the feeding and teaching scales and 90 percent for the home environment scale for live assessments.

The validity of the parent-child interaction construct was determined by factor analysis (Child Health Assessment, 1979) when maternal-child variables had higher loadings than either set of variables alone. The researchers caution against unconditional acceptance of the findings due to the small subjects-to-variables ratio, however.

Little information is provided relative to the validity of the tools. The home environment scale correlated 0.60 ($p < 0.01$) with the 4-year Stanford-Binet test, lending some support to its predictive validity. The construct validity of the home environment subscales was estimated by factor analysis. This resulted in the hierarchical placement of the items in the subscales, with items loading highest on the subscales appearing first.

Uses: The tools have potential for early diagnosis and management of developmental difficulties. One of several studies demonstrating their utility is Snyder, Charlene, Sandra J. Eyres, and Kathryn Barnard: "New Findings About Mothers' Antenatal Expectations and Their Relationship to Infant Development." *MCN: American Journal of Maternal Child Nursing.* 4:6, November/December, 1979, pp. 354–357.

Comments: Interrater reliability should be assessed at regular intervals. Pairs of raters should be changed periodically to avoid a unique response set between raters.

Additional References: In addition to the major source cited at the beginning of this section, material was also gained from the following:

_____ : *Child Health Assessment, Part 2: The First Year of Life.* Kathryn E. Barnard and Sandra J. Eyres, Eds. DHEW Publication No. HRA 79-25, Washington, D.C.: U.S. Government Printing Office, 1979. Bradley, Robert and Bettye M. Caldwell: "Early Home Environment and

Changes in Mental Test Performance in Children 6–36 Months." *Developmental Psychology.* 12:3, March, 1976, pp. 93–97.

Bradley, Robert and Bettye M. Caldwell: "The Relation of Infants' Home Environments to Mental Test Performance at Fifty-Four Months: A Follow-up Study." *Child Development.* 47:4, December, 1976, pp. 1172–1174.

Copyright: Kathryn E. Barnard
                University of Washington School of Nursing
                Seattle, Washington 98195

THE NURSE PRACTITIONER RATING FORM (NPRF).

Source: *The Nurse Practitioner Rating Form: A Primary Care Process Measure.* Wakefield, Mass.: Nursing Resources, 1981.

Authors: Ada K. Jacox, Patricia A. Prescott, Maureen K. Collar, and Laura D. Goodwin

Variable: The *dimensions of the direct patient care role* of the nurse practitioner in ambulatory care settings.

Description: This primary care process measure is divided into two parts:

Part I.   Observation schedule with two major subsections:
    A.   Activity area (p. 20)
         1. History
         2. Physical exam
         3. Treatments
         4. Advice, directions, or instructions
         5. Factual information
         6. Explanation
         7. Demonstration
         8. Consultation
         9. Out of room
        10. Other
    B.   Content of teaching (p.21)
         1. Somatic aspects of existing problems
         2. Psychosocial aspects of existing problems
         3. Somatic aspects of health promotion
         4. Psychosocial aspects of health promotion

Part II. Global (multidimensional) scales to rate:
    A.   Communication style of the nurse practitioner.
    B.   Participation of the client.

Also included is a face sheet to categorize the type of visit observed.

Development: After a review of the literature revealed that the ability of nurse practitioners to perform physical examinations and to take medical histories (cure-oriented activities) had been adequately documented, attention was focused on the care-oriented components of the nursing role, particularly client teaching, as the conceptual basis for the tool. Definitions of the categories were repeatedly revised as a result of input from experienced nurse practitioners and educators who were asked to react to and to test the tool.

Format: The observation schedule provides for trained observers to make judgments at 30-second intervals regarding the predominant type of activity the nurse practitioner is performing. Each category is defined and specific examples are given which illustrate the particular category. The global scales consist of a 7-point rating scale with cues for scale points 2, 4, and 6, which serve as behavioral anchors for the scale. Cues are also given for the global scales to assist the rater in scoring.

Application: The instrument may be used by observer-raters to rate the type of activity performed by the nurse practitioner, the communication style of the nurse practitioner, and the participation of the client in the visit. Because the categories are fairly general, it may also be used in settings other than ambulatory care sites.

Administration: The instrument was designed to be used by observer-raters following a training period of approximately four hours. Live client visits may be observed or audio tapes may be rated with equal success, provided explicit instructions are given to the nurses being rated. However, interchanging raters and stimuli (live vs. taped visits) is not recommended due to questionable interrater stability.

Scoring: Each subpart is scored separately. The observation scale can be scored by counting the frequency of each category. However, it is more meaningful to determine the proportion or percentage of time spent in each category (frequency of a category ÷ total number of time intervals × 100) (p. 104). Each global scale generates an overall score ranging from 1 to 7. For the communication scale, lower scores represent stereotyped communication with the client and the higher scores reflect a more interactive and individualized approach on the part of the nurse. For the client participation scale, lower scores represent a low level of participation on the part of the client while higher scores indicate a more active or participatory client.

A number of additional approaches to scoring and handling the data obtained with this instrument are discussed (e.g., using alternative units of analysis and creating new variables).

Interpretation: The intent of the tool (i.e., the identification of the dimensions of the patient care role) and the format of the global scales suggest a norm-referenced interpretation of scores.

Reliability and Validity: Three reliability studies were conducted using different combinations of rater pairs to estimate interrater reliability for each of the four subparts of the tool. Both direct observation and taped visit ratings were obtained. When visits were rated by pairs of raters from the project staff, reliability coefficients ranging from 0.70 to 0.86 were obtained, except in the case of correspondence between direct observation and taped ratings by different raters which yielded low reliability (0.17). The interrater reliability of the global scales ranged from 0.06 to 0.65 and was subsequently revised.

When pairs of newly trained external raters with different specialties were used, interrater reliability coefficients ranging from 0.53 to 0.86 were obtained for the observation scale and from 0.21 to 0.77 for the global scales. A third study yielded substantial reliability estimates when two new raters were paired (0.75 to 0.85) but less substantial (0.54 and 0.55 on the observation scales and 0.33 and 0.35 for the global scales) when an experienced rater was paired with a new rater.

Content validity was addressed by the method of tool development. The lack of suitable external criteria precluded establishing concurrent validity. To estimate construct validity, hypothesis-testing was employed. Seven of the nine hypotheses were supported (three were weakly supported and four strongly supported). Further testing is recommended by the authors.

Uses: Some of the projected uses of this instrument are to measure selected provider activities, for formative and summative evaluation of nurse practitioner and student performance, as one component in a quality assurance program and as a device for content analysis of curricular materials used in the preparation of nurse practitioners.

Comments: According to the authors, interchanging of both raters and stimuli (live vs. taped ratings) should be avoided, since this tends to lower interrater agreement. In order to guard against a unique response set among pairs of raters, raters should be periodically rotated so that new pairs are formed.

Instrument Copyright: Nursing Resources
                                  12 Lakeside Park
                                  Wakefield, Mass. 01880

SPECIAL PROCEDURES TO ORGANIZE A NURSING DATA BASE

Two procedures that are particularly useful to organize a data base in nursing are the critical-incident technique and the problem-oriented medical record. Brief descriptions will highlight some of the features and potential uses of the procedures.

PROBLEM-ORIENTED MEDICAL RECORD.

Source: *Medical Records, Medical Education and Patient Care.* Chicago: Year Book Medical Publishers, Inc., 1971.

Author: Lawrence L. Weed

Description: The problem-oriented medical record (POMR) is a systematic approach to the organization of patient data that facilitates dealing with the complexities of patient care. The procedure is derived from the scientific method and has four phases:

    1. Establishment of a data base (patient profiles, history, physical, and psychosocial assessment),

    2. Identification of patient problems according to a classification system (e.g., active/resolved, medical/nursing, physical/nonphysical),

    3. Development of initial plans to deal with each problem (diagnostic, therapeutic, and educational plans),

    4. Written progress notes for each problem, using the SOAP method of charting (SOAP = subjective, objective, assessment, plan).

The technique may be used in any agency in which the collection and organization of patient data are necessary. The system is updated regularly (often daily) to maintain a current list of problems and relevant plans for handling them.

Uses: The problem-oriented medical record has been useful in the implementation of total care for patients with multiple care providers. It has particular utility for formulating nursing care plans and has also been used as a framework to evaluate the quality of patient care. Numerous examples of its use are illustrated in Hurst, J. Willis and H. Kenneth Walker, Eds.: *The Problem-Oriented System.* New York: Medcom Press, 1972.

Reliability and Validity: The type of reliability and validity required depends upon the use to which the technique is put. If, for example, the patient record is used to assess the quality of care, interrater reliability between content analysts or data retrievers is critical. If the patient record is being compared with certain standards of care, content experts should validate the standards.

CRITICAL-INCIDENT TECHNIQUE.

Source: "The Critical-Incident Technique." *Psychological Bulletin.* 51:4, July, 1954, pp. 327–358.

Author: John C. Flanagan

Description: The critical-incident technique employs a set of flexible principles for collecting data on observable human activity. Initially, the general aims of the activity are identified, the content and characteristics of the activity are precisely defined, and plans are made for data collection (i.e., who will collect the data, what methods will be employed, who constitutes the sample). Data may be collected by a variety of methods including interviews, questionnaires, records, observation, or self-report obtained from persons most closely involved with the activity.

Analysis of the data involves classifying the incidents into specific but simple categories such as effective or ineffective incidents. The categories should be submitted to content experts for validation. Statistical analysis of the data may be done after content analysis of the incidents is completed.

The critical-incident technique has been adapted for use in nursing and is described in Fivars, G. and D. Gosnell: *Nursing Evaluation: The Problem and the Process.* Pittsburgh: Psychometric Techniques Associates, 1966.

Uses: The technique may be used to collect data on any activity deemed relevant to nursing. A study that illustrates the use of the critical-incident technique to collect data on activities performed by nurses with different educational preparation is Jacobs, Angeline M.: *Comparison of Critical-Incidents About Baccalaureate, Associate Degree and Diploma Nurses.* Chicago: National Council of State Boards of Nursing, Inc., 1981.

Reliability and Validity: It is necessary to determine the degree of interrater reliability between pairs of observers or content analysts. If the data are collected by self-report, precise definitions of the content and characteristics of the activity must be provided, these having been validated by content experts. Evidence of content validity of the categories is recommended also.

SUMMARY

The use of existing methods and devices to measure nursing phenomena can be an effective and efficient approach to the collection of data, resulting in the accumulation of a body of nursing knowledge. Several theoretical models were presented which may serve as frameworks for education, practice, or research. Compendia that describe or list instruments of possible relevance to nursing were reviewed, and selected instruments and procedures for the collection of data or the organization of a nursing data base were discussed. Although this material is not exhaustive, it does serve to illustrate the wide variety of available resources that may be used for data collection in nursing.

REFERENCES

JOHNSON, DE: "The Behavioral System Model for Nursing." In REIHL, JP AND ROY, C: *Conceptual Models for Nursing Practice*, ed. 2. Appleton-Century-Crofts, New York, 1980, pp. 207–215.

KING, I: *A Theory for Nursing: Systems, Concepts, Process.* John Wiley and Sons, New York, 1981.

NEWMAN, M: *Theory Development in Nursing.* FA Davis, Philadelphia, 1979.

OREM, DE: *Nursing: Concepts of Practice*, ed. 2. McGraw-Hill, New York, 1980.

ROGERS, ME: *An Introduction to the Theoretical Basis of Nursing.* FA Davis, Philadelphia, 1970.

ROGERS, ME: "Nursing: A Science of Unitary Man." In REIHL, JP AND ROY, C: *Conceptual Models for Nursing Practice*, ed. 2. Appleton-Century-Crofts, New York, 1980, pp. 329–337.

ROY, C, Sr.: "The Roy Adaptation Model." In REIHL, JP AND ROY, C: *Conceptual Models for Nursing Practice*, ed. 2. Appleton-Century-Crofts, New York, 1980, pp. 179–188.

INDEX

Page numbers in *italics* indicate figures; page numbers followed by a *t* indicate tables.

mutually exclusive, defined, 44
Central tendency, measures of, 50–53, 51, 52
  distribution shape and, 52–53, 52
  in scoring, 123
CGDI. *See* Criterion-groups difference index.
Chance error. *See* Random error.
Change score(s)
  raw
    alternatives to, 81
    defined, 80
    reliability of, 80–82
Characterization by a value or value concept, in taxonomy of affective domain, 95t
Chart, profile
  defined, 129
  in standardized measures, 236–238, 237, 238
Checklist(s)
  as cognitive measures, 6
  as structured observational approaches, 253
  performance, for psychomotor measures, 10
Chi square value, in item response chart, 152–153, 155
Clarity, in evaluating operationalization of concepts, 39
Classical measurement theory. *See* Measurement theory.
Clinical outcomes, 324
Clinical performance, blueprint for measure of, 99t
Closed-ended question(s)
  in interview, 266–267
  in questionnaires, 276
Cluster, in selection-type format, 105t
Cluster sampling
  in establishing norms, 223, 225
  multistage, 223, 225
  stratified, 225, 225
Code for Nurses, 325
Coefficient
  alpha
    factors affecting, 138
    formula for determining, 136–137
  of correlation. *See* Pearson Product-Moment Correlation Coefficient.
  reliability, defined, 72–73
  validity, criterion-related, 149–151
Cognition in nursing research course, Mager's approach to stating behavioral objectives in, 87, 88
Cognitive domain, Bloom's taxonomy of, 88, 90t–93t, 98
Cognitive measures, defined, 6–7
Cognitive phase, in Fitts's phases of complex skill development, 96t
Cohen's K, in test-retest criterion-referenced procedures, 189–191

Collegial relationships, variable dimensions of, 33
Combined question and explanation, in multiple choice item format, 109t
Combined response, in multiple choice item format, 108t
Communicating Nursing Research, 343
Comprehension, in taxonomy of cognitive domain, 90t
Computer(s), interactive, in Delphi technique, 282
Concept(s). *See also* Nursing concepts.
  definition of, 1, 19
    purpose of, 25
  meaning space of, mapping and, 29
  nonvariable, variable concept vs., 32–33
  observables vs., 20
  variable
    frequency as dimension and, 33
    nonvariable concept vs. 32–33
Conceptual framework, defined, 20
Confidentiality, 330–331
Connotative meaning, semantic differential measuring, 9–10
Consensus, in evaluating operationalization of concepts, 39
Consent, informed, 326–328
Consistency
  in evaluating operationalization of concepts, 39
  in standardized measures, 234
Construct validity
  contrasted groups approach to, 143
  multitrait-multimethod approach to, 145–149, 146, 147, 148
  of criterion,-referenced measurement, 200–201
    experimental methods and contrasted groups approach to, 201
Contamination, criterion, 150
Content, in content analysis, 256
Content analysis, 255–262
  advantages of, 262
  defined, 256
  disadvantages of, 262
  example of, 257–258
  objectivity in, 256
  procedure for
    defining the universe of content to be examined, 258–259
    developing a sampling plan for, 260
    developing a scheme for categorizing the content of, 260
    developing explicit coding and scoring instructions for, 261
    identifying the characteristics or concepts to be measured in, 259
    performing the analysis, 262
    pretesting the categories and coding instructions in, 261
    selecting the unit of analysis to be employed in, 259

Heterotrait-heteromethod coefficients, 146, *148*
  in construct validity procedures, 146, *147*
Histogram(s)
  defined, 47, *48*
  for scoring, 122, *123*
  standards for constructing, 122
Hollinghead's Two-Factor Index of Social Position, 23t
Holtzman Inkblot test, 287t
Homogeneous responses, in multiple choice item format, 111t
Human Rights Guidelines for Nurses in Clinical and other Research, 325
Human subjects, ethical issues related to measurement in. See Measurement, ethical issues in.

IDEAL-sort, 300
IGI. *See* Individual gain index.
Illness, in selected theories/conceptual frameworks for nursing measurement, 346t
Imperfect matching, in selection-type format, 106t
Index, reliability, defined, 72
Index of Content Validity, defined, 142, 143t
Index of item-objective congruence, 196
Indicator(s)
  defined, 20
  empirical
    random errors in, reliability and, 65
    validity of, systematic error and, 66–67
  examples of, 23t
  observable
    either-or vs., variable, 36–37
    identifying, literature and, 37–38
    indicating, for concept, 35–38, 35t 36t, *37*
Indirect nursing practice, defined, 2
Indirect observation, in psychomotor measures, 12–13
Individual gain index, in validity assessment of criterion-referenced measurement, 206–207, 208t
Infant development
  concept of, indicators of, 36
  meaning categories and indicators for, *37*
Informal devices, measuring, person constructing, 16–17
Informed consent, 326–328
Instrument(s)
  existing
    conceptual basis for, 314–315
    evaluating, 312–316
    purpose of evaluating

norm- vs. criterion-referenced mode, 313–314
  population, 314
  setting, 314
  stated aim of measurement tool, 313
  time perspective, 314
psychometric properties of, 315–316
selection and use of, 311–317
use and reporting with, 316–317
resource books on, specific to nursing, 354–355
theoretical definition and, 38
Instrumentation, defined, 1–2
Internal consistency reliability
  alpha coefficient in, determination of, 136–137
  in norm-referenced measurement, 136–140, 137t
  KR 20 and KR 21 in, determination of, 138–139
Interpretation
  in selection-type item formats, 114t
  in taxonomy of cognitive domain, 91t
Interrater agreement, determination of, in assessment of content validity by content specialists in criterion-referenced measurement, 198–200, 199t
Interrater agreement procedures, for reliability in criterion-referenced measurement, 193
Interrater reliability
  checking for, in interview, 272
  in norm-referenced measurement, 140–141, 140t
  in projective techniques, 293
Interval scale measurement, defined, 45
Interview(s)
  advantages and disadvantages of, 274–275
  as cognitive measures, 6
  as self-report measures, 8
  closed-ended questions in 266–267
  defined, 263
  demand characteristic effects and, validity and, 273
  example of, 273–274
  face-to-face, 263
    disadvantages of, 274
  factual information reported by respondents and, 273
  filter questions in, 267
  funnel questions in, 267
  inconsistencies in, validity and, 273
  interviewer bias in, 265
  limits on utility of, 263–264
  open-ended questions in, 266–267
  probes in, 264
  procedure for developing the schedule for

Orem's theory of self-care — *continued*
  framework for measurement in, 350*t*
  goal of nursing in, 346*t*
  health and illness in, 346*t*
  key concepts in, 347*t*–349*t*
  measurement devices and techniques in, 351*t*
  unit of analysis in, 350*t*
Organization, in taxonomy of affective domain, 95*t*
Outcome(s)
  clinical, 324
  defined, 321
Outcome measurement, 321–322, 323–325
Outcome variables
  and criterion-referenced measurement frameworks, 4
  in operationalizing nursing concepts, 3

P LEVEL, item, 151–152
Parallel form procedures, 135–136
  for reliability in criterion-referenced measurement, 192–193
Parallel measures, model of
  domain-sampling model and, relationship of, 75
  reliability coefficient and, 73–74
Paraphrase, in linguistic transformation approach, to criterion-referenced measurement, 175
Participant observer roles, in observational methods, 249
Patient's Bill of Rights, 328
Peakedness, defined, 48, 49
Pearson Product-Moment Correlation Coefficient, 56–63, 59, 60
  computation of, from raw scores, 62
  effects of restriction of range on, 61–62, 62
  in intrarater reliability, 141
  in Q-Sort, 303
  measurement error affecting, 62
  other coefficients related to, 63, 64*t*
Peer utilization surveys, as cognitive measures, 6
Percentage anchors, in selection-type item formats, 112*t*
Percentage of explained variance, defined, 60–61
Percentage score, determination of, in criterion-referenced measurement, 177
Perfect matching, in selection-type format, 105*t*
Performance, types of, measurement of, 15, 16*t*
Performance checklist, for psychomotor measures, 10
Performance measure
  maximum, 15

  typical, 15, 16*t*
Percentile, defined, 129
Percentile rank, defined, 129
Percentile scores
  defined, 128
  in establishing norms, 228
Phaneuf's Nursing Audit, 322, 368–370
Phenomenon(a), defined, 1
Phi, Pearson Product/Moment Correlation Coefficient related to, 63, 64*t*
Physical measurements, 242–244, 244
  bioinstrumentation in, 243–244
    problems with, 244
  display equipment used in, 243
  relationship between subject and instrument system in, 244
  transducers used in, 243
Physiologic measurement, 241
  advantages and disadvantages of, 247–248
  as objective measures, 14
  as self report measures, 8
  defined, 13
  instrument compendia/resource books on, 360–362
  reliability and validity of, 246–247
  types of, 242–248, 244
    biochemical measurements, 244–246
      sources of error in, 247
    microbiologic/microscopic measurement, 246
      sources of error in, 247
    physical measurements, 243–244, 244
Picture interpretation, as self-report measure, 8
Piles, arrangement of, in Q-Sort, 300–303, 302
Platykurtic curve, defined, 49, 50
Play techniques, 291*t*
Policy Delphi, 283–284
Polygon
  frequency
    for scoring, 122
    of criterion-referenced test scores for masters and nonmasters, 178, 179
  standards for constructing, 122
Populations, specific, measures for, instrument compendia/resource books on, 364–366
Potency, semantic differential scales measuring, 10, 11*t*
Pragmatist view, vs. fundamentalist view, of measurement, 45–46
Precision
  in biochemical measurements, defined, 246
  in evaluating operationalization of concepts, 39
  reliability and, relationship of, 246
Prediction-sort, 300

Scores(s) — *continued*
  converted to standard scores, 125
  defined, 46
  in establishing norms, 228
  Pearson-Product-Moment Correlation
    Coefficient affected by, 62
  variance calculated using, 55
residualized change, defined, 81
standard
  change, defined, 81
  defined, 125
  in establishing norms, 228
  T, in establishing norms, 228
true
  defined, 68
  observed scores and, hypothetical dis-
    tribution of, 69, *70*
variance in, sources of, 78–82. See also
  Score variance.
variation in between measurements,
  79–80
Z
  defined, 125–127
  in establishing norms, 228
Score variance
  item difficulty and, 103
  observed, 70–72, *71*
  reliability and, statistical definition
    of, 72–73
Scoring
  derived score in, 128
  frequency polygon for, 122
  histogram for, 122, *123*
  in norm-referenced measurement, 115,
    120–130, 121*t*, 122*t*, *123*, *124*,
    125, *127*
  measures of central tendency in. See
    Measure(s), of central tendency.
  percentile in, defined, 129
  percentile rank in, defined, 128, 129
  percentile score in, defined, 128
  profile chart in, defined, 129
  quartile in, defined, 129
  standard deviation units in, 127–128
  standard scores in, defined, 125
  stanines in, 130
  symmetric distribution in, defined, 124,
    125
  theory of personal influence and, 115
  unit normal curve in, 127, *127*
  Z scores in, defined, 125–127
Scoring responses, methods of, 13–15
Selection-type items, in norm-referenced
    measures, 102, 104*t*–114*t*,
    116*t*–118*t*
Selective recall, in multiple choice item
    format, 108*t*
Self-care, Orem's theory of. See Orem's
    theory of self-care.
Self-evaluation measures, as cognitive
    measures, 6–7

Self-ideal-sort, 300
Self-report measures, 8
Self-sort, 300
Semantic differential scales, 8–10, 11*t*
Sentence completion, 290*t*
  as cognitive measure, 6
  as self-report measure, 8
Sex role identity, as nursing concept, 23*t*
Simplification, in content analysis, 257
Skewed distribution, defined, 47, *49*
Skewness
  degree of
    defined, 47
    measures of central tendency, 52–53,
      52
  in binomial model, 76
Slater Nursing Competencies rating scale,
  370–372
Social dependence
  as nonvariable concept, 33
  defined, 31–32
Socioeconomic class, as nursing concept,
  23*t*
Sociologic/occupational measures, instru-
    ment compendia/resource books
    on, 362–364
Spearman rank-order correlation, in
    Q-Sort, 303
Spearman Brown formula, 156–158
Special attributes, measures of, instrument
    compendia/resource books on,
    366–367
Specific populations, measures of, re-
    source books on, 364–366
Specimen collection, in biochemical mea-
    surements, 245
Sphygmomanometer, defined, 13
S-Procedure, 300
S-sort, 300
Standard(s)
  in biochemical measurements, 245–246
  in criterion-referenced measures, meth-
    ods for setting, 176–182, *179*, *180*
Standard deviation
  as units along a baseline of normal dis-
    tribution, 57
  defined, 53, 55
Standard deviation units, defined, 127–
  128
Standard error of measurement
  defined, 70
  in binomial model, 76
Standard score(s)
  defined, 125
  in establishing norms, 228
  interpretation of, consistency of, 229
Standardized change scores, defined, 81
Standardized interview, 264–265
Standardized measures, 223–239. See also
  Norms.
  administration and scoring of, 216–217,